IADVL

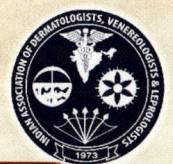

Manual on Management of
Dermatophytoses

Chief Editor

Kabir Sardana MD, DNB, MNAMS

Professor
Department of Dermatology and STDs
PGIMER, Dr Ram Manohar Lohia Hospital
New Delhi

Associate Editor

Ananta Khurana MD, DNB, MNAMS

Associate Professor
Department of Dermatology and STDs
PGIMER, Dr Ram Manohar Lohia Hospital
New Delhi

Assistant Editors

Shilpa Garg DNB (Dermatology and Venereology)
Consultant, Department of Dermatology
Sir Ganga Ram Hospital, Rajinder Nagar
New Delhi

Shital Poojary MD, DNB
Professor and Head
Department of Dermatology
KJ Somaiya Medical College, Mumbai

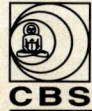

CBS

CBS Publishers & Distributors Pvt Ltd

New Delhi • Bengaluru • Chennai • Kochi • Kolkata • Mumbai
Hyderabad • Jharkhand • Nagpur • Patna • Pune • Uttarakhand

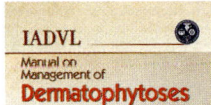

ISBN: 978-93-87742-88-8

First Edition: 2018

Published by Satish Kumar Jain and Produced by Varun Jain for

CBS Publishers & Distributors Pvt Ltd
4819/XI Prahlad Street, 24 Ansari Road, Daryaganj, New Delhi 110 002, India.
Ph: 23289259, 23266861, 23266867   Fax: 011-23243014   Website: www.cbspd.com
e-mail: delhi@cbspd.com; cbspubs@airtelmail.in.
Corporate Office: 204 FIE, Industrial Area, Patparganj, Delhi 110 092
Ph: 4934 4934   Fax: 4934 4935   e-mail: publishing@cbspd.com; publicity@cbspd.com

Branches

- **Bengaluru:** Seema House 2975, 17th Cross, K.R. Road,
  Banasankari 2nd Stage, Bengaluru 560 070, Karnataka
  Ph: +91-80-26771678/79   Fax: +91-80-26771680   e-mail: bangalore@cbspd.com
- **Chennai:** 7, Subbaraya Street, Shenoy Nagar, Chennai 600 030, Tamil Nadu
  Ph: +91-44-26680620, 26681266   Fax: +91-44-42032115   e-mail: chennai@cbspd.com
- **Kochi:** Ashana House, No. 39/1904, AM Thomas Road, Valanjambalam,
  Ernakulam 682 016, Kochi, Kerala
  Ph: +91-484-4059061-65   Fax: +91-484-4059065   e-mail: kochi@cbspd.com
- **Kolkata:** 6/B, Ground Floor, Rameswar Shaw Road, Kolkata-700 014, West Bengal
  Ph: +91-33-22891126, 22891127, 22891128   e-mail: kolkata@cbspd.com
- **Mumbai:** 83-C, Dr E Moses Road, Worli, Mumbai-400018, Maharashtra
  Ph: +91-22-24902340/41   Fax: +91-22-24902342   e-mail: mumbai@cbspd.com

Representatives

• Hyderabad	0-9885175004	• Jharkhand	0-9811541605	• Nagpur	0-9021734563
• Patna	0-9334159340	• Pune	0-9623451994	• Uttarakhand	0-9716462459

Printed at Magic International Pvt. Ltd., Greater Noida, UP, India

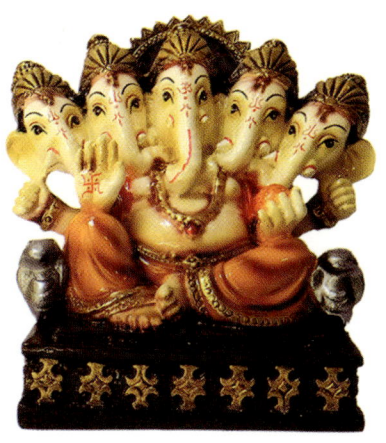

वक्रतुण्ड महाकाय सूर्यकोटि समप्रभ।
निर्विघ्नं कुरु मे देव सर्वकार्येषु सर्वदा॥

I meditate on
Sri Ganesha
Who has a Curved Trunk, Large Body,
and
Who has the Brilliance of a Million Suns,
O Lord
Please make all my Works Free of Obstacles,
Always

Contributors

Ananta Khurana MD, DNB, MNAMS
Associate Professor
Department of Dermatology and STDs
PGIMER, Dr Ram Manohar Lohia Hospital
New Delhi

C Janaki MD (Derm), DD, MAMS
Professor (Retd), Department of Dermatology
Madras Medical College, Chennai 600 003

Chander Grover MD, DNB, MNAMS
Professor, Department of Dermatology and STD
University College of Medical Sciences and GTB Hospital
Delhi, India
Honorary Secretary, IADVL-Delhi State Branch-2017
Founder Secretary, Nail Society of India

Deepak Jakhar MD
Senior Resident
Department of Dermatology and STD
University College of Medical Sciences and GTBH

Devi S Menon MBBS
Postgraduate student
Department of Skin and VD
Medical College, Vadodara

G Sentamilselvi MD, DD, Ph.D, FAMS
Professor and Head (Retd)
Department of Dermatology
Madras Medical College, Chennai

Kabir Sardana MD, DNB, MNAMS
Professor
Department of Dermatology and STDs
PGIMER, Dr Ram Manohar Lohia Hospital
New Delhi

Manjunath Shenoy M MD, DNB
Professor and Head, Department of Dermatology
Yenepoya Medical College
Mangalore

Namrata Chhabra MD
Assistant Professor
Department of Dermatology and Venereology
All India Institute of Medical Sciences, Raipur
Chhattisgarh

Pooja Arora Mrig MD, DNB, MNAMS
Associate Professor
Department of Dermatology and STDs
PGIMER, Dr Ram Manohar Lohia Hospital
Delhi

Prachi Kawthekar MD
Consultant Dermatologist
Indore, Madhya Pradesh

Premanshu Bhushan MD
Senior Consultant
PN Behl Skin Institute and School of Dermatology
New Delhi

Madhu Rengasamy MD (Derm), DCH
Senior Assistant Professor
Department of Dermatology (Mycology)
Madras Medical College, Chennai 600 003

Richa Anjleen Tigga MBBS
Postgraduate Resident (3rd year)
Department of Microbiology
UCMS and GTB Hospital
Dilshad Garden, Delhi

Sanjay Kr Rathi MD
Consultant Dermatologist
Siliguri

Shilpa Garg DNB (Dermatology and Venereology)
Consultant, Department of Dermatology
Sir Ganga Ram Hospital, Rajinder Nagar
New Delhi

Shital Poojary MD, DNB
Professor and Head, Department of Dermatology
KJ Somaiya Medical College, Mumbai

Shukla Das MD, DNB, MNAMS
Director Professor
Department of Microbiology
UCMS and GTB Hospital
Dilshad Garden
Delhi

Shyam Verma MBBS, DV and D, FRCP (London)
Consultant Dermatologist, Nirvana Skin Clinic, Vadodara

Sidharth Sonthalia MD, DNB
Medical Director, Senior Consultant, Dermatologist
Skinnocence: The Skin Clinic and Research Center
Gurugram

Sucheta Sharma MD
Senior Resident, Department of Dermatology and
Venereology
LHMC and Associated Hospitals, New Delhi

Taru Garg MD
Professor, Department of Dermatology and Venereology
LHMC and Associated Hospitals
New Delhi

Yogesh S Marfatia MD
Professor of Skin and VD
Medical College
Vadodara

Foreword

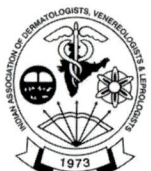

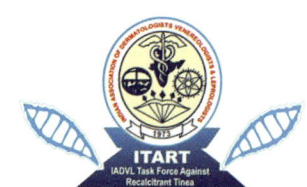

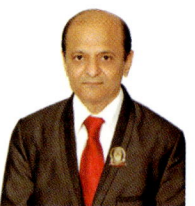

Management of tinea has become challenging and needs multipronged approach based on a lot of considerations. A comprehensive manual on practical aspects of management of chronic and recalcitrant tinea was a felt need.

I am grateful to all IADVLites for giving consent to go ahead with a manual on tinea, focusing on current issues and serving the purpose of a ready reckoner.

While going through content, I realized that all issues related to management of tinea are comprehensively covered.

Inclusion of topics like epidemiologic transformation, dermoscopy, rational use of antifungal agents in chronic and recurrent tinea, corticosteroid modified tinea, special procedures like LASER PDT treatment for dermatophytoses and a chapter on role of powders, soaps and washes, make the manual very rich in content. Discussion on management of challenging cases by experts is a welcome addition. I hope the users will find it very helpful while managing challenging cases of tinea.

I acknowledge efforts of members of IADVL Task-force Against Recalcitrant Tinea (ITART) as well as Academy Chair and Convener, for facilitating this project resulting into a unique scientific publication.

I am indebted to Kabir Sardana, Ananta Khurana, Shilpa Garg, Shital Poojary and editorial team for transforming my idea into reality.

I am sure that this will be a milestone publication.

Best wishes
Let us create brilliance together

Yogesh S Marfatia
Immediate Past National President IADVL

Foreword

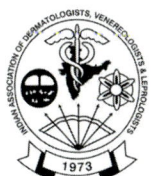

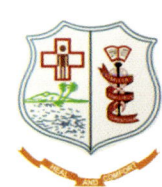

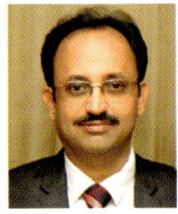

Management of dermatophytoses has become a challenge nowadays. The epidemic of superficial fungal infection has not only presenting with varied clinical and microbiological presentation but also difficult to treat. IADVL has taken steps to conduct research and disseminate knowledge about these aspects through IADVL Task-force Against Recalcitrant Tinea (ITART). This textbook on dermatophytoses edited by Dr Kabir Sardana will help dermatologists in understanding the varying clinical manifestations and management.

Ramesh Bhat M
President IADVL National
Professor
Fr Muller Medical College
Mangalore, Karnataka

Preface

The *IADVL Manual on Management of Dermatophytoses* comes at a very appropriate time, when dermatologists all over the nation are grappling with the issue of recalcitrant dermatophytic infections. Though the issue continues to perplex us and scientific reasoning for it is still awaited, we have made an attempt to bring out a comprehensive text covering all aspects of dermatophytoses, to update the reader of existing literature and possible directions for the future.

This project has many "creators" and we were the accidental editors. It was originally the brain child of Dr Yogesh S Marfatia and the ITART and was then handed over to the IADVL Academy who under Dr Ameet Valia, Dr Kolalapudi Seetharaman and Dr Deepika Pandhi invited nomination for the book and its team. We thank them for assigning us this task. The contents were largely their suggestions and the idea of scenarios was of Dr Yogesh S Marfatia.

The manual begins with a detailed analysis on the changing patterns of dermatophytoses both clinically and mycologically. It is evident that the clinical morphologies we are witnessing now reflect a shift in the host–pathogen relationship, with hitherto rare and unusual forms being commonly encountered. This is well illustrated by Dr Manjunath Shenoy M in the concerned chapter. A possible species-shift as a reason for the present situation is discussed at length by Dr Shital poojary. The author puts forward numerous references, both old and new, from across the country, exploring this possibility. Dr Shukla Das, an accomplished mycologist, provides useful insights into the laboratory confirmation techniques and antifungal susceptibility testing. Dermoscopy, an upcoming tool in diagnostic assessment of dermatophytoses, is covered with ample illustrations by Dr Ananta Khurana and Dr Deepak Jhakar. Dr Namrata Chhabra has contributed a large part covering general measures, topical therapies and role of ancillary treatments. Chapter 8 by Dr Madhu Rengarajan, provides an in-depth knowledge of the various systemic drugs for dermatophytoses, covering pharmacokinetics, pharmacodynamics and adverse effects of each. This is taken further in Chapter 9 focussing specifically on the rationale of use of antifungal drugs based on skin pharmacokinetics. The topic has been succinctly covered by Dr Pooja Arora Mrig and Dr Kabir Sardana. An elaborate overview on steroid modified tinea has been presented by Dr Yogesh S Marfatia, bringing to forefront the ill effects of topical steroids and the ramifications thereof. An in-depth review of the possible causes of the present scenario of recalcitrant infections and treatment options is presented by Dr Kabir Sardana and Dr Ananta Khurana. Separate sections on management of dermatophytic infections of the hair and nail have been done full justice by Dr Taru Garg and Dr Chander Grover respectively. Treatment in certain special patient groups, an often ignored aspect, is covered in detail by Dr Ananta Khurana. In the last section, Dr Ananta Khurana covers the emerging, though yet lacking quality evidence backing, therapies for onychomycosis in the form of lasers and PDT.

The end of the book has clinical scenarios which is an important part as it gives views of various practitioners across India and also gives an idea of the different approaches to the problem. The one unique aspect is that clinicians have used various oral drugs, including fluconazole, terbinafine, griseofulvin and itraconazole with good results, which goes against the theory of *in vitro* resistance, which discredits all drugs except itraconazole. It has insights into novel interventions including ciclopirox olamine which certainly holds potential.

A big thanks to CBS Publishers & Distributors, Mr SK Jain CMD, and Mr YN Arjuna Senior Vice President—Publishing, Editorial and Publicity, and their team, Mrs Ritu Chawla Assistant General Manager—Production, Mr Vikrant Sharma, Mr Sanjay Chauhan, Mr Neeraj Prasad, Mr Prasenjit Paul, and Mr SK Verma, apart from the great support staff at their easily accessible office. Also as Chief Editor a big thanks to my team including Dr Shilpa Garg and Dr Shital Poojary, who took out time from their schedules to pay attention to this book. Needless to say a big thanks to Dr Ananta Khurana who manages to take out hidden energy and inexplicable time from her already over encumbered academic and personal schedules for her assigned tasks. And thanks to the academy for such great co-editors.

Hope the book and its contents are useful for the readers.

Kabir Sardana
Chief Editor

Contents

1

Epidemiological Transformation of Dermatophytes in India: Changing Morphological Patterns

Manjunath Shenoy M

INTRODUCTION

Dermatophytes are keratinophilic fungi belonging to three genera: Trichophyton, Microsporum and Epidermophyton. Dermatophytes infect humans (anthropophilic), other mammals (zoophilic), or are found in soil (geophilic). They can invade the skin, hair and nails leading to pruritus, alopecia and dystrophic nails. Though majority of infections respond well to treatment, some are chronic and refractory in nature. Tropical climate, obesity, tight-fitting clothes, sharing of clothes, sport activities and overcrowding are known risk factors for fungal infections. Dermatophytoses, commonly referred to as "tinea", are commonly seen in practice, but in recent years there has been an alarming increase in the incidence of this infection. The clinical presentation of dermatophytoses has also undergone major transformation.

Classical Presentation of Dermatophytosis

Classically, dermatophytosis presents with involvement of the glabrous skin with erythematous annular scaly plaques with active borders, popularly known as the "ringworm".

Tinea Corporis and Cruris

Tinea corporis is superficial dermatophytic infection of the glabrous skin (i.e. skin other than scalp, groin, palms, and soles) and tinea cruris is the infection of the groins (Figs 1.1 and 1.2). Infected patients generally have variable pruritus but can rarely be asymptomatic. Annular plaque with an advancing border is the characteristic lesion. It can involve any part of the body but occluded areas like the waist line, inframammary region and gluteal region are more commonly affected. Tinea cruris can extend to the adjoining skin and is usually associated with severe pruritus and burning sensation.

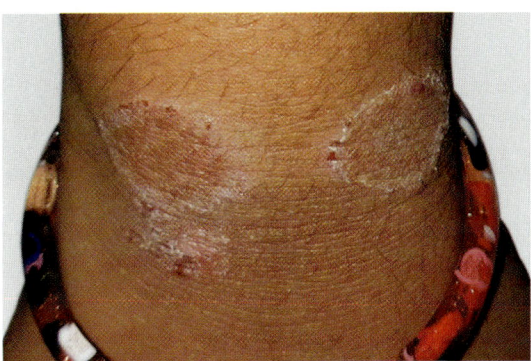

Fig. 1.1: Classical tinea corporis

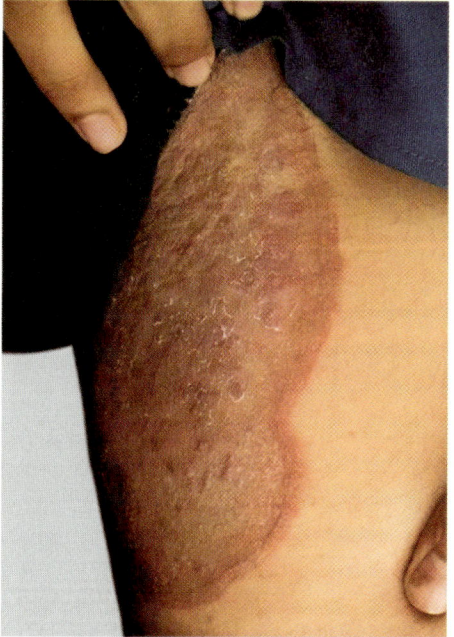

Fig. 1.2: Classical tinea cruris

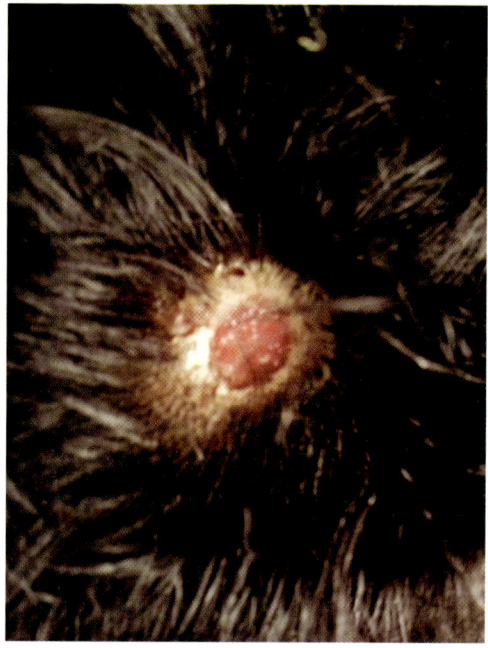

Fig. 1.4: Classical tinea capitis (inflammatory)

Tinea Capitis

It can manifest as noninflammatory and inflammatory types.

a. *Noninflammatory type:* Grey patch, black dot and seborrheic dermatitis-like pattern are seen (Fig. 1.3).

b. *Inflammatory type:* Kerion refers to the inflamed, thickened, abscess-like lesions

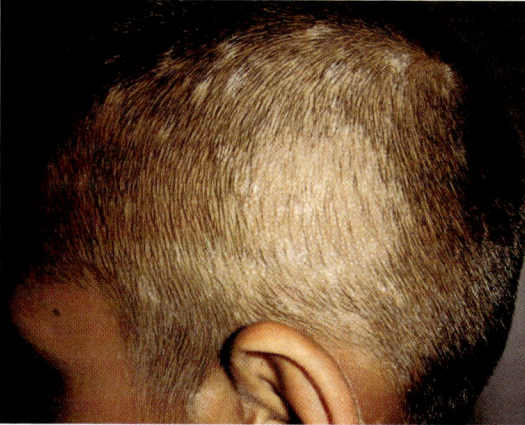

Fig. 1.3: Classical tinea capitis (noninflammatory)

over the scalp due to the host inflammatory response to infection of the hair follicles (Fig. 1.4). Favus is a rare form of tinea capitis characterised by chronic crusted plaques, usually found in endemic areas of Jammu and Kashmir in India.

Tinea Pedis

It can manifest as scaly soles or maceration and fissuring between the toes (Figs 1.5 and 1.6). Uncommonly vesicular or ulcerative lesions can also be seen.

Tinea Unguium

Also known as onychomycosis, it typically presents with subungual hyperkeratosis with discoloration of nail plate, known as the distal lateral subungual onychomycosis (DLSO). Proximal subungual onychomycosis (PSO) is less commonly seen. True nail plate involvement with chalky white plaques on nail plate is known as superficial white onychomycosis (SWO). Total nail dystrophy (TDO) can occur in advanced cases (Fig. 1.7).

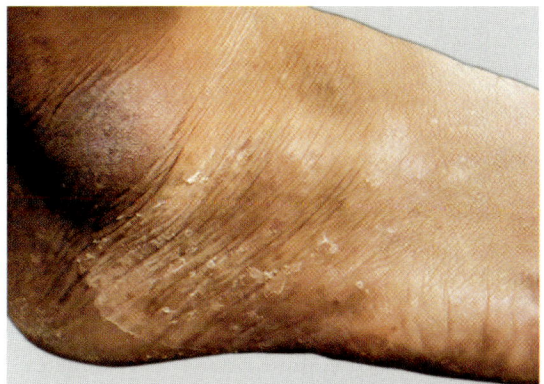

Fig. 1.5: Tinea pedis

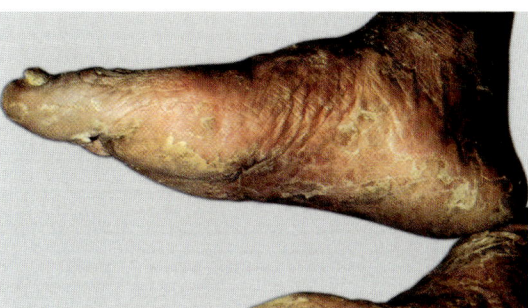

Fig. 1.6: Tinea pedis

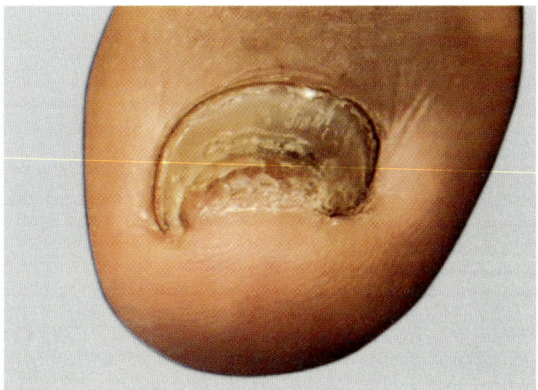

Fig. 1.7: Onychomycosis

Changing Morphological Patterns

Dermatophytoses presenting in an atypical manner has always been reported but such occurrences have become more frequent in the recent times. It is common in immunocompromised patients but healthy individuals

may also present with atypical tinea which may cause diagnostic challenges. Pattern of presentation has been changing in the recent past due to certain known and unknown factors. Morphology, extent of involvement and association with other dermatoses can cause diagnostic dilemmas.

Extent

Dermatophytoses can present as large patches, multiple lesions, distant site involvement and extensive disease (Figs 1.8 and 1.9). Extension

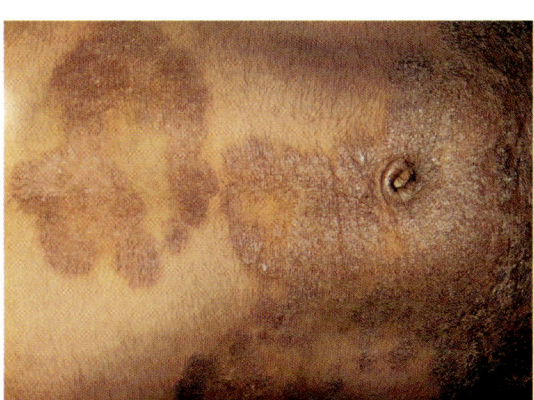

Fig. 1.8: Extensive tinea corporis

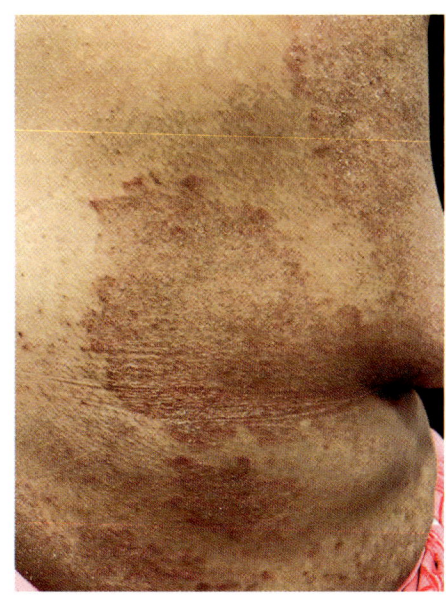

Fig. 1.9: Extensive tinea corporis

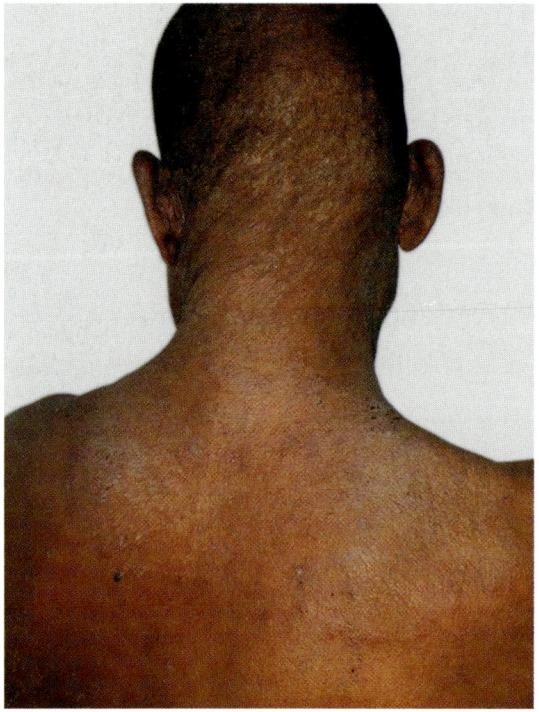

Fig. 1.10: Tinea extending to scalp

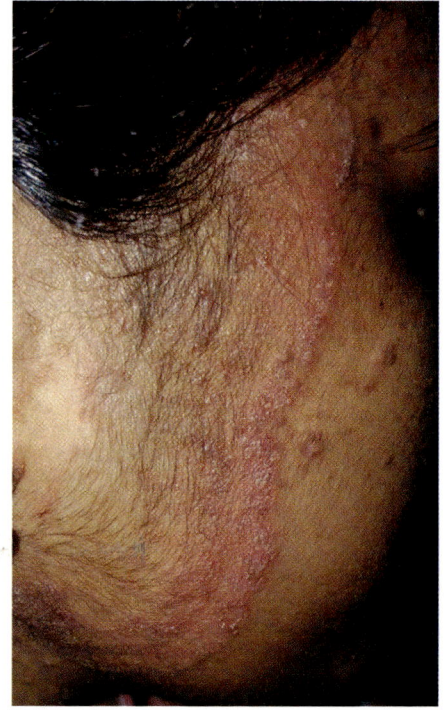

Fig. 1.11: Tinea faciei

of disease from back, chest and neck on to the face and scalp has been frequently noticed (Fig. 1.10). Very extensive disease accounting for erythroderma has also been reported. Such involvement can occur in a relatively short duration of time.

Location

Uncommon locations such as face, scalp, genital and hand involvement has been noticed more frequently than before (Figs 1.11 and 1.12). Such involvement may be seen as an isolated lesion or as a part of extensive disease.

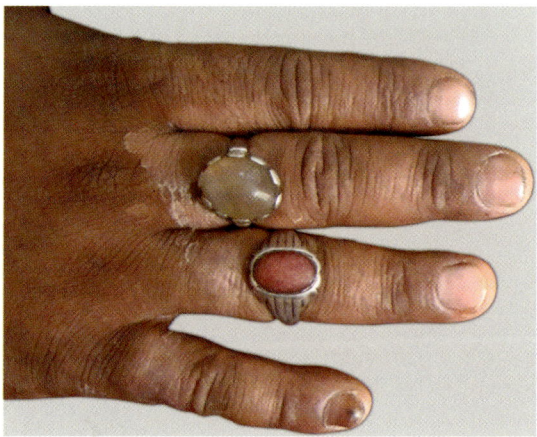

Fig. 1.12: Tinea of hand

Morphology

Tinea manifesting with unusual morphology including pseudoimbricata, pustular lesions, eczematous lesions, follicular lesions and nodular lesions can be seen (Figs 1.13 to 1.15). Many of these manifestations are due to topical steroid abuse.

Dermatophytosis with other Dermatoses

Currently dermatophytosis is the commonest disease seen in the dermatology outpatient. It is seen in association with other common and uncommon dermatoses like acne, eczemas, psoriasis, lichen planus, etc. (Figs 1.16 to 1.18).

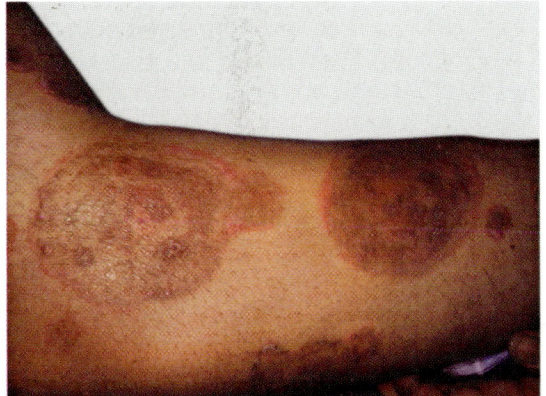

Fig. 1.13: Tinea pseudoimbricata

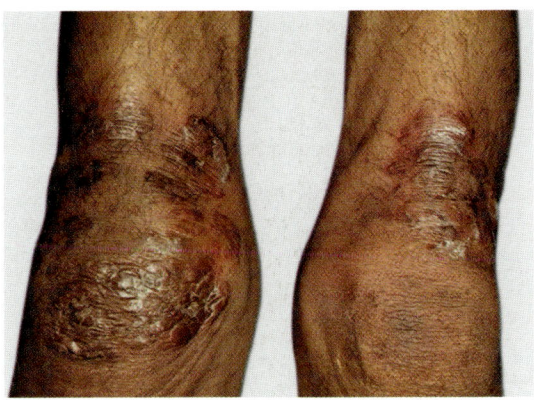

Fig. 1.16: A case of psoriasis with tinea

Many such dermatoses require topical steroids which may aggravate dermatophytosis or lead to tinea incognito.

Steroid Modified Tinea and Tinea Incognito (Also see in Chapter 10)

Steroid modified tinea presents as a distinct entity with an extensive and modified clinical presentation. Tinea incognito manifests with lack of inflammatory advancing margins. Similar changes have been reported with topical calcineurin inhibitors. Cutaneous atrophy and striae may also accompany where there is steroid abuse (Fig. 1.17).

Differential Diagnosis

Tinea on the body may resemble psoriasis, eczema and other dermatoses (Fig. 1.18). Tinea faciei may resemble other facial dermatosis like rosacea, seborrheic dermatitis and lupus erythematosus. Noninflammatory tinea capitis may resemble seborrheic dermatitis. Inflammatory lesions may resemble psoriasis and other inflammatory scalp dermatoses. Kerion resembles a scalp abscess.

Reasons for Transformation

Reasons for the changing morphological presentation are not clearly understood. Topical steroid abuse is a known factor but there are many other poorly understood factors. These may include host factors like

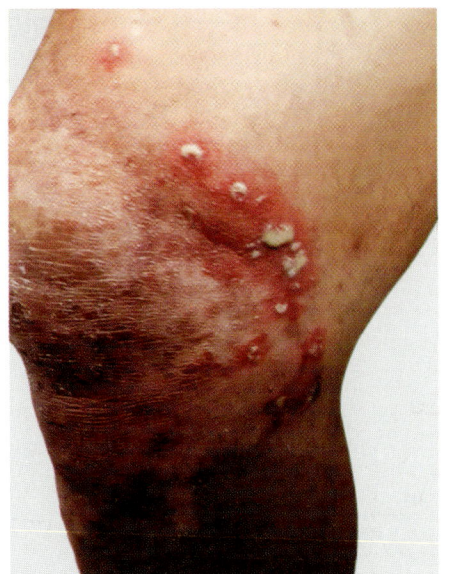

Fig. 1.14: Pustular tinea

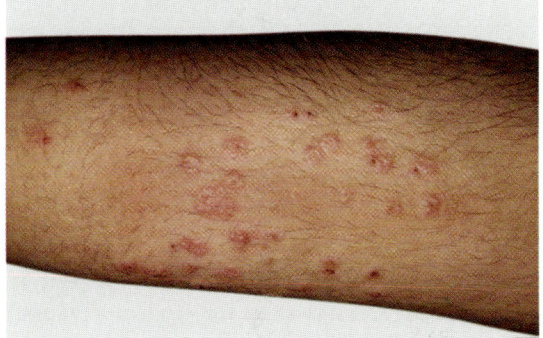

Fig. 1.15: Follicular tinea

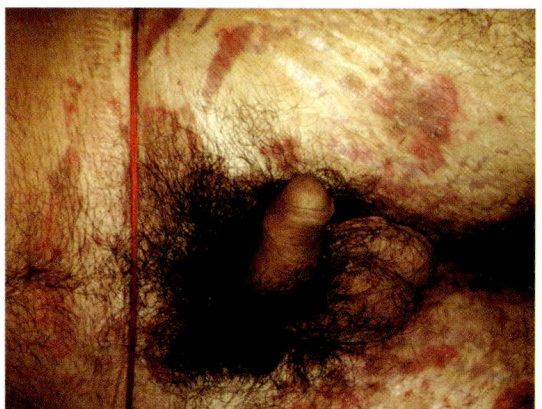

Fig. 1.17: Tinea incognito due to steroid abuse

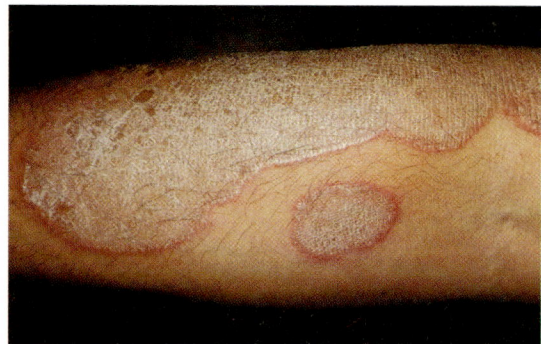

Fig. 1.18: Psoriasiform tinea

immune suppression, changing immune status like atopy, clothing patterns, travels, contact with pets and hygiene. Pathogen related factors like changes in species may also contribute. Environmental changes such as global warming may also have a role to play.

Bibliography

1. Dogra S, Narang T. Emerging atypical and unusual presentations of dermatophytosis in India. Clin Dermatol Rev 2017;1, Suppl S1:12–8.

2. Shenoy MS, Shenoy MM. Fungal nail disease (Onychomycosis); Challenges and solutions. Arch Med Health Sci 2014;2:48–53.

3. Verma S. Tinea pseudoimbricata. Indian J Dermatol Venereol Leprol 2017;83:344–5.

2

Epidemiological Transformation of Dermatophytes in India: Mycological Evidence

Shital Poojary

INTRODUCTION TO DERMATOPHYTES AND THEIR CLASSIFICATION

Dermatophytes are Ascomycetes with septate hyphae most closely related to *Coccidioides immitis*. There are three genera of dermatophytes: Trichophyton, Microsporum and Epidermophyton, based on morphology and physical attributes.[1]

Four decades ago, the sexual state of dermatophytes was not known. The species for which the sexual state was identified were later classified into a single genus Arthroderma in the phylum Ascomycota. As the sexual states are not routinely identified, most of the times the names of the asexual anamorph states have been used in practice. *Arthroderma benhamiae* is the sexual anamorph of *T. mentagrophytes*.[1] Increasing use of molecular techniques in identification of species has further changed the nomenclatures of the dermatophytes and a multilocus phylogenetic taxonomy has been proposed by De Hoog et al.[2]

Dermatophytes are also classified into anthropophilic, zoophilic and geophilic types (Table 2.1). Geophilic species generally cause acute and severe disease. Anthropophilic species are usually associated with long-term

Table 2.1: Ecological classification of dermatophytes	
Type	*Name of species*
Anthropophilic	*Epidermophyton floccosum*
	Microsporum audouinii
	Microsporum ferrugineum
	Trichophyton concentricum
	Trichophyton interdigitale
	Trichophyton rubrum
	Trichophyton schoenleinii
	Trichophyton soudanense
	Trichophyton tonsurans
	Trichophyton violaceum
Geophilic	*Microsporum gypseum*
	Microsporum praecox
Zoophilic	*Microsporum canis*
	Microsporum canis var. *distortum*
	Microsporum gallinae
	Microsporum nanum
	Microsporum persicolor
	Trichophyton equinum
	Trichophyton mentagrophytes
	Trichophyton simii
	Trichophyton verrucosum

chronic disease. Zoophilic species also cause acute disease but lesser inflammation as compared to anthropophilic species. However, classification of the dermatophytes according to the ecological niches may not always be sharply demarcated. Geophilic species can contaminate or infect animals and subsequently infect the humans via an intermediate animal host.

Factors Affecting Distribution of Species Throughout the World

1. Socioeconomic behavior and environment of humans
2. Migration of individuals or groups
3. Occupation
4. Evolution of new genotypes
5. Transfer or adaptation of species indigenous to animal populations to parasitism in humans.

Thus, the distribution of species is not static and can change rapidly or gradually depending on the factors involved.

Why is it Essential to know the Epidemiological Distribution of Species?

Epidemiological transformation has great bearings on the prevalence of infection, chronicity of infections, severity of infections and also treatment response.

A change in species can result in epidemics confined to specific geographic areas and later spread to other areas due to migration. As mentioned above, geophilic and zoophilic species are likely to cause more inflammatory lesions as compared to anthropophilic species and by corollary shorter course of infections. Identification of species may have a bearing on treatment, e.g. terbinafine was found to be more effective against *T. tonsurans* as compared to *Microsporum canis*. However, in practice antifungals are not yet prescribed according to the isolated species. However, in the current scenario of recalcitrant dermatophytosis, this point may be needed to be taken into account.

Distribution of Dermatophyte Species in India

Distribution of dermatophyte species in India prior to present epidemic of recalcitrant

dermatophytosis: before 2012 and after 2012 have been depicted in Tables 2.2 and 2.3, respectively.[3–31]

Prior to the present epidemic, most studies show that *T. rubrum* was the predominant dermatophyte isolated except in cases of *T. capitis* where *T. tonsurans* and *T. violaceum* have been predominant species.[22]

On close perusal of the studies, it is observed that at least one study in the series of studies after 2012 shows predominance of *T. mentagrophytes* (22.8%) as compared to *T. rubrum* (5.86%).[26] Two studies showed a relatively higher proportion of *T. mentagrophytes* in comparison with earlier studies, although *T. rubrum* still retained predominance.[24, 28] The study by Parmeshwari et al shows *T. mentagrophytes* at 35.7% which is definitely more compared to the average prevalence of earlier studies. Study by Ramaraj et al showed proportion of *T. mentagrophytes* to be 44.75% almost equalling the proportion of *T. rubrum*. These findings also find an echo in the personal observations of Dr Miskeen who has found similar findings in his laboratory.[32]

An interesting observation can be made from the group of studies prior to 2012: two studies show an increased proportion and preponderance of *T. mentagrophytes* as compared to *T. rubrum*.[12,16] The study by Agarwal et al from Jaipur is of particular significance as is a similar study by Jain et al from Jaipur in 2008, both of which showed predominance of *T. rubrum*.[13]

All these observations are a definite indication that a shift is occurring in the predominance of causative species from *T. rubrum* to *T. mentagrophytes*. In some areas, the shift probably set in even before the epidemic became clinically apparent on ground (as is evident from the Jaipur studies).

The cause for these can only be speculated upon, depending on personal observations, as no definite studies are there in literature defining the causes of the shift. Following factors may be responsible for the gradual shift in species:

1. Increasing misuse of topical steroid combinations in Indian scenario could have caused alteration in the local immunity creating a fertile ground for adaptation of new species. The substitution of betamethasone based combinations with clobetasol based combinations could have accelerated the shift.

2. Global warming may provide the necessary warm temperatures for the spores to survive in the environment. However, this theory would not explain why the phenomenon is confined to India.

Implications of Epidemiological Transformation and Shift in Species

Is the gradual change in predominant causative species responsible for the present epidemic of recalcitrant dermatophytosis? As of now, there are no definite studies published to show that *T. mentagrophytes* is less susceptible to antifungals as compared to *T. rubrum*. Personal observations do suggest that *T. mentagrophytes* have a higher range of minimum inhibitory concentration as compared to *T. rubrum* but multicentric studies are required to confirm these observations.

Authors	Year	Region	Type of dermatophytoses	No. of patients	Predominant species isolated with percentage
Karmakar et al	1995	Jodhpur	All types T. cruris, predominant (34.4%) T. capitis (16.8%) Tinea corporis (24.0%)	250 (105 culture positive)	T. violaceum (55.76%) from all clinical types followed by T. rubrum (42.3%)
Patwardhan and Dave	1999	Aurangabad	All types T. corporis, predominant	175	T. rubrum (28.12%) T. mentagrophytes (25%)
Singh S et al	1999–2000	Baroda	All types T. corporis, predominant	260 (44.62% culture positivity)	T. rubrum (73.27%) T. mentagrophytes (17.24%) E. floccosum (7.75%) T. violaceum (1.72%)
Grover and Roy	1999–2001	Northeast India	T. pedis, predominant T cruris: 2nd most common	103	T. tonsurans (20.3%) T. rubrum (8.7%) M. ferruginum (5.8%) T. mentagrophytes (2.9%) NDM: 34%
Bindu V, Pavithran K	2002	Calicut	All types T. corporis, predominant	150	T. rubrum, predominant species in all types (66.2%) T. mentagrophytes (25%) T. tonsurans (5.9%) E. floccosum (2.9%)
Kannan et al	2001–2002	Chennai	All types T. corporis, predominant	80 (66.3% culture positivity)	T. rubrum (39.6%) T. mentagrophytes (16.7%) T. violaceum (39.6%)

Table 2.2: Studies of epidemiology of dermatophytes up to 2012 (pre-dermatophyte epidemic)

(Contd.)

Authors	Year	Region	Type of dermatophytoses	No. of patients	Predominant species isolated with percentage
			Table 2.2: Studies of epidemiology of dermatophytes up to 2012 (pre-dermatophyte epidemic) *(Contd.)*		
Peerapur et al	2004	Bijapur	All types T. corporis, predominant	102 (64% culture positivity)	*T. rubrum* (43.7%) *T. mentagrophytes* (18, 28.1%) *E. floccosum* (7.8%) *M. audouinii* (6.2%)
Surendran et al	2006–2008	Mysore	All types T. corporis, predominant	100 (39% culture positivity)	*T. rubrum* (67.5%) *T. mentagrophytes* (20%) *E. floccosum* (5%)
Venkatesan et al	2007	Chennai	All types T. corporis, predominant	90 (78.9% culture positivity)	*T. rubrum* (73.3%) *T. mentagrophytes* (19.7%) *E. floccosum* (4.2%) *M. gypseuem* (2.8%)
Noronha et al	2007–2008	North Karnataka	All types T. corporis, predominant	150 (40% culture positivity)	*T. mentagrophytes* (48.3%) *T. rubrum* (38.3%) *T. verrucosum* (8.3%) *T. violaceum* (5%)
Jain et al	2008	Jaipur	All types T. corporis, predominant T. capitis: 2nd most common	120 (58.33% culture positivity)	*T. rubrum* (45.71%) *T. mentagrophytes* (14.29%) *T. violaceum* (10%) *T. tonsurans* (8.57%) *T. schoenleinii* (4.29%)
Bhagra et al	2008–2009	Shimla	All types T. corporis, predominant	100 (68% culture positivity)	*T. rubrum* (66.17%) *T. mentagrophytes* (19.11%) *T. violaceum* (7.35%) *T. tonsurans* (2.94%)
Surekha et al	2011	Tirupati	All types T. corporis, predominant	138 culture positivity: 18.1%	*T. rubrum*: 64% *T. mentagrophytes*: 20% Rest: *T. verrucosum* and *T. tonsurans*
Agarwal US et al	2011–2012	Jaipur	All types T. corporis, predominant	300 (80% culture positivity)	*T. mentagrophytes* (37.9%) *T. rubrum* (34.2%) *T. violaceum* (11.3%) *T. tonsurans* 8.3% *M. audouinii* (6.2%) *M. canis* (1.7%), *T. verrucosum* (0.4%)
Bhavsar et al	2011	Ahmedabad	All types	377 (20.1% culture positivity)	*T. rubrum* (55.26%) *T. mentagrophytes* (27.63%)
Hanuman-thappa et al	2012	Mysore	All types T. corporis, predominant	150	*T. rubrum* (58.9%) *T. mentagrophytes* (24.6%)

Table 2.3: Studies of epidemiology of dermatophytes after 2012 (during epidemic)					
Authors	Year of study	Region	Type of dermatophytoses	No. of patients	Species isolated with percentage
Mallik A et al	2011–2013	Aligarh	All types T. corporis, predominant	123	T. rubrum (58.5%) T. mentagrophytes (21.1%) E. floccosum (8.1%) M. gypseuem (4.1%) T. tonsurans (5.6%)
Kaur et al	2012–2013	New Delhi	All dermatomycoses	215	NDMs (36.1%), Trichophyton rubrum (4.6%) T. mentagrophytes (2.1%) T. verrucosum (3.2%)
Lakshmanan et al	2013–2014	Chengalput, TN	All types T. corporis, predominant	277 (22.38% culture positivity)	T. rubrum (79%) T. mentagrophytes (14.5%) M. canis, M. gypseum (3.2% each)
YJ Bhat et al	2014	Kashmir	Tinea capitis	150 (84% culture positivity)	T. tonsurans (61.11%) T. rubrum (13.48%) T. violaceum (10.32%) T. schoenleinii (6.35%) T. verrucosum (4.76%)
Sarkar et al	2014–2015	Kolkata	Onychomycosis	118 (52.54% culture positivity)	T. rubrum (13.63%) T. tonsurans (09.09%) T. soudanense (07.57%) T. schoenleinii (04.5%) NDM (24.19%) Candida (33.87%)
Parmeshwari et al	2015	Kakinada	All types T. corporis, predominant	150 (55% culture positivity)	T. rubrum (50%) T. mentagrophytes (35.7%) T. violaceum (8.6%) M. gypseum (4.3%) E. floccosum (1.4%)
Poluri et al	2015	Telangana	All types T. corporis, predominant	110 (56.36% culture positivity)	T. rubrum (58.06%) T. mentagrophytes (22.58%) T. violaceum (6.54%) E. floccosum (6.45%) T. tonsurans (3.22%) T. schoenleinnii (3.22%)
Venkatesh et al	2014–2016	Karwar	All types T. corporis, predominant	1590 (59% culture positivity)	T. mentagrophytes (22.8%) T. rubrum (5.86%) T. mentagrophytes var interdigitale (5.97%) NDM and Phaeoid species (25.58%)

(Contd.)

Authors	Year of study	Region	Type of dermatophytoses	No. of patients	Species isolated with percentage
Manjunath et al	2016	Shimoga	All types T. corporis, predominant	130 (53.8% culture positivity)	T. rubrum (38.57%) T. mentagrophytes (22.85%) M. audouni (21.42%) M. gypseum (11.43%) T. violaceum (4.28%) E. floccosum (1.43%)
Ramaraj et al	2016	Chennai	All types	210	T. rubrum (48.95) T. mentagrophytes (44.75%) Other isolates: T. tonsurans (3.50%) isolates M. gypseum (1.40%)
Majid et al	2016	Kashmir	All types	100	Trichophyton rubrum (55%) Trichophyton tonsurans (20%) T. mentagrophytes (12%)
Janardhan B et al	2017	Telangana	All types T. corporis, predominant	200 (72% culture positivity) T. corporis, predominant	T. rubrum (52%) T. mentagrophytes (14%) T. violaceum (4%) M. audounii (2%) (T. capitis)
Aruna et al	2017	Chitradurga	All types	135 (93/135)	T. rubrum (67.74%) E. floccosum (16.12%) T. mentagrophytes (10.75%) M. canis (4.93%) and M. gypseum (1.23%)

Table 2.3: Studies of epidemiology of dermatophytes after 2012 (during epidemic) (Contd.)

References

1. Hay RJ, Ashbee HR. Fungal infections in Griffiths CEM, Barker J, Bleiker T, Chalmers R, Creamer D Eds. Rook's Textbook of Dermatology, Wiley Blackwell 9th ed 2016;32:18–32,53.

2. De Hoog GS, Dukik K. Monod M, Packeu A, Stubbe D. Towards a Novel Multilocus Phylogenetic Taxonomy for the Dermatophytes. Mycopathologia 2017; 182:5–31.

3. Karmakar S, Kalla G, Joshi KR. Dermatophytoses in a desert district of Western Rajasthan. Indian J Dermatol Venereol Leprol 1995;61:280–3.

4. Patwardhan N, Dave R. Dermatomycosis in and around Aurangabad. Indian J Pathol Microbiol 1999; 42:455–62.

5. Singh S, Beena PM. Profile of dermatophyte infections in Baroda. Indian J Dermatol Venereol Leprol 2003; 69:281–3.

6. Grover SC, Roy PC. Clinicomycological profile of superficial mycosis in a hospital in Northeast India. Med J Armed Forces India 2003;59:114–6.

7. Bindu V, Pavithran K. Clinicomycological study of dermatophytosis in Calicut. Indian J Dermatol Venereol Leprol 2002; 68: 259–61.

8. Kannan P, Janaki C, Selvi GS. Prevalence of dermatophytes and other fungal agents isolated from clinical samples. Indian Journal of Medical Microbiology 2006; 24:212–5.

9. Peerapur BV, Inamdar AC, Pushpa PV, Srikant B. Clinicomycological Study of Dermatophytosis in

Bijapur. Indian J Med Microbiol 2004; 22: 273–4.

10. Surendran K, Bhat RM, Boloor R, Nandakishore B, Sukumar D. A clinical and mycological study of dermatophytic infections. Indian J Dermatol 2014;59:262–7.

11. Venkatesan G, Ranjit Singh A JA, Murugesan AG, Janaki C, Shankar SG. *Trichophyton rubrum*—the predominant etiological agent in human dermatophytoses in Chennai, India. Afr J Microbiol Res 2007;9–12.

12. Noronha TM, Tophakhane RS, Nadiger S. Clinico-microbiological study of dermatophytosis in a tertiary care hospital in North Karnataka. Indian Dermatol Online J 2016;7:264–71.

13. Jain N, Sharma M, Saxena VN. Clinico-mycological profile of dermatophytosis in Jaipur, Rajasthan Indian J Dermatol Venereol Leprol 2008; 74:274–5.

14. Bhagra S, Ganju SA, Kanga A, Sharma NL, Guleria RC. Mycological pattern of dermatophytosis in and around Shimla hills. Indian J Dermatol 2014;59: 268–70.

15. Surekha A, Ramesh Kumar G, Sridevi K, Murty DS, Usha G, Bharathi G. Superficial dermatomycoses: a prospective clinicomycological study. J Clin Sci Res 2015;4:7–15.

16. Agarwal US, Saran J, Agarwal P. Clinico-mycological study of dermatophytes in a tertiary care centre in Northwest India. Indian J Dermatol Venereol Leprol 2014;80:194.

17. Bhavsar HK, Modi DJ, Sood NK, Shah HS. A study of superficial mycoses with clinical mycological profile in tertiary care hospital in Ahmedabad, Gujarat national journal of medical research 2012; 2:160–4.

18. Hanumanthappa H, Sarojini K, Shilpashree P, Muddapur SB. Clinicomycological Study of 150 Cases of Dermatophytosis in a Tertiary Care Hospital in South India. Indian J Dermatol 2012 Jul-Aug; 57(4): 322–3.

19. Abida Malik, Nazish Fatima, Parvez Anwar Khan. A Clinicomycological Study of Superficial Mycoses from a Tertiary Care Hospital of a North Indian Town. Virol Mycol 2014;3: 135.

20. Kaur R, Panda SP, Sardana K, Khan S. Mycological Pattern of Dermatomycoses in a Tertiary Care Hospital. J Tropical Medicine 2015;157828.

21. Lakshmanan A, Ganeshkumar P, Mohan SR, Hemamalini M, Madhavan R. Epidemiological and clinical pattern of dermatomycoses in rural India. Indian J Med Microbiol 2015;33:S134–6.

22. Bhat YJ, Zeerak S, Kanth F, Yaseen A, Hassan I, Hakak R. Clinicoepidemiological and mycological study of tinea capitis in the pediatric population of Kashmir valley: A study from a tertiary care centre. Indian Dermatol Online J 2017;8:100–3.

23. Sarkar M, Ghosh RR, Halder P, Ghosh AP, Chatterjee M. Clinicomycological Profile of Onychomycosis: A Study in a Tertiary Care Hospital in Kolkata. IOSR Journal of Dental and Medical Sciences 2016;15: 78–83.

24. Parameswari K, Prasad Babu KP. Clinicomycological study of dermatophytosis in and around Kakinada. Int J Med and Dent Sci 2015; 4:828–33.

25. Poluri LV, Indugula JP, Kondapaneni SL. Clinicomycological Study of Dermatophytosis in South India. J Lab Physicians 2015; 7(2): 84–9.

26. Venkatesh V N, Swapna Kotian. Dermatophytosis: A Clinicomycological profile from a tertiary care hospital. Journal of International Medicine and Dentistry 2016;3: 96–102.

27. Manjunath M, Mallikarjun K, Dadapeer Sushma. Clinicomycological study of dermatomycosis in a tertiary care hospital. Indian J Microbiol Res 2016;3:190–193.

28. Ramaraj V, Vijayaraman RS, Rangarajan S, Kindo AJ. Incidence and prevalence of dermatophytosis in and around Chennai, Tamil Nadu, India. International Journal of Research in Medical Sciences 2016, 4:695–700.

29. Majid I, Sheikh G, Kanth F, Hakak R. Relapse after oral terbinafine therapy in dermatophytosis: A clinical and mycological study. Indian J Dermatol 2016;61:529–33.

30. Janardhan B, Vani G. Clinicomycological study of dermatophytosis. Int J Res Med Sci 2017;5:31–9.

31. Aruna GL, Ramalingappa B. A Clinico-mycological Study of Human Dermatophytosis in Chitradurga, Karnataka, India. JMSCR 2017;5: 2573–2574.

32. Miskeen AK, Uppuluri P. Laboratory diagnosis of fungal infections: A primer in Sardana K, Mahajan K, Mrig PA (Eds). Fungal infections: Diagnosis and treatment. CBS Publishers, New Delhi. 2017;23–39.

3

Investigations for Diagnosing Dermatophyte Infection

Shukla Das, Richa Anjleen Tigga

The laboratory diagnosis of superficial fungal infections relies first on the direct microscopic observation of the pathogen in samples from the affected area. This is usually followed by culture and the specific identification of the fungus. For the laboratory to provide the optimum performance, the quantity and the quality of the material examined are critical.

Because for most samples, both culture and microscopic examination will be performed, it is essential that as much clinical material as possible is submitted to the laboratory to allow both diagnostic methods to be carried out.[1] Table 3.1 lists the various species of fungus which are known to infection skin, nails and hair.

Table 3.1: Fungal species causing infection of skin, nail and hair	
Clinical types	*Causative dermatophyte species*
Tinea corporis	*Trichophyton rubrum*
	Trichophyton mentagrophytes
	Trichophyton verrucosum
	Trichophyton tonsurans
	Epidermophyton spp.
	Microsporum gypseum
	Microsporum audouinii
Tinea cruris	*Epidermophyton floccosum*
	Trichophyton rubrum
	Trichophyton mentagrophytes
Tinea imbricata	*Trichophyton concentricum*
Tinea mannum	*Trichophyton rubrum*
	Trichophyton mentagrophytes
	Epidermophyton floccosum
Tinea pedis	*Trichophyton rubrum*
	Trichophyton mentagrophytes
	Epidermophyton floccosum

(Contd.)

Table 3.1: Fungal species causing infection of skin, nail and hair (Contd.)	
Clinical types	*Causative dermatophyte species*
Tinea barbae	*Trichophyton verrucosum* *Trichophyton mentagrophytes* *Trichophyton violaceum* *Trichophyton rubrum*
Onychomycosis	
Dermatophytic fungi	*Trichophyton rubrum* *Trichophyton mentagrophytes* *Epidermophyton floccosum*
Non-dermatophytic fungi	*Acremonium* species *Alternaria* species *Aspergillus* species *Fusarium* species *Botryodiplodia theobromae* *Onycochola canadensis* *Pyrenochaeta unguis-hominis* *Scytalidium dimidiatum* *Scopulariopsis* species *Scytalidium hyalimum*
Yeast	*Candida albicans* *Non-albicans Candida*

Tinea capitis		*Organism*
Based on types of hair invasion	Ectothrix	*Trichophyton mentagrophytes* *Microsporum canis* *Microsporum gypseum* *Microsporum audouinii* *Trichophyton verrucosum* *Trichophyton rubrum*
	Endothrix	*Trichophyton schoenleinii* *Trichophyton tonsurans* *Trichophyton violaceum* *Trichophyton soudanense*
Based on types of tinea capitis	Kerion	*Trichophyton verrucosum* *Trichophyton mentagrophytes* *Microsporum canis* *Microsporum gypseum*
	Favus	*Trichophyton schoenleinii* *Trichophyton violaceum* *Microsporum gypseum*
	Black dot	*Trichophyton tonsurans* *Trichophyton violaceum*

SPECIMEN COLLECTION FOR FUNGAL TESTING

Skin Scraping

1. Cleaning the skin with 70% alcohol may be useful if the patient has applied any ointment or powder[1]

2. Scaping for fungus is done by using disposable scalpel blade which is held vertical to the skin scrapings. Alternatively, one can use:
   i. Heat-sterilized, blunt, banana-shaped scalpels[1]
   ii. Blunt edge of glass slide

3. If the lesion has a definite edge, the material should be taken from the active margin, otherwise a general scraping is adequate (Fig. 3.1).[1]

4. When scaling is less, sample is taken by pressing a strip of sticky tape on to the lesion and then on to a drop of mounting fluid on a slide (Fig. 3.2).[1]

5. Strongly macerated skin between toes can be removed by forceps.

6. Gentle deroofing can be done for vesicles.

SAMPLE COLLECTION OF NAIL

Collecting the Nail Specimen[2]

The first step of the sample collection process is thorough cleansing of the nail area with alcohol to remove debris and contaminants such as bacteria.

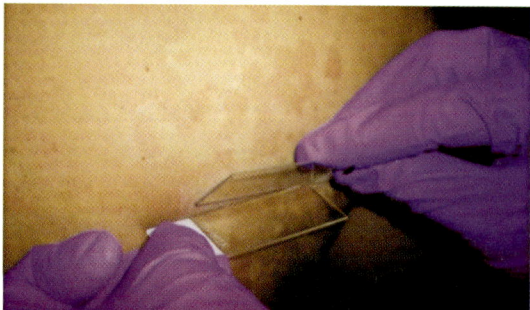

Fig. 3.1: General scraping from an annular erythematous skin lesion with minimal scaling
(*Source:* Usatine Richard P. "Watch and Learn: KOH Preparation." 19 June 2015, youtu./be LUwNQI_0BWU?t=49s.)

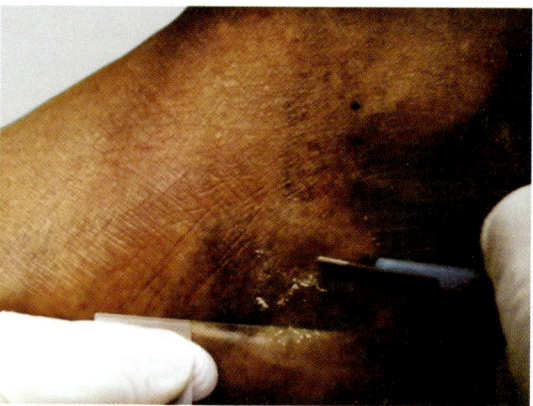

Fig. 3.2: Scraping from the active definite edge of the lesion using a disposable scalpel blade
(*Source:* Usatine, Richard P. "Watch and Learn: KOH Preparation." 19 June 2015, youtu.be/LUwNQI_0BWU?t=1m.)

Because the sites of invasion and localization of the infection differs in different types of onychomycosis, different approaches, depending on the presumptive diagnosis, are necessary to obtain optimal specimens and are as follows (Figs 3.3, 3.4 and 3.7):

a. **Distal subungual onychomycosis (DSO)**

- Because dermatophytes in patients with DSO invade the nail bed rather than the nail plate, the specimen must be obtained from the nail bed, where the concentration of viable fungi is greatest.

- The nail should be clipped short with nail clippers, and the specimen should be taken from the nail bed as proximally to the cuticle as possible with a small curette or a scalpel blade number 15.

- If debris is insufficient, material should be obtained from the nail bed.

- Material should also be obtained from the underside of the nail plate, with emphasis placed on sampling from the advancing infected edge most proximal to the cuticle (Fig. 3.4). This is the area most likely to contain viable hyphae and least likely to contain contaminants.

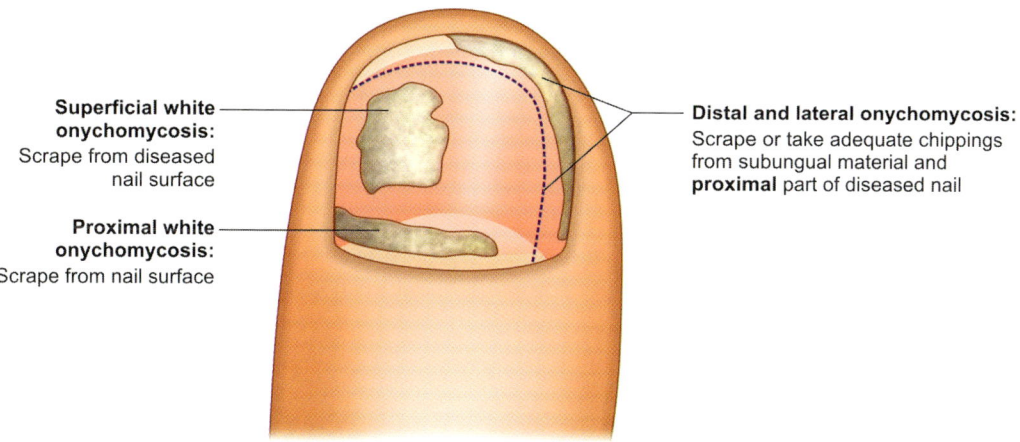

Superficial white onychomycosis:
Scrape from diseased nail surface

Distal and lateral onychomycosis:
Scrape or take adequate chippings from subungual material and **proximal** part of diseased nail

Proximal white onychomycosis:
Scrape from nail surface

Fig. 3.3: Pictorial depiction of sampling techniques from affected part of nail
(*Source:* "Recommended Sites for Nail Specimens." Collecting Specimens for the Investigation of Fungal Infections, Best Tests, Mar. 2011, www.bpac.org.nz/BT/2011/March/img/nail.jpg.)

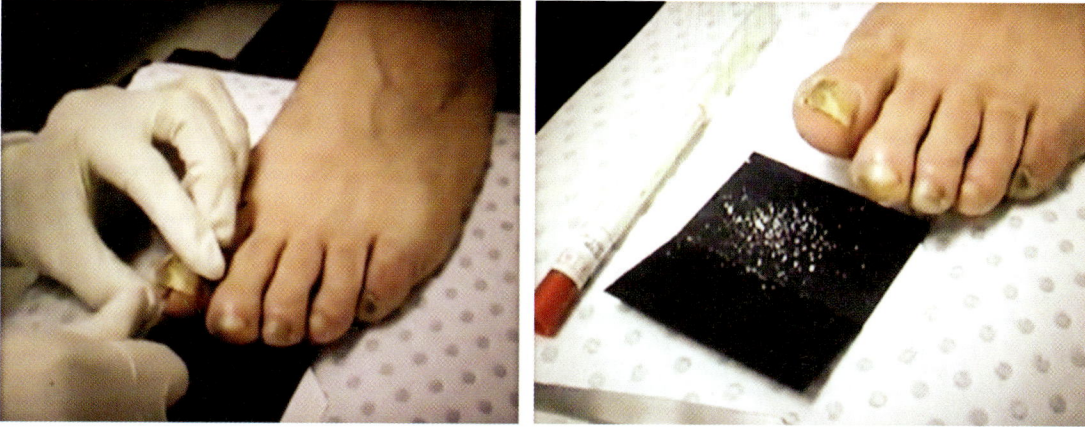

Fig. 3.4: Scraping of nail sample from the undersurface of nail plate for suspected distal and lateral onychomycosis
(*Source:* Fucay Luis. "Mycology Nail Specimen Collection." Mycology Specimen Collection Part 2, 5 Nov. 2010, youtu.be/wy2GAKcTZ54?t=3m52s.)

b. **Proximal subungual onychomycosis**
- Because the fungus invades under the cuticle before settling in the proximal nail bed while the overlying nail plate remains intact, the healthy nail plate should be gently pared away with a scalpel blade number 15.
- A sharp curette can then be used to remove the material from the infected proximal nail bed as close to the lunula as possible.

c. **White superficial onychomycosis**
- Since the infection affects the surface of the nail plate, a scalpel blade (number 15) or a sharp curette can be used to scrape the white area and remove the infected debris.

d. **Candidal onychomycosis**
- Specimen has to be collected from the proximal and lateral nail edges.
- If candidal onycholysis is suspected, the lifted nail bed should also be scraped.

- Scrapings can be taken from the under-surface of the nail if insufficient debris is present in the nail bed.

e. **Endonyx or total dystrophic onychomycosis**
   - Since the nail plate is primarily affected, nail clipping is required.

COLLECTION OF HAIR SPECIMEN[1]

The lesion can be decontaminated with 70% alcohol. Small scales are scrapped off from the margins by rounded scalpel.

1. Hair to be examined for the presence of black or white piedra may be simply cut off at the level of the skin.

   a. If dermatophytosis is suspected, the hair should be removed with the roots intact using epilation forceps (Fig. 3.5); cut hairs are unsuitable.

   b. In many instances, the affected hair may be recognized because they are dull and broken, but if not, the fact that they slip out easily with fine forceps may also help in selecting the right material. This is particularly useful in examining scalp or beard kerions caused by *Trichophyton verrucosum*, where relatively a little fungus may provoke a severe reaction, and it may be necessary to test many hair before an infected hair is found.

   c. In those instances where the hair breaks off at a very short distance from the scalp, as in black dot infections, scraping from scalp will yield the best material, with the infected roots appearing as tiny stumps among the skin scales.

   d. In tinea incognito the examination of vellus hairs may be the easiest method of diagnosis as, although fungi such as *T. rubrum* rarely invade the hair shaft, they may colonize the hair follicle.

2a. In addition to collecting scales and hair, brush samples are an excellent method for the culture of scalp infections, and may

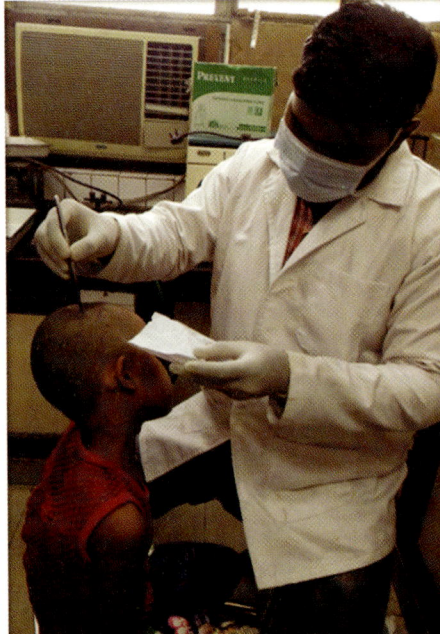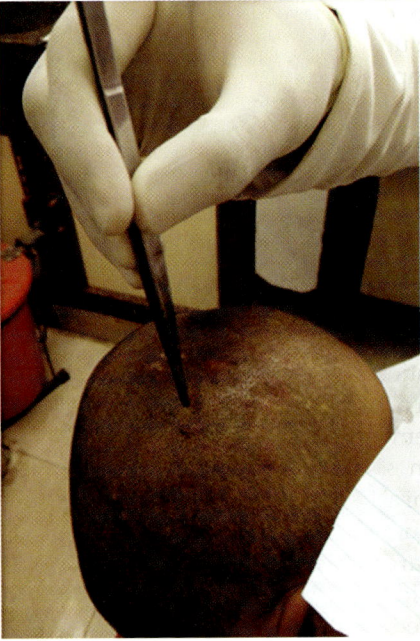

Fig. 3.5: Collection of hair samples from the affected lesion using epilation forceps
(*Source:* Dr Shukla Das, Incharge of Mycology Lab, UCMS, Delhi)

also be useful in testing suspected animal sources of infection, however microscopy cannot be performed on them.

  i. For brush samples, a sterile plastic scalp massager or disposable toothbrush is brushed firmly through the hair at least 10 times.

  ii. It is then pressed against the culture medium in a 90 mm Petri dish.

  b. This simple technique is an extremely sensitive culture method, and is invaluable when screening large numbers of children.

  c. Several hundred children may be examined in a day by performing a Wood's light examination and taking a brush sample from each child, which can then be taken back to the laboratory for culture.

  d. Cultures from infected children produce a fungal colony from many of the inoculation points; contacts of infected children usually yield only a few colonies.

3. In cases of kerion, when brush sampling may be unsuitable and painful, a transport swab wiped over the lesion will usually pick up enough conidia to give a positive culture.

TRANSPORT OF SPECIMEN

• The scrapings should be collected (Fig. 3.6) and transported in a folded paper, which keeps the specimen dry, thus preventing over-growth of bacterial contaminants.

  – Plastic containers are unsuitable, as the skin adheres to the sides and is difficult to remove. The use of glass slides, which then should be transported to the laboratory, is hazardous as they are frequently broken.

  – Squares of brightly colored paper card are ideal; these may then be carefully folded and secured by a paper clip.

  – Sterilized glass plates can be used to collect the scraping and transport them.

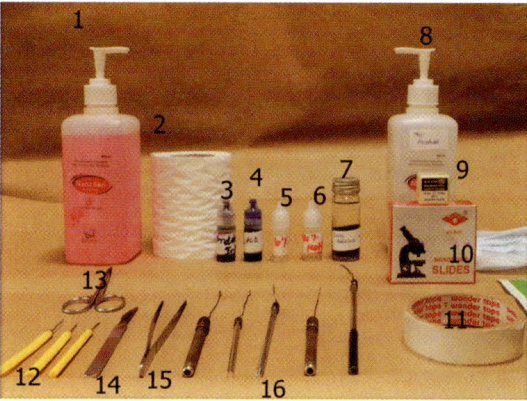

Fig. 3.6: Pieces of equipment are used in sample processing:

1. Hand sanitizer	2. Tissue roll
3. India ink	4. LPCB
5. 10% KOH	6. 40% KOH
7. Sand alcohol	8. 70% Alcohol
9. Coverslips	10. Microscope slides
11. Cellotape	12. Teasing needles
13. Scissors	14. Blunt scalpel and holder
15. Epilation forceps	16. Inoculating loops: L-shaped/straight wire/round

(*Source:* Dr Shukla Das, Incharge of Mycology Lab, UCMS, Delhi)

• The details of the patient, exact site of the lesion, and time of sampling, animal contact or recent travel should then be clearly recorded.

• If the processing is to be delayed for more than several hours, it is recommended that the dermatological sample be stored at 15–30°C.

• Dermatophytes in skin scrapings may remain viable for months, and yeasts for several weeks.

MICROSCOPY

1. **Preparation of specimen:** A few minutes spent carefully preparing the specimen are well spent. Clinical specimens must be processed as soon as possible on the appropriate isolation media and temperature.

  a. For routine examination, specimens are usually mounted in 10–30% potassium hydroxide (KOH); the higher the percentage, the faster the specimen will dissolve (Fig. 3.7iii).

b. For skin scrapings and nails, gently warming the specimen over the pilot light of a Bunsen burner (Fig. 3.7v) will speed up the process, but boiling should be avoided, as this tends to encourage the formation of artefacts, which may confuse the inexperienced observer.

c. It is important to soften skin and nail samples, as thinner the specimen, easier it is to observe the fungal elements.

d. The coverslip should be pressed down firmly to obtain a monolayer of cells before microscopic observation.

e. Excess potassium hydroxide will etch microscope lenses, so it must be removed by blotting with small squares of filter paper or tissue.

f. Nail specimens take longer to dissolve than skin, but if small pieces and debris are taken, they will usually soften within 10 min. In those instances where the nails do not soften satisfactorily, the slide may be put in a 37°C incubator for 1 hour, and the material can then be flattened.

g. Tube KOH preparation (40%) kept overnight for hard nail can be beneficial. A drop from the tube can be used for KOH slide mount next day.

h. In contrast to skin and nail samples, infected hairs are very delicate, and if heated or left in mounting fluid for more than a few minutes tend to disintegrate, obscuring the characteristic arrangement of the arthroconidia. They should therefore be examined as soon as possible after mounting.

2. **Examination of specimen** (Fig. 3.7vii)

a. The lighting is critical; over illumination, particularly when scanning the slide under low power (40X), will render the fungal elements invisible.

The various special stains used are detailed in Box 3.1.

b. The light should therefore be low initially and then raised when the presence of fungus is confirmed by

Box 3.1: Direct microscopy stains	
Wet mount	*Stains*
1. KOH (10–40%)	1. Grocott-Gomori's
2. Calcofluor white	methenamine silver
3. Chlorazol black E	(GMS)
4. Parker blue-black ink	2. Periodic acid–Schiff
5. Chicago sky blue stain	(PAS)

examination with a higher power lens (20X or 40X).

c. An alternative clearing agent, which does not require warming of the specimen, is 10% sodium sulphide solution.

i. In onychomycosis, direct microscopy is the most efficient screening technique with a rapid turn around time.

- The specimen can be mounted in a solution of 40% KOH or NaOH mixed with 5% glycerol, heated to emulsify lipids (1 hour at 51 to 54°C), and examined under 400X.

- An alternative formulation consists of 40% KOH and 36% dimethyl sulfoxide (DMSO) for faster clearing of debris and rapid visualization.

- Tetraethylammonium hydroxide (TEAH) can also be used.

- It is important to understand the limitations of direct microscopy in diagnosing the cause of onychomycosis.

  – The test serves only as a screening test for the presence or absence of fungi but cannot differentiate among the pathogens.

  – Direct microscopy is often time-consuming, because nail debris is thick and coarse and hyphae are usually only sparsely present.

  – The clinician should be aware of the possibility of false-negative results, which occur at a rate of approximately 5 to 15%.

- A final caveat concerns the common practice of treating nail infections

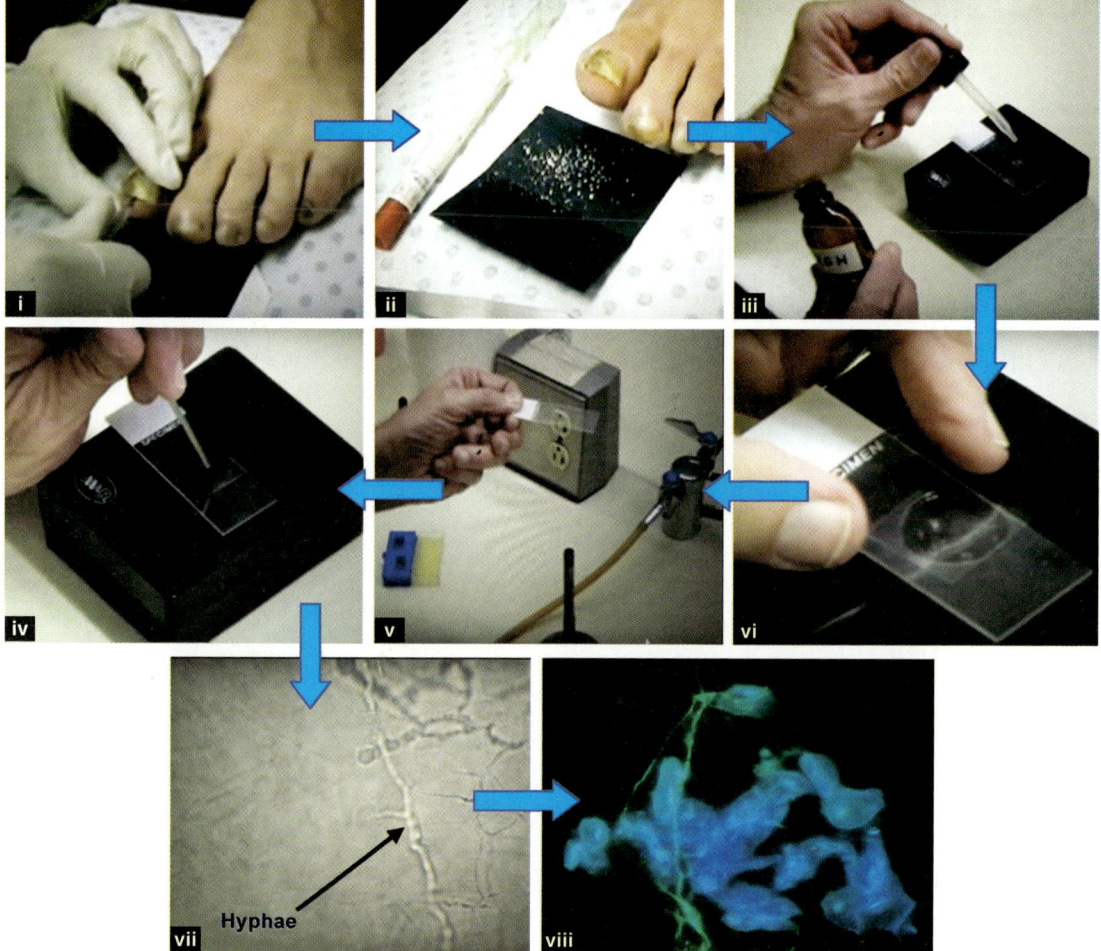

Fig. 3.7: Steps in detection of fungal element in sample: i. Scraping of nail sample; ii. Collection of sample on a sterile black paper; iii. A portion of scraping is put on clean glass slide and a drop of 10% KOH is added; iv. A coverslip is put on KOH preparation; v. The slide is gently warmed (not boiled); vi. Coverslip gently pressed to make a single layer of cells; vii. Detection of fungal element (hyphae) in sample when observed under 40X in bright field microscopy; and viii. Use of calcofluor—highlights the apple green fluorescence of hyphal elements

i-ii (*Source:* Fucay, Luis. "Mycology Nail Specimen Collection." Mycology Specimen Collection Part 2, 5 Nov. 2010, youtu.be/wy2GAKcTZ54?t=3m52s.)

iii-vii (Source: Usatine Richard P. "Watch and Learn: KOH Preparation." 19 June 2015, youtu.be/LUwNQI_0BWU?t = 1m.

viii (*Source:* Dr Shukla Das, Incharge of Mycology Lab, UCMS, Delhi)

based on a microscopic preparation alone without culturing the putative pathogen.

- Almost half of all specimens taken from onychomycotic nails fail to yield a pathogen in culture.

ii. Use of contrast enhancement dyes:
  - The specimen may be counterstained with chitin-specific Chlorazol black E to accentuate hyphae that are present; this is of value if the number of fungal elements is small. This stain is

especially useful because it does not stain likely contaminants such as cotton or elastic fibers, which can help prevent false-positive identifications.

- Parker blue-black ink also can be added to the KOH preparation to improve visualization, but this stain is not chitin specific.
- Chicago sky blue stain highlights the fungal hyphae and spores blue against a purplish background.

iii. Fluorescent staining with optical brighteners (diaminostilbene) like Blankophor® or Calcofluor® which bind to chitin, the main cell wall component of fungi, and cellulose produce a chalk white or apple green fluorescence. This is the most sensitive method for detection via microscopy, i.e. fluorescent microscopy (Fig. 3.7viii)

- Although histological processing of samples has been shown to yield a higher rate of positivity than culture, the rates were similar to those obtained with potassium hydroxide microscopy. As the facilities for histopathological processing may not be available in a small laboratory, routine microscopy using a fluorescent technique is still the method of choice.

iv. When examining a KOH preparation, it is important to observe the hyphae closely to determine if they are typical of dermatophyte fungi or have features of non-dermatophyte molds or yeasts.

v. Although direct microscopy can provide clues about the identity of the micro-organism, careful matching of microscopic and culture results is necessary for the clinician to be confident of the diagnosis.[9]

WOOD'S LIGHT EXAMINATION

The recognition that hair infected by certain dermatophytes produces a characteristic fluorescence in ultraviolet (UV) light filtered by Wood's glass was an important advancement in medical mycology.

a. Wood's glass, which consists of barium silicate containing about 9% nickel oxide, transmits rays of wavelength above 365 nm. Most sources of UV light are suitable. The nature and source of the fluorescent substances in infected hairs are not fully understood, but tryptophan metabolites produced by dermatophytes may be involved. The hair remains fluorescent after the fungus has ceased to be viable, and the fluorescent material can be extracted from the hair in hot water or in a cold solution of sodium bromide. The color of the fluorescence is influenced by the pH of the solution. Because fungi growing in culture or on hair *in vitro* do not fluoresce in this way, the phenomenon must be attributed to some substance produced by the interaction of the fungus and the growing hair. Its chemical nature has not been defined, and the suggestion that it may be a pteridine has been challenged.

b. Only some of the dermatophytes capable of invading hair will induce fluorescence. These include members of the genus *Microsporum* (e.g. *M. audouinii* and *M. canis*), which are common in many densely populated parts of the world. Hairs infected by these species produce a brilliant green fluorescence, easily recognized in a darkened room. Only the fully invaded portions of the shaft develop this property. In recent infections or at the spreading margin of early lesions, the fluorescent part of the hair may not have emerged from the follicle, and can be detected only after the hair is plucked.

c. Among other Microsporum species and variants, only *M. canis* var. *distortum* and *M. ferrugineum* regularly induce fluorescence, and *M. gypseum* and *M. nanum* occasionally do so.

d. *Trichophyton schoenleinii* causes a paler green fluorescence of infected hair.

e. In favus, the fluorescent hairs tend to be long, in contrast to the short, broken stumps characteristic of *Microsporum* infections.

f. In areas where *Microsporum* infections are prevalent, the Wood's light is an essential tool in the diagnosis and treatment of the individual patient, and in the control of epidemics. The lamp is easily transportable and can be taken to schools or institutions for the rapid examination of contacts.

g. The most common sources of error are:

  i. The bluish or purplish fluorescence produced by ointments containing petrolatum, scales, serum or exudate.

  ii. An insufficiently darkened room.

  iii. Light reflected from the examiner's white coat.

  iv. Failure to remember that not all fungi cause fluorescence.

Correctly performed and interpreted, the test is virtually specific, but absence of fluorescence in some infections with *M. audouinii* and *M. canis* has been reported. The lamp can be used in the detection of subclinical infection, and to assess response to treatment or spontaneous cure.

ONYCHOSCOPY

Onychoscopy is dermatoscopic examination of nail unit and its components, namely the proximal nail fold, lateral nail fold, hyponychium, nail plate and nail bed. It is a potential link between naked eye examination (clinical onychology) and nail histopathology, opening a valuable second front with a potential to prevent biopsy. Further details are covered in the chapter on dermoscopy of dermatophytic infections.

Regarding mycological assessment of the affected nail, onychoscopy aids to proper selection of affected area for collection of nail specimen.

CULTURE

- Culture is the only method by which the causative microorganism can be identified and its viability confirmed.[2]

- It is a valuable complement to direct microscopic examination and histological analysis, which do not provide identification at the species level.[3]

- Precise identification indeed is useful, since prophylactic measures may vary depending on the dermatophyte species.[3] Biosafety level 2 (BSL-2) and animal biosafety level 2 (ABSL-2) practices, containment equipment, and facilities are recommended for handling cultures (Fig. 3.8).

1. Specimens should be plated on two different media (Figs 3.9 and 3.10):

   a. A primary medium that is selective against most non-dermatophytic molds and bacteria.

   b. A secondary medium that allows the growth of non-dermatophytic molds and bacteria.

2. Cycloheximide inhibits the growth of non-dermatophytes and is incorporated into media such as:

   a. Dermatophyte test medium (DTM)

   b. Dermatophyte identification medium (DIM) (DTM + incubation at 35°C and the use of an increased concentration of cycloheximide.[4]

   c. Sabouraud peptone—glucose agar (Emmons' modification) with cycloheximide—glucose/peptone agar, either with 4% sugar, 1% peptone and an acid pH (Sabouraud's dextrose agar) or with 2% sugar, 1% peptone and a neutral pH.

3. Cycloheximide-free media that are commonly used include:

   a. Sabouraud's glucose agar,

   b. Littman's oxgall medium

   c. Inhibitory mold agar (Sabouraud's glucose agar with the addition of antibiotics).

4. Antibacterial antibiotics such as gentamicin (0.0025%) and/or chloramphenicol (0.005%) may be added to reduce contamination and, if a dermatophyte infection has been diagnosed, the addition

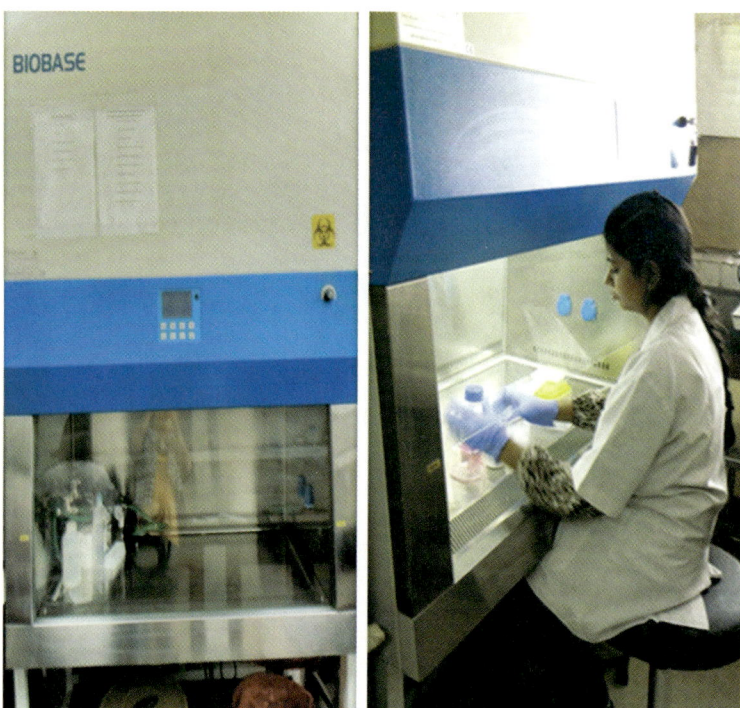

Fig. 3.8: Biosafety Cabinet (Biobase): Used for handling of cultures, antifungal susceptibility tests and preparation of isolates prior to molecular techniques.
(*Source:* Dr.Shukla Das, Incharge of Mycology Lab, UCMS, Delhi)

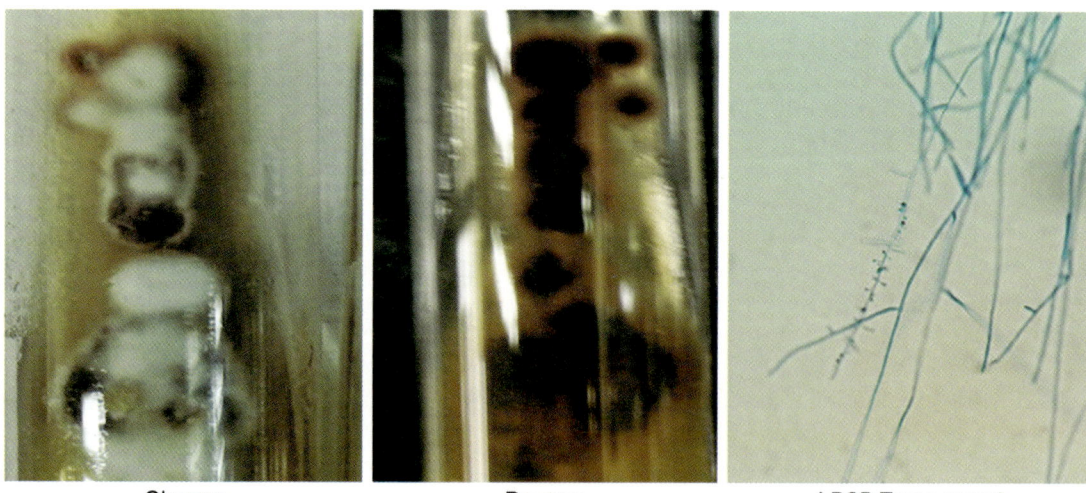

| Obverse | Reverse | LPCB Tease mount |

Fig. 3.9: Growth of *Trichophyton rubrum* on Sabouraud dextrose agar from skin sample:
Obverse: colonies of white downy growth with tinge of cinnamon color.
Reverse: Wine red color.
LPCB tease mount: Scanty slender, clavate microconidia.
(*Source:* Dr Shukla Das, Incharge of Mycology Lab, UCMS, Delhi)

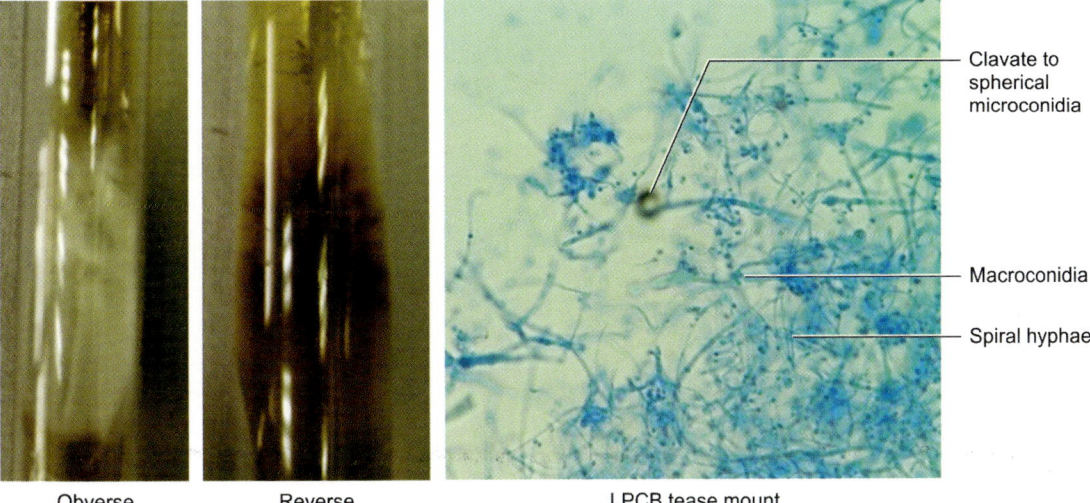

| Obverse | Reverse | LPCB tease mount |

Fig. 3.10: Growth of *Trichophyton mentagrophytes* on SDA from skin sample:
Obverse: Colonies of white, cottony growth
Reverse: Orange reverse.
LPCB tease mount: Showing clavate to spherical microconidia, macroconidia and spiral hyphae
(*Source:* Dr Shukla Das, Incharge of Mycology Lab, UCMS, Delhi)

of cycloheximide at 0.04% will inhibit the growth of non-dermatophyte molds.

5. The media is inoculated with the material and incubated at room temperature, i.e. 22–33°C for the period ranging 1–6 weeks. In majority of dermatophytes, growth and sporulation occurs in 7–10 days. When growth becomes evident on the primary culture media, it is examined and the differentiation of dermatophytes, yeasts, and molds is predicated on:

a. Macroscopic characteristics (upper and bottom side of colonies as well as pigmentation) (Fig. 3.9).

b. Microscopic characteristics (formation of macro- and microconidia, respectively other growth forms) by lactophenol cotton blue (LPCB) tease mounts (Fig. 3.10).

c. Physiological tests:
   i. *Biochemical properties (Christensen urea agar for urea hydrolysis):* Filter-sterilized urea agar base (Difco) is mixed with sterile molten agar and allowed to set. The medium is then inoculated with the test organism. After incubation at 26°C for 7 days, if urea is degraded, the color turns from yellow to magenta red.

   ii. Nutritional tests: Vitamin and amino acid supplemented Trichophyton agars: Trichophyton agars 1–7 (Difco) are used to determine vitamin requirements. Agar 1 is a casein-based, vitamin-free control; agar 2 is supplemented with inositol; agar 3 with thiamine and inositol; and agar 4 with thiamine alone. Agar 5 contains nicotinic acid. Agar 6 is an ammonium nitrate vitamin-free control for agar 7, which is supplemented with histidine. Small, agar-free inocula are transferred from Sabouraud's agar plates and incubated for 2–3 weeks at 26°C.

iii. *In vitro* hair perforation tests: Sterile human hair is suspended in sterile distilled water supplemented with yeast extract. The test organism is inoculated onto the hairs. After 2 weeks' incubation at 26°C, hairs are mounted to look for wedge-shaped penetrations perpendicular to the hair axis.

iv. Growth on rice grains: Ordinary white rice is covered with distilled water and autoclaved. The test organisms are then inoculated straight onto the surface, and growth is assessed after 2–3 weeks' incubation at 26°C.

v. Growth on 1% peptone agar: On this sugar-free medium *Microsporum persicolor* will produce a pink surface color, in contrast to *Trichophyton mentagrophytes* var *mentagrophytes*, which remains white.

6. If growth occurs on both types of media, the infective agent is probably a dermatophyte, whereas growth only on the cycloheximide-free medium indicates that the infective agent may be a non-dermatophyte such as *Scopulariopsis brevicaulis, Scytalidium dimidiatum,* or *Scytalidium hyalinum.*

7. However, growth of a non-dermatophyte alone from a specimen that has tested positive for fungi on direct microscopy does not prove conclusively that the infective agent is a non-dermatophyte.

   a. Part of the difficulty in evaluating the role of non-dermatophyte fungi cultured from the nail arises because the same fungi that can be laboratory contaminants are also occasionally found to be pathogens.

   b. Reference laboratories should provide data on whether the isolated fungus was a likely pathogen or an unlikely one.

i. All dermatophytes should be considered pathogens.

ii. All other isolated organisms are probably laboratory contaminants unless KOH or microscopy indicates they have the atypical frond-like hyphae associated with non-dermatophyte molds or if the same organism is repeatedly isolated.

c. NDM identification:[5] Walshe and English recommended considering any fungus causal if

   i. compatible elements were detected by direct microscopy, and

   ii. the fungus grew from 5 or more of 20 inoculum pieces (that is, pieces of nail material planted on fungal growth medium) in the absence of a dermatophyte. The fungal agent should grow at least 3 times from 3 different sites sampled from the affected nail.

   iii. This criterion was based on the premise that an established nail invader would consistently colonize a substantial proportion of the nail material, whereas contaminants would usually consist of one or a few scattered propagules, with any consistency being coincidental and hence unlikely.

   iv. The criterion was later restricted to filamentous fungi by English,[11] since widely dispersed yeast contamination had been found to be common.

d. As an additional confirmatory technique, definitive identification of non-dermatophytic invasion in nails may require the isolation of the agent from successive specimens from the infected region.

If the infective pathogen is a dermatophyte, subsequent cultures will most probably grow out the dermatophyte itself, a second contaminant unrelated to the first, or no growth at all.

e. Some investigators believe that claims of an increasing proportion of mixed infections in onychomycosis are exaggerated and have gone so far as to state that non-dermatophyte molds and yeasts are usually contaminants secondary to dermatophyte onychomycosis and that their presence need not affect treatment outcome.

f. Caution should be used in analyzing culture results, because nails are non-sterile and fungal and bacterial contaminants may obscure the nail pathogen.

8. Cultures often lack sensitivity, they are time-consuming (7–28 days) and identification of filamentous fungi at the species level using morphological characteristics requires an experienced staff. Subcultures on specific media that stimulate the conidiation and/or the production of pigments are often necessary, when identification of dermatophyte isolates is not achievable directly from primary cultures. These are:
   i. Potato dextrose agar (Difco)
   ii. Brain-heart infusion (Sigma)
   iii. Borelli's lactrimel agar (SR2B) media.

9. Microscopic features may be observed using a needle mount, a sticky tape strip or a slide culture.
   - The simplest method is a needle mount, when a portion of the growth is removed with a stiff wire needle, and teased out in a drop of a suitable stain, such as lactophenol cotton blue. A coverslip is applied and the sample examined microscopically (Figs 3.9 and 3.10).
   - Inorder to retain more conidia, apply a piece of sticky tape, sticky surface down, onto the surface of the colony, and then mount this in a drop of stain and examine the preparation directly through the back of the tape. The sticky tape strip is extremely useful for the examination of colonies with many conidia.
   - The most successful but time-consuming method for examining the details of conidial structure and formation, however, is the slide culture. In this method, the fungus is inoculated onto the four sides of a square of agar, sandwiched between a glass slide and coverslip, and maintained in a sterile Petri dish with a moist atmosphere. The fungus grows out from the agar block directly onto the glass of the coverslip and slide, which may be used to prepare two undisturbed mounts of the growing fungus. When sealed with nail polish, these form permanent preparations.

HISTOLOGY[3]

For onychomycosis and deep mycosis, the "gold standard" method is histological examination of a nail plate with direct *in situ* visualization of fungal elements within the host tissue.

1. Achten's technique with Grocott-Gomori's methenamine silver (GMS)—hyphae appear grey-black.
2. Periodic acid–Schiff (PAS)—hyphae appear red colored. Hotchkiss and MacManus's technique, which is performed on nail clippings stained with PAS, stands for a good compromise between direct examination and histology.

It may be necessary to perform histopathologic analysis of the nail unit in cases in which the clinical appearance suggests the presence of a fungal nail infection, but the KOH preparation and culture are negative.

While the diagnosis of PSO or SWO usually requires a punch biopsy from the nail plate, simple nail clippings generally suffice in all other forms of onychomycosis.

Limitations

i. False-negative results may be observed in early nail infections.
ii. Histological analysis does not allow species identification.
iii. It does not determine the viability of fungi.

Accurate identification of the pathogen cannot be achieved through histology alone, and mycological cultures remain necessary.

Although histological processing of samples has been shown to yield a higher rate of positivity than culture, the rates were similar to those obtained with potassium hydroxide microscopy and, as the facilities for histopathological processing may not be available in a small laboratory, routine microscopy using a fluorescent technique is still the method of choice.

IN VIVO CONFOCAL MICROSCOPY[3]

In vivo confocal microscopy has been proposed for direct examination by Piérard. This non-invasive and specific method allows visualizing fungal hyphae *in vivo* using a microscope objective directly applied on nail surface, but its cost has hampered its use in clinical laboratories.

MOLECULAR TECHNIQUES

With recent advances in molecular techniques, direct detection of dermatophytes from infected sample is quick and reproducible, overcoming the observer's bias (Fig. 3.11).[7] Due to ongoing taxonomic revisions within dermatophytes, relying largely on DNA profiles and pathogenicity, rather than conventional morphological features, molecular methods detecting DNA signatures may

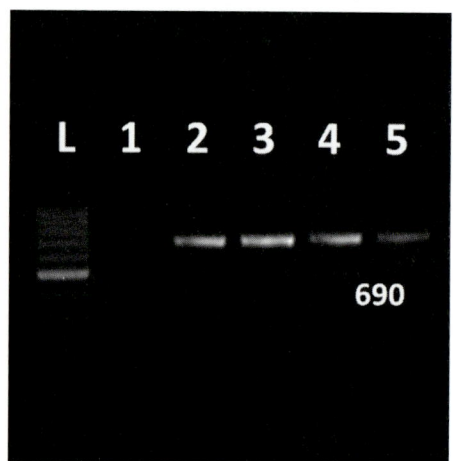

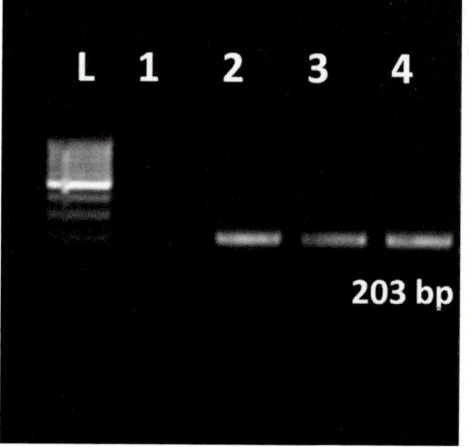

Lane 1: Negative control (no template DNA)
Lane 2: Positive control (ATCC)
Lanes 3–5: Amplification using pan fungal primer (ITS 1 and ITS 4) on clinical specimens (nail)

Lane 1: Negative control (no template DNA)
Lane 2: Positive control (ATCC)
Lanes 3–4: Amplification using *Trichophyton rubrum*-specific primer on clinical specimens (nail)

Fig. 3.11: Molecular techniques
Detection of the amplified products: The PCR amplified products were electrophoretically separated in a 2% agarose gel in 1X tris-acetate-EDTA buffer and they were visualized by using ethidium bromide, under a UV transilluminator (Bio-Rad Laboratories India Pvt. Ltd).

provide an even higher diagnostic advantage in the future.

Genotypic methods available for fungal identification are as follows:

1. Polymerase chain reaction (PCR)[8]
   a. PCR fingerprinting
   b. Random amplification of polymorphic DNA
   c. PCR and restriction fragment length polymorphism analysis
   d. Arbitrarily primed PCR
   e. Real-time PCR for dermatophyte DNA detection (Fig. 3.12)

The main targets have the following genes or DNA fragments:[9]
   i. The ribosomal DNA region
   ii. DNA topoisomerase II genes
   iii. Chitin synthase gene
   iv. Non-transcribed spacer (NTS) regions
   v. Metalloprotease gene
   vi. 11 tubulin gene
   vii. Promoter region within ribosomal intergenic spacer
   viii. Transcription elongation factor 1
   ix. Actin gene
   x. Calmodulin gene.
   xi. Microsatellite-marker, like GT-microsatellite repeat specific for strains of the *T. rubrum / Trichophyton violaceum* clade.[10]

2. Single-stranded conformation polymorphism (SSCP)
3. Restriction analysis of the mitochondrial DNA

Drawbacks of molecular techniques:
   i. Increased contamination
   ii. Failure to differentiate between pathogenic and non-pathogenic fungi.
   iii. Not practical for laboratories which are small scale or tightly budgeted.
   iv. Requires highly skilled personnel.
   v. Limited availability.
   vi. PCR methods are limited to only discovering targeted species.

Pan-dermatophyte PCR with Sanger sequencing, offers a simple strategy to both detect and identify dermatophytes.

Apart from direct fungal detection in clinical samples using molecular techniques such as PCR, larger laboratories have established MALDI-TOF (matrix-assisted laser desorption ionization-time of flight mass spectrometry) as culture confirmation test in the differentiation of dermatophytes. This procedure is immensely time saving, as it enables simultaneous identification of up to 64 dermatophyte strains, with results coming back within minutes. Although the test's specificity-based on protein mass fingerprint or mass spectrum is high, the plausibility of identified species should still always be verified.[11]

ROLE OF ANTIFUNGAL SUSCEPTIBILITY TESTS

Despite availability of many antifungal agents, antifungal clinical resistance occurs, perhaps because of an infecting organism found to be resistant *in vitro* to one or more antifungals tested. The role of the antifungal susceptibility testing is to determine which agents are likely to be effective for a given infection (Fig. 3.13).

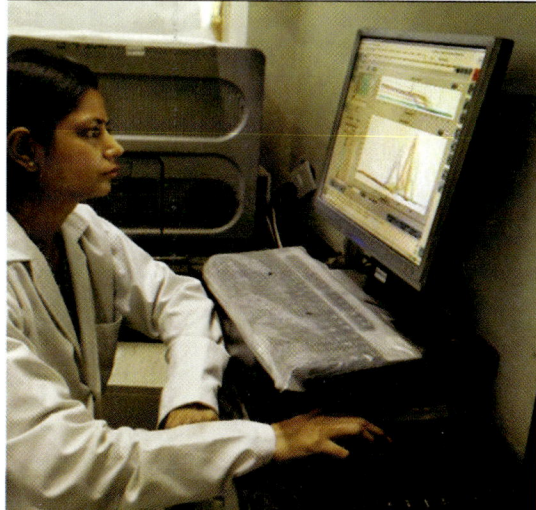

Fig. 3.12: Realtime analysis of RT PCR

(*Source:* Dr Shukla Das, Incharge of Mycology Lab, UCMS, Delhi)

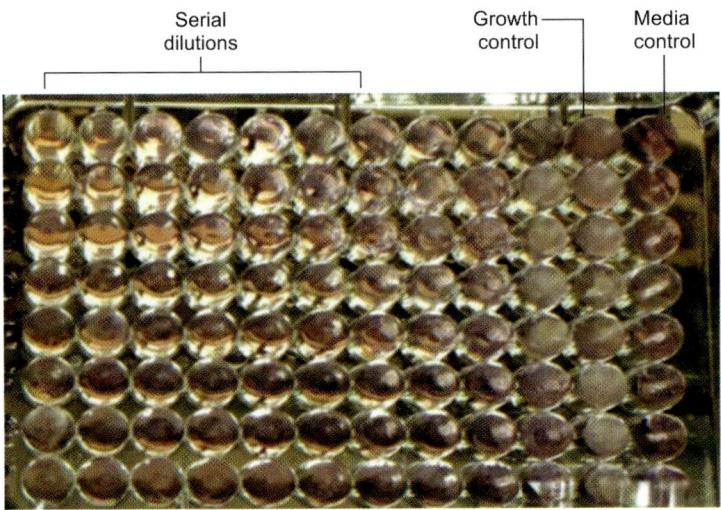

Fig. 3.13: Microdilution plate for determination of MIC

(*Source:* Dr Shukla Das, Incharge of Mycology Lab, UCMS, Delhi)

Thus, if antifungal susceptibility testing results are timely generated by the clinical micro-biology laboratory and communicated to clinicians, they can aid in the therapeutic decision making, especially for difficult-to-treat chronic dermatophytic infections.

Preparation of Antifungal Agents as per CLSI (M38-A)

Antifungal drugs: Fluconazole dissolves in sterile distilled water and other drugs dissolve in 100% dimethyl sulfoxide (DMSO).

Stock solutions of 1,000 µg/ml can be prepared for each drug and stored at –20°C till tests are performed. All the working solutions of water-insoluble drugs are further diluted to two-fold dilutions in DMSO before transferring onto microtiter plates, whereas two-fold serial dilutions of water-soluble drugs are prepared directly in microtiter plate. The final concentrations range from 0.0625 to 128 µg/ml for fluconazole, 0.0078 to 16 µg/ml for itraconazole, and 0.0156 to 16 µg/ml for terbinafine.

Preparation of inoculum: The minimal inhibitory concentration (MIC) determination is as per CLSI (M38-A) modified method in a polystyrene microtiter plates with U-bottom wells. Inoculum suspensions of dermatophytes are prepared from the seven-day subcultures grown on SDA at 25°C. The fungal colonies are covered with 10 ml of normal saline, and the suspensions are made by scraping the surface with the tip of a sterile loop. The mixture of conidia and hyphae fragments, withdrawn and transferred to sterile tubes, are left for 15 to 20 minutes at room temperature. The OD of this suspensions is read at 530 nm, adjusted to transmittance of 80% (1 to 4×10^6 cells/ml) and diluted with RPMI 1640 medium and MOPS (4-morpholinepropanesulfonic acid). Further a 1:50 dilution is prepared to obtain the final inoculum size of approximately 0.4×10^3 to 5×10^4 cells/ml. Inoculum density of the dermatophytes can be verified by quantitative colony counts on colony counter unit.

Test procedure (susceptibility testing): RPMI (100 µL) with antifungal drug is distributed in all wells and 200 µL of RPMI is taken as media control in the wells of U-bottom microtiter plate. Inoculum (100 µL) added in each well except media control well. Growth

Box 3.2: Antifungal testing values of common drugs

Range

(F): Fluconazole: 64–0.125 µg/ml
(A): Amphotericin B: 16–0.0313 µg/ml
(I): Itraconazole: 16–0.0313 µg/ml
(T): Terbinafine: 16–0.0313 µg/ml
(G): Griseofulvin: 128–0.0313 µg/ml

and drug sterility control wells are also maintained for each assay (Fig. 3.13).

Quality control ATCC strains used are:
- *T. rubrum*: ATCC 4438
- *Candida parapsilosis*: ATCC 22019
- *Candida krusei*: ATCC 6258
  Plates are incubated for 96 hours at 35°C.

Endpoint determination: Endpoint determination values are performed visually every 24 hours until the indication of growth in control, drug-free well up to 96 hours. The lowest dilution of the drug, which inhibits the fungal growth, is taken as the MIC (Box 3.2). For itraconazole, MICs correspond to the lowest drug concentration that results in a 100% reduction in growth as compared with the growth control. Terbinafine and fluconazole MICs correspond to the lowest drug concentration that gives a reduction in growth of 80%.

References

1. Burns T, Breathnack S, Cox N, Griffiths C. Rook's Textbook of Dermatology. 8th ed. A John Wiley and Sons Ltd., Publication 2010; 36:1–36.

2. Elewski BE. Onychomycosis: Pathogenesis, Diagnosis, and Management. Clin Microbiol Rev 1998;11:415–29.

3. Pihet M, Le Govic Y. Reappraisal of Conventional Diagnosis for Dermatophytes. Mycopathologia 2017;182:169–80.

4. Gromadzki S, Ramani R, Chaturvedi V. Evaluation of new medium for identification of dermatophytes and primary dimorphic pathogens. J Clin Microbiol 2003;41:467–8.

5. Gupta AK, Cooper EA, Donald PMAC, Summerbell RC. Utility of Inoculum Counting (Walshe and English Criteria) in Clinical Diagnosis of Onychomycosis Caused by Nondermatophytic Filamentous Fungi 2001;39:2115–21.

6. Ellis D, Davis S, Alexiou H, Handke R, Bartley R. Descriptions of medical fungi. North 2007; p. 1–198.

7. Chander J. In: Textbook of Medical Mycology. 3rd ed. Mehta Publishers 2009; p. 122–42.

8. Brillowska-da A, Saunte DM, Arendrup MC. Five-hour Diagnosis of Dermatophyte Nail Infections with Specific Detection of *Trichophyton rubrum*. J Clin Microbiol 2007;45:1200–4.

9. Emam SM, El-salam OHA. Real-time PCR: A rapid and sensitive method for diagnosis of dermatophyte induced onychomycosis, a comparative study. Alexandria J Med [Internet] 2016;52:83–90.

10. Kupsch C, Ohst T, Pankewitz F, Nenoff P, S, Winter I, et al. The agony of choice in dermatophyte diagnostics performance of different molecular tests and culture in the detection of *Trichophyton rubrum* and *Trichophyton interdigitale*. Clin Microbiol Infect J 2016;22:11–7.

11. Nenoff P, Krüger C, Schaller J, Ginter-Hanselmayer G, Schulte-Beerbühl R, Tietz H-J. Mycology—an update Part 2: Dermatomycoses: Clinical picture and diagnostics. J Dtsch Dermatol Ges [Internet] 2014;12:749–77.

12. Fucay, Luis. "Mycology Nail Specimen Collection." Mycology Specimen Collection Part 2, 5 Nov. 2010, youtu.be/wy2GAKcTZ54?t=3 m52s.

13. Piraccini BM, Balestri R, Starace M, Rech G. Nail digital dermoscopy (onychoscopy) in the diagnosis of onychomycosis. J Eur Acad Dermatol Venereol 2013; 27:509–13.

14. De Crignis G, Valgas N, Rezende P, Leverone A, Nakamura R.Dermatoscopy of onychomycosis. Int J Dermatol 2014;53: e97–9.

4

Dermoscopy of Dermatophytoses

Ananta Khurana, Deepak Jakhar

INTRODUCTION

The diagnosis of fungal infections is aided by direct microscopic examination with potassium hydroxide and fungal culture. These conventional mycological tools, however, are rather complex, time-consuming and require trained personnel and laboratory setting. In addition, the sensitivity is often low, especially for nails. Dermoscopy is a simple, cost-effective and non-invasive diagnostic technique which now has an established role in diagnosing tinea capitis. It is being increasingly utilized in diagnosing onycho-mycosis (OM) and especially in differentiating it from other common onychopathies. Role in cutaneous dermatophytotsis is, however, less well defined.

Onychomycosis

Dermoscopy has become an important adjunctive tool in the diagnosis of nail disorders. It assumes a special importance for the diagnosis of OM, where the laboratory techniques have a significant false negative rate.[1] Dermoscopy largely just magnifies what

is visible to the naked eye, but some specific signs have been described over past few years which can aid in establishing the clinical diagnosis with conviction and may negate the need for routine KOH microscopy and culture in many cases.

Technique

Onychoscopy is application of dermatoscope for the study of onychopathies. It is essential to know the basic anatomy and parts of nail unit before performing onychoscopy. Digit should be kept on a dull non-refractile surface and any undue pressure by the patient or physician should be avoided.[2] As the entire nail unit cannot be visualized in a single field, the instrument needs to be moved back and forth, as well as transversally to choose the field of interest.[2] Whereas dry onychoscopy reveals information about the surface abnormalities, wet onychoscopy is better suited for pigmentation and vasculature.[2] Figure 4.1 shows the stepwise approach in utilization of dermatoscope and linkage fluid for the study of onychomycosis.[2] We prefer to

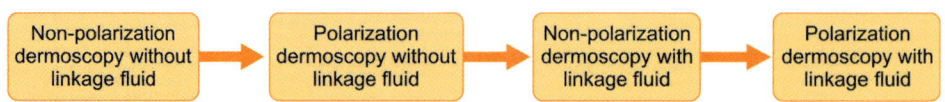

Fig. 4.1: Stepwise approach to utilization of dermatoscope and linkage fluid in dermoscopy

use ultrasound gel as the linkage fluid for onychoscopy. Other options for the same include antiseptic gels (e.g. alcohol itself or alcohol-based hand sanitizers) or oils (e.g. mineral oil).[2]

Onychoscopic Features of Onychomycosis

Pirracini et al described 2 characteristic signs for distal lateral subungal onychomycosis (DLSO) from their analysis of 57 dermoscopic images, compared with mycology findings.[3] Jagged proximal margin of the oncholytic area with sharp longitudinal whitish indentations, corresponding to the proximal progression of the fungi, showed a sensitivity of 100% for DLSO (Fig. 4.2). Traumatic onycholysis and nail psoriasis, clinically seen as onycholysis with subungal hyperkeratosis, similar to DLSO, are often difficult differentials. The jagged margin differentiates onychomycotic onycholysis from a traumatic onycholysis, which would have a smooth linear proximal margin. Onycholysis in nail psoriasis has an erythematous border proximal to onycholytic band with or without dilated fusiform nail bed vessels.[2] Pirracini et al reported that the 'linear edge' sign had 100% specificity for traumatic onycholysis.[3] The other specific pattern seen with onychomycosis

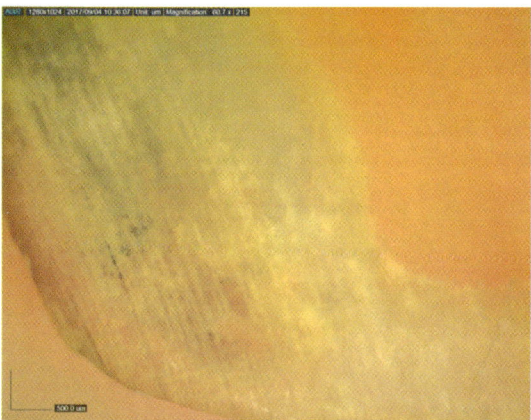

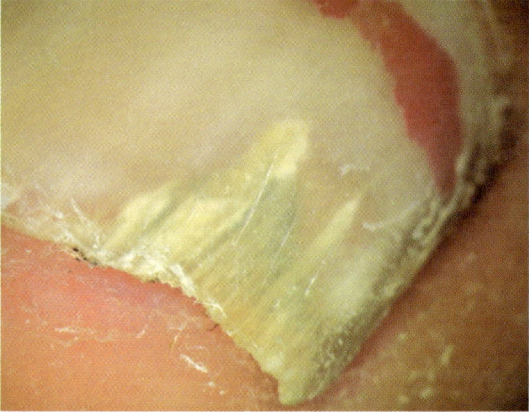

Figs 4.3 and 4.4: 'Aurora borealis' pattern characterized by longitudinal striae of different colors (60X)

is the presence of longitudinal striae with different colors (i.e. white, yellow, orange, and brown) giving an impression similar to aurora borealis ('aurora pattern')[3] (Figs 4.3 and 4.4). This sign was shown to have a sensitivity of 86.5% in DLSO. Blackish dots and globules (due to subungual hemorrhage) (Fig. 4.5) and yellow–orange homogenous colors of the affected nail plate are less commonly seen (Fig. 4.6), and are not considered specific.[4] Based on these, a working algorithm for diagnosis of DLSO has been proposed. The first step is an evaluation of the edge: If it is linear, onychomycosis can be excluded, while if it is jagged, the presence of spikes must be looked for: If they are present and are associated with striae, the diagnosis of DSO is confirmed.[3]

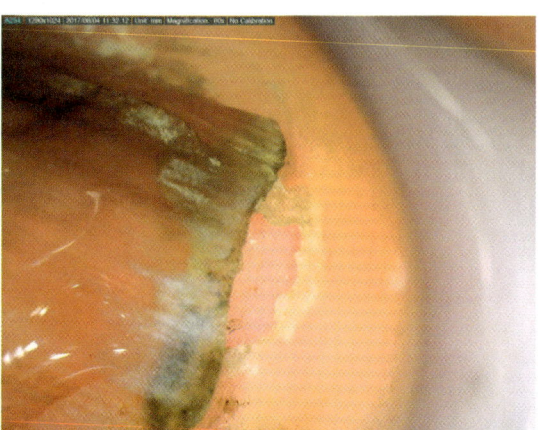

Fig. 4.2: Polarizing dermoscopy showing jagged proximal margin of the onycholytic area with sharp longitudinal whitish indentations (60X)

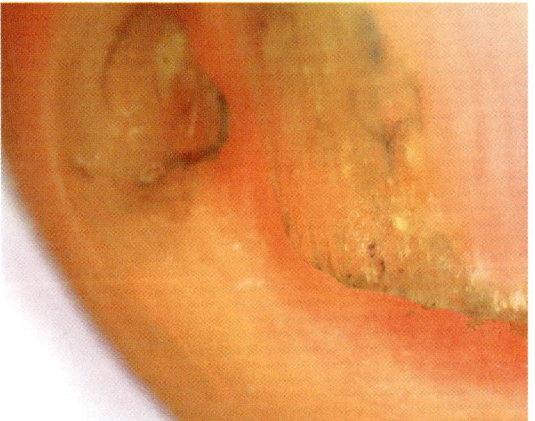

Fig. 4.5: Black dots and streaks within the onycholytic area suggestive of subungual hemorrhage (60X)

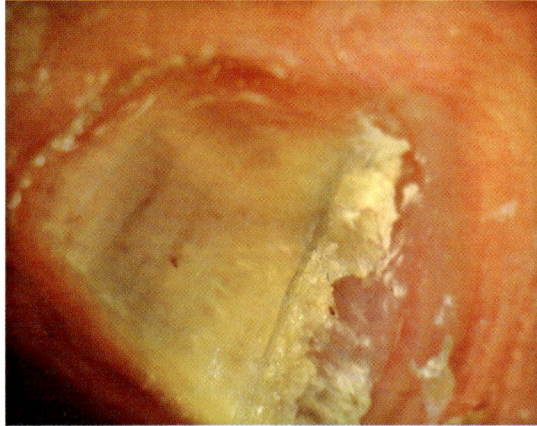

Fig. 4.7: 'Ruin pattern' characterized by distal pulverization and thickening of the nail plate as well as separation of the nail plate from the nail bed (60X)

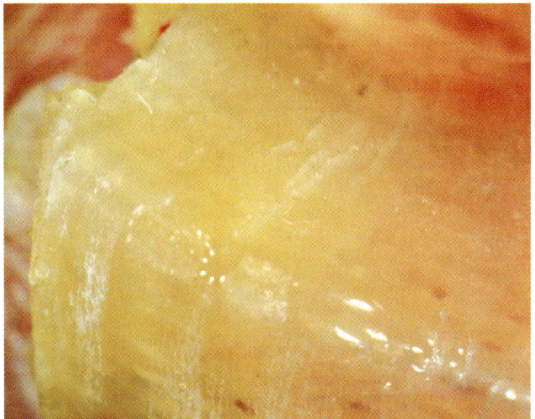

Fig. 4.6: Yellowish homogenous discoloration of the onychomycotic nail plate (60X)

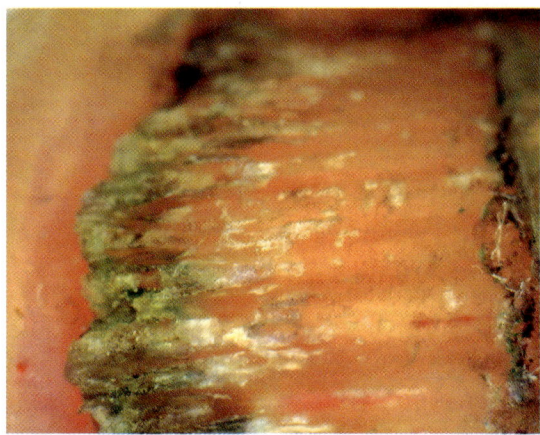

Fig. 4.8: Onychomycotic nail plate showing distal irregular termination (60X)

Nakamura et al performed dermoscopic study of 500 cases of common onychopathies (onychomycosis; ungual psoriasis; ungual lichen planus, and nail fragility syndrome) and identified four most frequent dermoscopic characteristics of OM—chromonychia, onycholysis, opacity and longitudinal spikes.[5] They also described 'ruin appearance' of subungual hyperkeratosis (Fig. 4.7) and presence of dermatophytomas as round yellow–orange subungual areas.[5,6] Similarly, Jesús-Silva et al described the appearance of four signs in 155 KOH positive patients of OM.[4] Longitudinal striae were the most commonly seen

pattern, being present in 94 patients (54% of these had total dystrophic onychomycosis (TDO) and 44% had DLSO). Distal irregular termination of the thickened nail plate (Fig. 4.8) was seen in 67 patients (61%: TDO and 38%: DLSO). Spiked appearance of proximal edge was seen in 39 patients (56%: TDO and 43%: DLSO). And, contrary to the description by Pirracini et al, a smooth linear edge was present in 34 patients (58%: TDO and 38%: DLSO) (Fig. 4.9).

Fungal melanonychia is characterized by homogenous pigmented bands with pigment

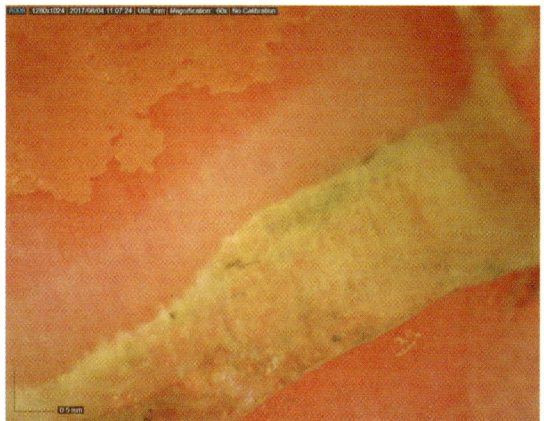

Fig. 4.9: Distal smooth edge of onycholysis in a KOH and culture positive onychomycosis (60X)

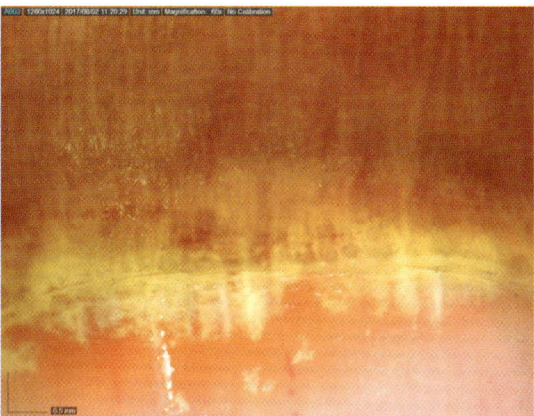

Fig. 4.10: 'Spiked pattern' seen in PSO, similar to that described in DLSO (60X)

clumps or granules, corresponding to the fungal colonies, within the bands. Another characteristic feature is that these bands are wider distally and narrow proximally.[7]

No specific pattern has been described with superficial white onychomycosis (SWO) and proximal subungual onychomycosis (PSO). We, however, have observed a similar spiked pattern in cases of PSO as well (Fig. 4.10).

Dermatophytosis of Skin

Dermoscopy of tinea of the skin is uncommonly described and largely non-specific. There is often an erythematous background without any specific vascular pattern, with scales and micropustules (Fig. 4.11). Knopfel et al described presence of brown spots surrounded by white-yellowish halo, with short non-pigmented vellus hair in the center of some, suggesting fungal invasion of the hair follicle.[8] Other described signs are translucent hair (possibly due to massive fungal invasion) (Fig. 4.12), broken hair, corkscrew hair (result of subsequent cracking and bending of a hair shaft filled with hyphae), black dots and

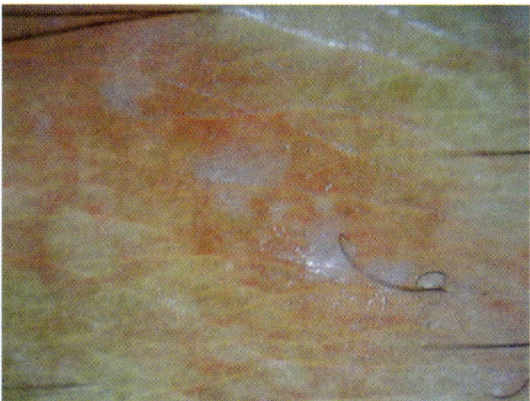

Fig. 4.11: Dermoscopy of tinea corporis showing pustules (white areas) and scaling over an erythematous background (60X)

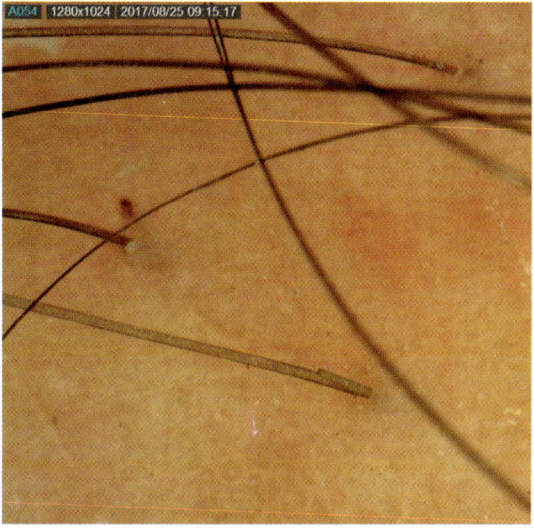

Fig. 4.12: Translucent hair due to fungal invasion of the hair. Note an adjoining broken hair (200X)

dystrophic hair.[9] Morse code-like hair or bar code-like hair, showing multiple white bands across the hair shaft (Fig. 4.13), were initially described in tinea capitis at high magnifications.[10,11] Similar findings have now been described in tinea of the vellus body hair as well.[9,12] Bar code-like hairs must be differentiated from the interrupted medulla of normal hairs, in which the band covers <50% of the thickness of the hair shaft (Fig. 4.14). Fungal involvement of vellus hair is likely to have important therapeutic and prognostic implications as it may predict from the outset

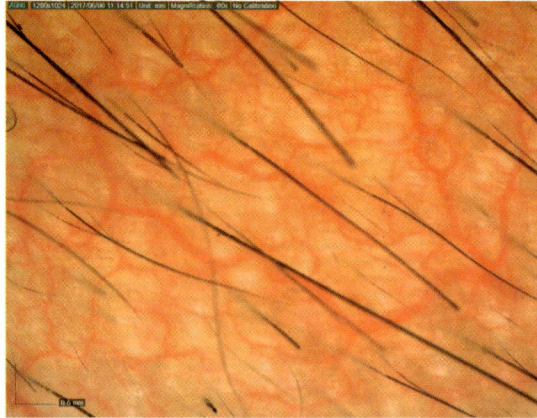

Fig. 4.15: Thick tortuous blood vessels in a patient with a prolonged history of application of clobetasol containing combination creams over a patch of tinea (60X)

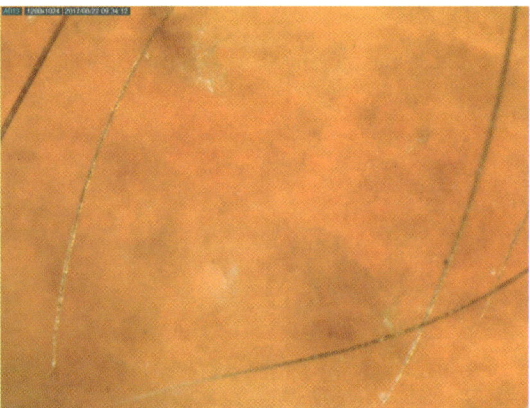

Fig. 4.13: Body hair invasion seen as alternating white and black bands (Morse code or Bar code hair) (200X)

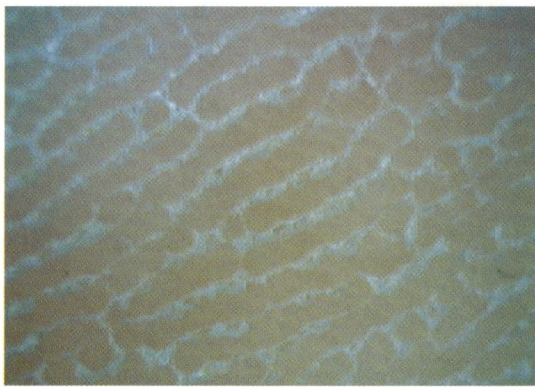

Fig. 4.16: Dermoscopy of tinea pedis showing scaling characteristically localized to the plantar creases (20X)

patients who are likely to respond poorly or not at all to topical therapy.[12,13] Lastly, signs of topical steroid abuse may be seen in tinea incognito, in the form of broad tortuous vessels in the background (Fig 4.15). In authors' personal observation, tinea mannum and pedis have localization of scales to the palmar and plantar creases (Fig. 4.16).

Tinea Capitis

Tinea capitis is probably the most studied fungal infection with dermatoscope. A number of studies has described dermoscopic

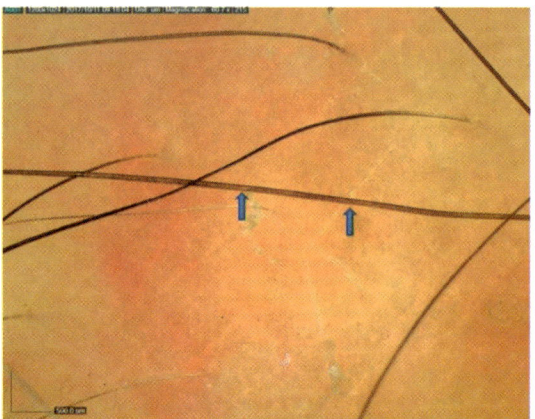

Fig. 4.14: Interrupted medulla seen as lighter colored areas covering less than 50% of the width of the hair shaft (200X)

features of tinea capitis in the form of 'comma' hair (C-shaped hair shaft with a sharp, slanting end and homogeneous thickness) (Fig. 4.17), 'corkscrew' hair (twisted or coiled, short, broken hair fragments) (Fig. 4.18), "zigzag" hair (hair shaft bent at multiple points) and "Morse code" hair (presence of multiple transverse bands throughout the hair shaft).[14–17] Comma hair and corkscrew hair are said to be specific for tinea capitis and presence of perifollicular scaling further increases the specificity.[14–17] Nonspecific dermoscopic features include broken and dystrophic hair, i-hair, black dots, yellowish dots, erythema and scaling. Flame-shaped hair are typically described with trichotillomania, but in our personal experience flame-shaped hair can also be seen in tinea capitis (Fig. 4.19). In addition, pustules and elongated blood vessels with underlying erythema are seen in kerion (Fig. 4.20). Favus may show large yellow wax colored perifollicular areas.

Trichoscopy has also been employed to monitor the therapeutic response in tinea capitis. Disappearance of corkscrew hairs and dystrophic hairs marks the successful therapeutic response to antifungals.[18] Scaling disappears late and this should not be considered as treatment failure.[18]

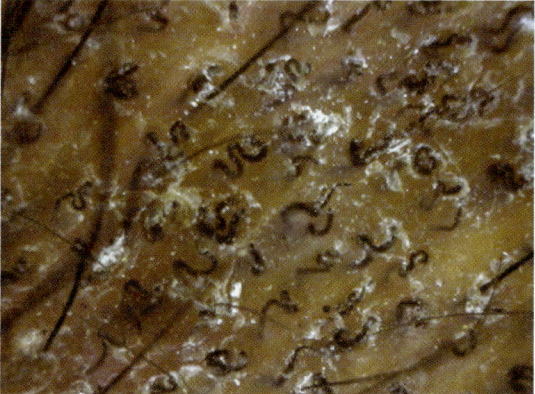

Fig. 4.17: Trichoscopy of tinea capitis showing comma hair and corkscrew hairs. Also note the perifollicular scaling (50X)

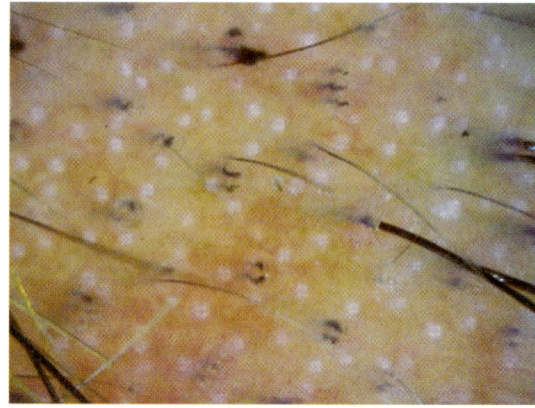

Fig. 4.19: Flame-shaped hairs seen in a case of KOH and culture positive tinea capitis (50X)

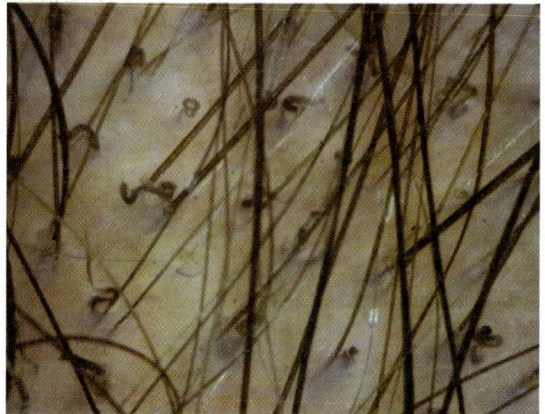

Fig. 4.18: Trichoscopy showing dystrophic and broken hairs (50X)

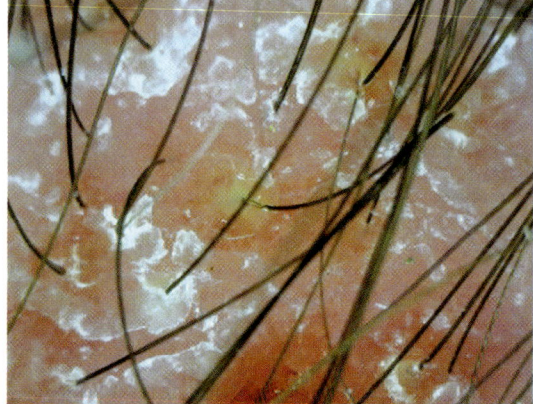

Fig. 4.20: Trichoscopy of kerion showing perifollicular pustules and erythematous background (50X)

CONCLUSION

Preliminary findings in dermoscopy of fungal infections are promising. Dermoscopy has opened up an exciting front where not only the visible clinical features are magnified but the invisible subsurface features can also be explored. It can serve as an auxillary tool for the diagnosis and management of dermatophytic infections of the hair and nail. Further research is however needed in delineating specific dermoscopic features of dermatophytosis of the skin.

References

1. Shenoy MM, Teerthanath S, Karnaker VK, et al. Comparison of potassium hydroxide mount and mycological culture with histopathologic examination using periodic acid–Schiff staining of the nail clippings in the diagnosis of onychomycosis. Indian J Dermatol Venereol Leprol 2008;74:226–9.

2. Grover C, Jakhar D. Onychoscopy: A practical guide. Indian J Dermatol Venereol Leprol 2017; 83:536–49.

3. Piraccini B, Balestri R, Starace M, et al. Nail digital dermatoscopy (onychoscopy) in the diagnosis of onychomycosis. J Eur Acad Dermatol Venereol 2013;27:509–13.

4. Jesús-Silva MA, Fernández Martínez R, Roldán Marín R, et al. Dermoscopic patterns in patients with a clinical diagnosis of onychomycosis: results of a prospective study including data of potassium hydroxide (KOH) and culture examination. Dermatol Pract Concept 2015;5: 39–44.

5. Nakamura RC, Costa MC. Dermatoscopic findings in the most frequent onychopathies: Descriptive analysis of 500 cases. Int J Dermatol 2012;51:483–5.

6. De Crignis G, Valgas N, Rezende P, et al. Dermatoscopy of onychomycosis. Int J Dermatol 2014;53:e979.

7. Kilinc Karaarslan I, Acar A, Aytimur D, et al. Dermoscopic features in fungal melanonychia.

8. Knöpfel N, Del Pozo J, Escudero MM, et al. Dermoscopic visualization of vellus hair involvement in tinea corporis: a criterion for systemic antifungal therapy. Pediatric Dermatol 2015;32:e226–22.

9. Gómez-Moyano E, Crespo Erchiga V, Martínez Pilar L, et al. Using dermoscopy to detect tinea of vellus hair. Br J Dermatol 2016;174:636–8.

10. Lacarrubba F, Verzì AE, Micali G. Newly described features resulting from high-magnification dermoscopy of tinea capitis. JAMA Dermatol 2015;151:308–10.

11. Wang HH, Lin YT. Bar code-like hair: dermoscopic marker of tinea capitis and tinea of the eyebrow. J Am Acad Dermatol 2015;72:S41–42.

12. Moyano EG, Erchiga VC, Pilar LM, et al. Correlation between dermoscopy and direct microscopy of morse code hairs in tinea incognito. J Am Acad Dermatol 2016;74:e7–8.

13. Gómez-Moyano E, Crespo-Erchiga V. Tinea of vellus hair: an indication for systemic antifungal therapy. Br J Dermatol 2010;163:603–6.

14. Slowinska M, Rudnicka L, Schwartz RA, et al. Comma hairs: a dermatoscopic marker for tinea capitis: a rapid diagnostic method. J Am Acad Dermatol 2008; 59(5 Suppl.):S77–9.

15. El-Taweel AE, El-Esawy F, Abdel-Salam O. Different trichoscopic features of tinea capitis and alopecia areata in pediatric patients. Dermatol Res Pract 2014;2014:763–848.

16. Ekiz O, Sen BB, Rifaioðlu EN, Balta I. Trichoscopy in paediatric patients with tinea capitis: a useful method to differentiate from alopecia areata. J Eur Acad Dermatol Venereol 2014;28:1255–8.

17. Brasileiro A, Campos S, Cabete J, et al. Trichoscopy as an additional tool for the differential diagnosis of tinea capitis: a prospective clinical study. Br J Dermatol 2016;175:208–9.

18. Vazquez-Lopez F, Palacios-Garcia L, Argenziano G. Dermoscopic corkscrew hairs dissolve after successful therapy of *Trichophyton violaceum* tinea capitis: A case report: dermoscopy in tinea capitis. Australas J Dermatol 2012;53:118–9.

Clinical and experimental dermatology 2015; 40:271–8.

5

General Measures for Treating Fungal Infections

Namrata Chhabra

Dermatophytoses are commonly encountered infections in dermatology practice, especially in a tropical country like India, where warm and moist conditions support fungal survival. Patient counseling is important for prevention of dermatophytosis and transmission of infection to healthy individuals.

General Measures for Tinea Corporis/Cruris/Pedis

1. In patients with dermatophytosis, infection from animals/pets should be considered.
2. Humid areas such as floor and carpet of bathroom should be cleaned and kept dry.
3. Dusting, wet mopping or vacuuming the house followed by cleaning with detergent should be done on a regular basis so as to reduce the spore load in the immediate environment.
4. One should avoid walking barefoot especially in a public place. This may be a problem in religious places but after using public places like swimming pools, feet should be wiped with a towel or washed with a soap to prevent adhesion of dermatophytes to the feet.
5. The toe clefts and skin folds should be dried before wearing clothes/shoes.

6. Occlusive footwear such as gum boots should be avoided.
7. Antifungal powder applicated over the feet may also prevent toe cleft tinea pedis.
8. One should avoid sharing garments. Loose fitting garments and socks, preferably made of cotton should be preferred.
9. Clothes and bed linen should be washed in hot water and dried in sun preferably inside out in order to destroy dermatophytes. In the absence of sunlight, ironing the clothes would be beneficial. If ironing is not possible, well dried inner garments after 3–4 days of washing should be used.
10. Patients with tinea cruris should be instructed to wear "boxer shorts" instead of the tight fitting undergarments.
11. Sports that lead to prolonged close physical contact (e.g. wrestling) should be prohibited until the risk of infection no longer exists.

General Measures for Tinea Capitis

Patient should be educated regarding contagiousness of the disease. The infection often begins through contact with animals, and treatment of the latter may be necessary. Pets (e.g. dogs, cats) should also be examined and treated as necessary. As it is contagious, individuals living with infected patients should be examined and appropriately treated to avoid transmission of the infection from asymptomatic carriers in the family. Chronicity can develop if patient is continually re-exposed to untreated family members. Exclusion of affected children from school is not recommended once treatment is started. Scalp hygiene should be emphasized. One should avoid sharing combs, towels, scarves, hats and pillows with the affected individual. Antifungal shampoos such as selenium sulphide 2.5% or ketoconazole 2% three times weekly is also helpful in reducing the transmission by decreasing shedding of spores. For scalp kerion, careful removal of crust using wet compresses should be done.

General Measures for Tinea Unguium

All measures to prevent tinea pedis and tinea manuum as mentioned above would also prevent tinea unguium. Regular trimming of nails should be done to keep the nails short and avoid trauma to the fragile infected nail plate.

Bibliography

1. Elewski BE. Treatment of tinea capitis: beyond griseofulvin. J Am Acad Dermatol 1999; 40: S27–30.

6

Topical Therapies for Treatment of Dermatophytosis

Namrata Chhabra, Kabir Sardana

Topical therapy is generally effective for uncomplicated tinea corporis of small areas and of short duration. It is also used as an adjunct to oral antifungals for more extensive infection. An ideal topical agent used for superficial fungal infections should have the following prerequisites:

a. It should exhibit a broad-spectrum activity
b. High mycological cure rate
c. Convenient dosing
d. Low incidence of side effects
e. Low cost

Various topical antifungal agents are available for the treatment of localized tinea corporis, tinea cruris, tinea faciei, and tinea pedis.

NONSPECIFIC ANTIFUNGAL AGENTS

The *nonspecific* topical agents for dermatophytosis have been available for many years; these include *keratolytics* (salicylic acid, lactic acid, hydroxyl acid, Whitfield's ointment) and *antiseptics* (gentian violet, Castellani's paint, potassium permanganate). Since they cause irritation, staining and are minimally effective, with the advent of specific antifungal agents these non-specific agents have been replaced. However, these are still preferred in certain scenarios like:

- Moccasin type tinea pedis: Keratolytic agent is useful adjunct with topical antifungals.

- Interdigital type: In acute stage, Burow's wet dressings, saline compresses and hydrogen peroxide wash (1:1 dilution) is a useful adjunct.
- Castellani's paint is still used in some cases of inflammatory tinea pedis, particularly when bacterial infection coexists, although potassium permanganate followed by a topical antifungal is preferred.

In the present era, *Whitfield's ointment* has made a comeback and is now increasingly used, with many local companies manufacturing variants of the age-old compound. It has two advantages over specific topical antifungals, one it obviates the issue of "resistance" and also helps to exfoliate the stratum corneum where due to steroid abuse "persistence" of the dermatophytes is often an issue.

SPECIFIC TOPICAL ANTIFUNGALS

Topical treatment of fungal infections took a step forward in the 1960s with the introduction of biologically active agents with specific antifungal mechanism of action. The topical antifungals effective in dermatophytosis are mainly divided into polyenes, azoles, allylamines, and others.

Polyenes

These antifungal drugs were first described in 1950, and they are produced through fermentation of *Streptomyces* species. They have a higher affinity for ergosterol in the fungal cell membranes than for cholesterol in human cell membranes causing fungal cell leakage and permeability changes, which facilitate the destruction of fungi.[1] Polyenes can be fungistatic or fungicidal depending on the drug concentration and fungal sensitivity.

Amphotericin B

It is a broad-spectrum antifungal drug for intravenous use, not indicated in uncompli-cated superficial mycoses. Amongst the super-ficial mycoses, it is effective in candidiasis and for topical treatment of onychomycosis caused by nondermatophyte fungi. Recently, lipid-based amphotericin B gel has shown results in the treatment of various mucocutaneous fungal infections including dermatophytosis, with no adverse effects.[2] Its use for the treatment of superficial dermatophytosis should not be preferred, as it might promote its resistance in the community.

Azoles

At the end of the 60s and 70s, the discovery of imidazole derivatives with antifungal activity was an important milestone in the treatment of superficial and deep mycoses, due to their high efficacy and low toxicity, as well as immunomodulatory activity. Azole derivatives are the most promising group in terms of antifungal therapy, as they are highly effective and have a relatively low incidence of side effects.

There are two broad categories: Imidazoles and triazoles, having the same mechanism of action and practically the same range of antifungal uses. Azoles inhibit ergosterol synthesis by blocking 14α-demethylation of lanosterol, thus inhibiting fungal cell synthesis, leading to accumulation of 14α-methyl sterols (which damage the enzyme systems related to the membrane) and thereby block the growth of fungi.[3] They are fungistatic, except in high concentrations,

when they can also be fungicidal. In addition, they are also anti-inflammatory and anti-bacterial particularly for gram-positive organisms. The details regarding the use of these topical antifungals in dermatophytosisis discussed in Table 6.1.

Clotrimazole

It was the first imidazole derivative. The absorption rate of clotrimazole is less than 0.5% following application to intact skin. It is said to cure dermatophyte infections in 60–100% of cases but in India most dermatologists outside government hospitals do not prescribe this molecule. The adverse effects reported are occasional local irritation, hypersensitivity reaction, burning, erythema and pruritus.

Ketoconazole

Ketoconazole is a water-soluble imidazole derivative. It is a synthetic antimycotic with a broad spectrum of activity against dermato-phytes and yeasts. It is a *cheap* and *effective* drug, that is comparable with the newer azoles in clinical practice.

Econazole

Econazole is a deschloro derivative of miconazole. Absolute concentrations of econazole in the human stratum corneum after local application far exceeds the minimal inhibitory concentration for dermatophytes, and inhibitory concentrations are detected as deep as the mid-dermis.

Miconazole

Miconazole is a synthetic imidazole deriva-tive. It penetrates the stratum corneum well, and can be detected up to 4 days after a single application.

Oxiconazole

Oxiconazole was the first topical antifungal agent to be approved for *once daily* applica-tion. Because of the pharmacokinetic properties of oxiconazole, it persists in the epidermis at

Table 6.1: Topical antifungals used in the treatment of tinea corporis, cruris and pedis					
Topical antifungal	Formulation	Indication	Dosing regimen	Pregnancy category	Adverse effects
Clotrimazole	1% cream/ lotion/solution/ powder/spray	T. corporis/ cruris/pedis	BD for 4–6 weeks	B	Local irritation, hypersensitivity reaction, burning, erythema, pruritus
Ketoconazole	2% cream/ gel/shampoo	T. corporis/ cruris/pedis	BD for 2–4 weeks	C	Same as clotrimazole
Econazole	1% cream	T. corporis/ cruris/pedis	OD or BD for 4–6 weeks	C	Same as clotrimazole
Miconazole	2% cream/ lotion/powder/ gel	T. corporis/ cruris/pedis	BD for 4–6 weeks	B	Same as clotrimazole
Oxiconazole	1% cream/lotion	T. corporis/ cruris/pedis	OD/BD for 4 weeks	B	Same as clotrimazole
Bifonazole	1% cream	T. corporis/ cruris/pedis	OD	B	Same as clotrimazole
Sertaconazole	2% cream	T. corporis/ cruris/pedis	BD for 4 weeks	C	Same as clotrimazole
Eberconazole	1% cream	T. corporis/ cruris/pedis	OD for 2–4 weeks	C	Same as clotrimazole
Luliconazole	1% cream/ lotion	T. corporis/ cruris/pedis	OD for 1 week in T. corporis, 2 weeks for T. pedis	C	Same as clotrimazole
Terbinafine	1% cream/ powder	T. corporis/ cruris/pedis	BD for 2 weeks in T. corporis/ cruris, and 4 weeks in T. pedis	B	Redness, stinging, itching and contact dermatitis
Naftifine	1% cream/gel	T. corporis/ cruris/pedis	BD for 2 weeks in T. corporis/ cruris, and 4 weeks in T. pedis	B	Redness, stinging, itching and contact dermatitis
Butenafine	1% cream	T. corporis/ cruris/pedis	OD/BD for 2–4 weeks	C	Redness, stinging, itching and contact dermatitis

(Contd.)

Table 6.1: Topical antifungals used in the treatment of tinea corporis, cruris and pedis (*Contd.*)

Topical antifungal	Formulation	Indication	Dosing regimen	Pregnancy category	Adverse effects
Amorolfine	0.25% cream/ 5% nail lacquer	T. corporis/ unguium	BD for 4 weeks, once weekly nail lacquer for T. unguium up to 6–12 months	B	Erythema, pruritus, burning
Ciclopirox olamine	1% cream/ shampoo/8% nail lacquer	T. corporis/ cruris/pedis/ unguium	BD for 2–4 weeks, nail lacquer OD for 9–12 months in onychomycosis	B	Burning, pruritus, contact dermatitis, nail pigmentation, and onychocryptosis
Selenium sulfide	1%, 2.5% lotion/ shampoo	As adjuvant in treatment of T. capitis	OD for 7 days and then on the first and third days of the week for 6 months	C	Burning, pruritus, contact dermatitis, erythema dyschromicum perstans, photo-sensitivity, alopecia, and brittle hair

therapeutic levels for 7 days. This reservoir effect accounts for oxiconazole efficacy in fungus eradication with once daily dosing.

Bifonazole

Bifonazole has potent antifungal activity and is retained well in the stratum corneum. It is used in a once daily regimen.

Sertaconazole

Sertaconazole is relatively lipophilic compared to other azoles, leading to a greater *reservoir* effect in the stratum corneum. It possesses both fungistatic and fungicidal activity depending upon exact organism and its concentration.[4] One of the studies found sertraconazole to be highly efficient compared to other newer antifungals (luliconazole, eberconazole, terbinafine, amorolfine) in terms of efficacy and with lesser adverse effects.[5] It

also exhibits anti-inflammatory and anti-pruritic action. It inhibits the release of proinflammatory cytokines from activated immune cells. Sertaconazole also has antibacterial action.

Eberconazole

Eberconazole 1% cream is efficacious in the treatment of dermatophytoses, candidiasis, and pityriasis, with higher efficacy than clotrimazole cream in dermatophytosis.[6] Its clinical efficacy (clinical and mycologic cure) and safety are *equivalent* to those of miconazole 2% cream.[7]

Luliconazole

Luliconazole is an imidazole antifungal agent with a unique structure, as the imidazole moiety is incorporated into the ketene dithioacetal structure. Through this modification, high potency against filamentous fungi including dermatophytes has been achieved, while maintaining the broad antifungal spectrum of an imidazole. Although belonging to the azole group, it has demonstrated strong fungicidal activity at very low levels (minimum inhibitory concentration {MIC} of <0.001 µg/ml for *Trichophyton rubrum*), in both *in vitro* and *in vivo* studies, luliconazole has demonstrated potent and broad-spectrum activity against dermatophyte and non-dermatophyte pathogens, with reported MICs considerably lower than those of other antifungal drugs including terbinafine, bifonazole, clotrimazole, miconazole and amorolfine hydrochloride (Table 6.2).[8,9]

Like most fundamental research luliconazole 1% cream was approved in Japan in 2005 for the treatment of tinea infections, followed by approval in November 2013 by the US Food and Drug Administration for the treatment of interdigital tinea pedis, tinea cruris, and tinea corporis caused by *T. rubrum* and *E. floccosum* in patients 18 years of age and older. As a new antifungal drug, luliconazole1% cream is not only effective, but also can shorten the duration of therapy. Therefore, in clinical practice, luliconazole 1% with its stronger antifungal activity and good retention in skin, is in high demand.

A multicenter, randomized, single-blind, two-way, parallel-group study compared the clinical efficacy of luliconazole 1% cream applied once daily for 2 weeks with that of bifonazole 1% cream applied once daily for 4 weeks in patients with tinea pedis. Clinical efficacy at the end of 4 weeks was found to be similar for both groups, however, the clinical and mycologic efficacy of short-term (2-week) treatment with luliconazole was found to be at par with the standard 4 weeks of treatment with bifonazole for tinea pedis.[10] In another prospective study comparing luliconazole and terbinafine, luliconazole and terbinafine applied once daily for 2 weeks were found to be equally efficacious for tinea corporis/cruris.[11]

In one of the multicentric studies comparing sertaconazole 2%, terbinafine 1% and luliconazole 1% cream, four weeks of treatment with twice daily sertaconazole was concluded to be slightly more effective than 2 weeks of treatment with once daily luliconazole and terbinafine for tinea corporis/cruris. Sertaconazole was better than terbinafine and luliconazole in relieving signs and symptoms during study and follow-up period.[12]

The frequency of application (once daily) and duration of treatment (one week for tinea corporis/cruris and 2 weeks for interdigital

Table 6.2: Comparison of published minimum inhibitory concentrations (MIC) of antifungal agents against dermatophyte pathogens

	Luliconazole	Butenafine	Terbinafine	Bifonazole	Clotrimazole	Miconazole	Ketoconazole	Amorolfine hydrochloride
Trichophyton rubrum	≤0.00012–0.004	0.0039–0.031	0.002–>0.25 (0.0313–4)*	0.0078–>1	0.031–0.063	0.031–0.025	0.016–0.13 (0.0156–0.5)*	0.031
T. mentagrophytes	0.00024–0.002	0.0078–0.063	0.001–0.06 (0.0625–4)*	0.016–1	0.016–0.5	0.13–2	0.25–1 (0.0156–2)*	0.25
T. tonsurans	0.00024–0.00049	0.002–0.031	≤0.00098–0.016	0.063–1	0.13–0.25	0.13–1	0.13–1	0.063

*MIC values from Indian Study[16]

tinea pedis) with luliconazole is favorable when compared with other topical regimens used for the treatment of tinea pedis, such as 2–4 weeks of twice daily treatment with econazole, up to 4 weeks of twice daily treatment with sertaconazole, 1–2 weeks of twice daily treatment with terbinafine, 4 weeks of once daily application of naftifine, and 4–6 weeks of once daily treatment with amorolfine.[13] Furthermore, luliconazole has demonstrated potent activity against the dermatophyte isolates collected from patients with onychomycosis in one recent trial suggesting that luliconazole may be a suitable option for the treatment of this disease.[14]

Allylamines

Allylamines act by inhibiting the squalene epoxidase enzyme in the cytoplasmic membrane of the fungus, leading to ergosterol deficiency and intracellular toxic squalene accumulation. They are fungicidal for both dermatophytes and yeasts. The group also has anti-inflammatory and limited antibacterial action.

Terbinafine

Terbinafine is highly lipophilic, which results in high concentration and efficient binding to the stratum corneum, sebum and hair follicles, thereby reducing the probability of reinfection. Pharmacokinetic studies have demonstrated persistent concentrations well above the MIC for the common dermatophytes 7 days after topical application. The reported adverse effects are redness, stinging, itching and contact dermatitis. In India this drug has been found to be less effective than azoles and data on MIC has supported this trend.[15,16]

Naftifine

Naftifine, a topical allylamine, is fungicidal *in vitro* against a wide spectrum of dermatophyte fungi and has been shown to be highly effective against a variety of cutaneous dermatophyte infections. Rapid onset of clinical activity and favorable data on sustained clearance of infection has been documented with naftifine.

Butenafine

Butenafine is a benzylamine which is structurally related to allylamines. Butenafine cream has been the treatment of choice for tinea pedis, tinea corporis, tinea cruris, tinea versicolor, and cutaneous candidal infections in Japan since its introduction in 1992. Clinical trials conducted in Japan revealed 84–100% cure rates in tinea cruris, with only 2–3% of patients experiencing adverse effects, including erythema, irritation, and pruritus. This drug has a rapid efficacy within a week of treatment and, cure rates continued to increase 2 weeks after the end of treatment, suggesting that butenafine may possess residual therapeutic activity.

An Indian study comparing butenafine 1% and sertraconazole 2% found that butenafine 1% is more efficacious, cost effective, and equally safe as compared to sertaconazole 2% in tinea of skin. It also provides residual protection which may prevent relapse.[17]

Other Topical Antifungals

Amorolfine

It is a phenylpropyl morpholine derivative and acts by inhibiting ergosterol biosynthesis in the fungal cell membrane. Alterations in membrane sterol content lead to changes in membrane permeability and disruption of fungal metabolic processes. It acts on two different enzymes involved in the biosynthesis of the ergosterol, modifying the morphology of hyphae. This dual mechanism of action makes amorolfine a potent fungistatic and fungicidal agent.

Amorolfine can be useful in infections caused by dermatophytes, yeasts and non-dermatophytic molds. *In vitro* studies have demonstrated that at concentrations of 0.1–100 µg/ml, topical amorolfine induces varying degrees of damage to the nuclear, mitochondrial and plasma membranes of both *T. mentagrophytes and Candida albicans*.[18] A clinical study demonstrated comparable effectivity of amorolfine and bifonazole in the treatment of dermatomycosis.[19]

Somehow in India, the drug is not very effective, this is as a company had promoted this drug to GP for about 5 years before it was promoted to dermatologists.

Ciclopirox Olamine

Ciclopirox olamine acts by interrupting active membrane transport of essential cellular precursors disrupting cell function leading to fungal demise. Unlike most topical antifungal agents, ciclopirox does not appear to affect sterol biosynthesis, but acts by interfering with active membrane transport of essential macromolecular precursors, disrupting cell membrane integrity and inhibiting enzymes essential for respiratory processes. High affinity for trivalent cations, and subsequent blockade of enzymatic co-factors, is thought by most investigators to be the main mode of action. It has anti-inflammatory properties by inhibition of cyclooxygenase, 5-lipoxygenase, prostaglandins and leukotrienes.[20] It also has antibacterial properties against both gram-positive and gram-negative organisms.

In vitro, ciclopirox exhibits high inhibitory activity against dermatophytes, yeasts, and fungal saprophytes. In clinical trials, ciclopirox 1% cream (now re-labeled as 0.77%) was significantly more effective than its vehicle and clotrimazole 1% cream in the treatment of tinea pedis. This is also the case in the treatment of tinea corporis, tinea cruris, tinea versicolor, and cutaneous candidiasis. The gel formulation offers comparable efficacy with enhanced drying effect owing to its high alcohol content. The use of the nail lacquer to achieve complete resolution of onychomycosis requires prolonged daily use (9–12 months) and may not be the most advantageous maneuver from a pharmacoeconomic perspective, compared to oral antifungal therapy.

As this drug has not been extensively used in India except as a shampoo and a combination with steroid, this is a potentially useful drug in India. Surprisingly the two companies who have a shampoo and a topical steroid combination have not yet realized its untapped potential in dermatophyte infection of the skin.

Selenium Sulfide

It has cytostatic effect on keratinocytes, reduces corneocyte adhesion, thus allows shedding of fungi in the stratum corneum.

MISCELLANEOUS ASPECTS OF TOPICAL ANTIFUNGAL THERAPY

Role of Topical Antifungals in Tinea Unguium

Topical therapy is recommended in cases of onychomycosis where the nail matrix is not involved, when there are contraindications to systemic treatment, in white superficial onychomycosis, as an adjunct to oral therapy for resistant infection, and as post-treatment prophylaxis. Studies have shown that amorolfine 5% and ciclopirox 8% in the form of nail lacquer penetrates the nail plate and reaches the nail bed in higher concentration than the minimum inhibitory concentration for most fungi that cause onychomycosis. Nail sanding should be carried out weekly in both cases.

"The Rule of Two"

The topical antifungals should be applied 2 cm beyond the margin of the lesion for at least 2 weeks beyond clinical resolution. This recommendation of applying topical antifungals is called "The rule of Two", though there is no scientific logic in published data for this rule.

Role of Topical Steroids and Combination Creams

There are combined formulations available which contain imidazoles and corticosteroids. Furthermore, the irrational triple and quadruple combination creams (steroid-antifungal-antibacterial) are also easily available and are often the first cream used by the patient with tinea who buys them over-the-counter. Corticosteroids have been shown to stimulate fungal metabolism in low concentrations while they inhibit fungal metabolism in high concentrations due to their cytostatic effects.[21] Studies have also shown that addition of topical steroid increases the bioavailability of topical antifungals mostly imidazole groups. However, the precise role of these combined formulations is controversial.

They can occasionally be useful to accelerate resolution of symptoms when infected skin is very inflamed and pruritic. However, it is also possible that they may impair the response to the antifungal agent, and the familiar hazards of topical corticosteroids include the potential to mask a persisting infection. Further, most combination creams available in India use the superpotent steroid clobetasol, and this may outdo any expected benefit from these combinations.

Topical steroid abuse has also been implicated for the sudden outbreak of the complicated, atypical, chronic and recalcitrant dermatophytosis. Therefore, such practice should be strongly discouraged in countries like India where easy "over-the-counter" availability of irrational combination creams results in frequent misuse by patients who finally end up with tinea incognito.

Optimal Choice of Vehicle for Topical Treatment

The efficacy of topical agents in superficial mycoses depends not only on the type of lesion and the actual mechanism of action of the drug, but also on the viscosity, hydrophobicity and acidity of the formulation. Creams should be used for dry and scaly lesions. Lotions should be given for intertriginous areas, oozing lesions, and hairy areas. Ointments are cumbersome and overly occlusive to be used in macerated or fissured intertriginous lesions, and should be preferred for thicker, hyperkeratotic lesions. The use of powders, either in sprays or aerosol form, is limited in large part to the feet area and lesions in moist intertriginous areas.

Anti-inflammatory Effect of Topical Antifungals

Several topical antimycotic agents have demonstrated inherent anti-inflammatory properties. These properties are not only beneficial in reducing the inflammation associated with dermatomycoses, but also proved useful in the treatment of other inflammatory skin disorders. This may be of great importance in India and may help the atypical and occasionally inflammatory variants we see in practice.

Most of the azoles (clotrimazole, econazole, ketoconazole and miconazole) have demonstrated an ability to inhibit the chemotactic ability of PMN. Specifically *bifonazole* has also been shown to inhibit calmodulin, a protein integral to prostaglandin synthesis and histamine release from mast cells. *Sertaconazole* demonstrates *in vitro* anti-inflammatory activity in a Murine model of ear edema. Of the azoles, bifonazole and ketoconazole have demonstrated utility in a number of inflammatory skin conditions. *Ketoconazole* is able to inhibit 5-lipoxygenase in a dose-dependent fashion, which reduces the production of 5-HETE and leukotriene B4. This action may be related to inhibition of cytochrome P-450 enzymes, which may play a role in arachidonic acid metabolism.

Of the allylamines, *naftifine* has been found to be equipotent as clotrimazole 1%–hydrocortisone 1% combination. *Butenafine*, has demonstrated similar prevention of UVB-induced erythema. It has been postulated that this effect is mediated by the same anti-inflammatory mechanisms possessed by naftifine. *Ciclopirox olamine* also has anti-inflammatory properties.

CONCLUSION

Although there are many excellent topical antifungal agents, the number of sufferers has not decreased. In fact, the dermatophytosis with chronic, atypical, recalcitrant presentations are increasingly being reported. One of the hypotheses is the incomplete clearance of fungus in patients.

A majority of patients do not complete the therapy, and as soon as they find the clinical symptoms like pruritus, erythema, scaling are relieved, they stop the treatment. The symptomatic relief provided by the steroid combination creams translates into even shorter duration of treatment which is often repeated *ad libitum*. So, whenever we prescribe an antifungal, we should take the compliance of the patients into consideration. Although there is sufficient evidence to demonstrate the efficacy of topical antifungals in limited disease, there is scarce data on the frequency of relapse once topical monotherapy is discontinued.

It is possible that a small number of dermatophytes below the detection limit can survive in these partially treated lesions and/or surrounding tissues. As a result, the high rate of relapse in patients who were previously considered cured is one of the biggest challenges in the treatment of fungal infections. To tackle this, it is desirable to develop antifungals with fungicidal activity that attain mycologic negativity even after short-term use. It is likely that a once daily or shorter regimen may be associated with greater compliance and produce similar or probably higher efficacy in clinical practice. In addition, we also need to tackle the persistent problem of steroid abuse in our population, which might be adding to this load of unresponsive dermatophytosis, as mentioned earlier in this chapter.

Newer topical antifungals such as eberconazole and sertaconazole are found to be more efficacious compared to the older azoles like clotrimazole probably because they exert better anti-inflammatory effect.[12,22] Available in 1% cream formulation, luliconazole is effective as once daily application for 1–2 weeks for dermatophytic infection. In case of inflammation in tinea, topical antifungals with potent anti-inflammatory action such as sertaconazole or luliconazole may be a better option than an antifungal-steroid combination. Drugs with residual action like butenafine and unique actions like ciclopirox olamine should be considered in India.

In fact, we should think "out of the box" and drugs that are underutilized and with additional anti-inflammatory effects (butenafine, ketaconazole, luliconazole, ciclopirox olamine) are the need of the hour. Sadly though, companies look at ORG figures for launches.

While the Western data surmises that the allylamine/benzylamine type drugs are more potent *in vitro*, and have a higher efficacy *in vivo*, than the azole antifungal agents in the treatment of dermatophytoses, in India this may not be completely true and terbinafine, may not be as effective. A summary of data from India suggests that the *in vitro* anti-dermatophyte potency is:

Luliconazole > butenafine > ciclopirox = naftifine > other azoles > terbinafine.

References

1. Verma S, Heffernan MP. Superficial fungal infection: dermatophytosis, tinea nigra, piedra. In: Fitzpatrick TB, Eisen AZ, Wolff K, Freedberg IM, Austen KF, editors. Dermatology in general medicine.7th ed. New York: McGraw-Hill; 2008. p. 1807–21.

2. Sheikh S, Ahmad A, Ali SM, Paithankar M, Barkate H, Raval RC, et al. Topical delivery of lipid based amphotericin B gel in the treatment of fungal infection: A clinical efficacy, safety and tolerability study in patients. J ClinExpDermatol Res 2014; 5: 248.

3. Gilman AG, Molinoff PB, Hardman JG. FármacosAntimicrobianos; FármacosAntifúngicos. In: Hardman JG, Limbird LE, Molinoff PB, Ruddon RW, Gilman AG, editors. As bases Farmacológicas da Terapêutica: Goodman e Gilman. 9. ed. Santiago do Chile: McGraw-Hill; 1996; p. 864–75.

4. Carrillo-Munoz JA, Cristina T, Cárdenes DC, Estivill D, Giusiano G. Sertaconazole nitrate shows fungicidal and fungistatic activities against *Trichophyton rubrum, Trichophyton mentagrophytes,* and *Epidermophyton floccosum,* causative agents of tinea pedis. Antimicrob Agents Chemother 2011; 55: 4420–1.

5. Selvan A, Girisha G, Vijaybhaskar, Suthakaran R. Comparative evaluation of newer topical antifungal agents in the treatment of superficial fungal infections (tinea or dermatophytic). Int Res J Pharm 2013; 4: 224–8.

6. Del Palacio A, Ortiz FJ, Pérez A, Pazos C, Garau M, Font E. A double-blind randomized comparative trial: Eberconazole 1% cream versus clotrimazole 1% cream twice daily in Candida and dermatophyte skin infections. Mycoses 2001; 44: 173–80.

7. Repiso Montero T, López S, Rodríguez C, del Rio R, Badell A, Gratacós MR. Eberconazole 1% cream is an effective and safe alternative for dermatophytosis treatment: multicenter, randomized, double-blind, comparative trial with miconazole 2% cream. Int J Dermatol 2006;45: 600–4.

8. Koga H, Tsuji Y, Inoue K, Kanai K, Majima T, Kasai T, et al. *In vitro* antifungal activity of luliconazole against clinical isolates from patients with dermatomycoses. J Infect Chemother 2006;12: 163–5.

9. Koga H, Nanjoh Y, Makimura K, Tsuboi R. *In vitro* antifungal activities of luliconazole, a new topical imidazole. Med Mycol. 2009;47:640–7.

10. Watanabe S, Takahashi H, Nishikawa T, Takiuchi I, Higashi N, Nishimoto K. A comparative clinical study between 2 weeks of luliconazole 1% cream treatment and 4 weeks of bifonazole 1% cream treatment for tinea pedis. Mycoses 2006; 49: 236–41.

11. Lakshmi VC, Bengalorkar GM, Shiva Kumar V. Clinical efficacy of topical terbinafine versus topical luliconazole in treatment of tinea corporis/tinea cruris patients. Br J Pharm Res. 2013; 3: 1001–14.

12. Jerajani H, Janaki C, Kumar S, Phiske M. Comparative assessment of the efficacy and safety of sertaconazole (2%) cream versus terbinafine cream (1%) versus luliconazole (1%) cream in patients with dermatophytoses: a pilot study. Indian J Dermatol 2013; 58: 34–8.

13. Gupta AK, Einarson TR, Summerbell RC, Shear NH. An overview of topical anti-fungal therapy in dermatomycoses. A North American perspective. Drugs 1998; 55: 645–74.

14. Wiederhold NP, Fothergill AW, McCarthy DI, Tavakkol A. Luliconazole demonstrates potent *in vitro* activity against dermatophytes recovered from patients with onychomycosis. Antimicrob Agents Chemother 2014; 58: 3553–5.

15. Mahajan S, Tilak R, Kaushal SK, Mishra RN, Pandey SS. Clinico-mycological study of dermatophytic infections and their sensitivity to antifungal drugs in a tertiary care center. Indian J Dermatol Venereol Leprol 2017;83:436–40.

16. Bhatia VK, Sharma PC. Determination of minimum inhibitory concentrations of itraconazole, terbinafine and ketoconazole against dermatophyte species by broth microdilution method. Indian J Med Microbiol 2015;33:533–7.

17. Thaker SJ, Mehta DS, Shah HA, Dave JN, Mundhava SG. A comparative randomized open label study to evaluate efficacy, safety and cost effectiveness between topical 2% sertaconazole and topical 1% butenafine in tinea infections of skin.Indian J Dermatol 2013; 58: 451–6.

18. Müller J, Polak-Wyss A, Melchinger W. Influence of amorolfine on the morphology of *Candida albicans* and *Trichophyton mentagrophytes.* Clin Exp Dermatol 1992; 17:18–25.

19. Nolting S, Semig G, Friedrich HK, Dietz M, Reckers-Czaschka R, Bergstraesser M, et al. Double-blind comparison of amorolfine and bifonazole in the treatment of dermatomycoses. Clin Exp Dermatol 1992;17: 56–60.

20. Zhang AY, Camp WL, Elewski BE. Advances in topical and systemic antifungals. Dermatol Clin 2007; 25: 165–83.

21. Högl F, Raab W. The influence of steroids on the antifungal and antibacterial activities of imidazole derivatives. Mykosen 1980; 23: 426–39.

22. Moodahadu-Bangera LS, Martis J, Mittal R, Krishnankutty B, Kumar N, Bellary S, et al. Eberconazole-Pharmacological and clinical review. Indian J Dermatol Venereol Leprol 2012; 78: 217–22.

7

Role of Antifungal Powders, Soaps and Washes

Namrata Chhabra

Most of the dermatologists in their practice prescribe antifungal powders, soaps and washes in the treatment of tinea. Though there is not enough evidence regarding their efficacy in dermatophytosis, these can be useful as an adjuvant and their use can ensure the hygiene of the affected area.

Daily bath is almost a norm in India. By incorporating medications in soaps, the compliance can be ensured. Baths or compresses of potassium permanganate (1:10.000) can be used in cases of tinea pedis, when there is secondary infection.

Aggressive bathing though may actually damage the barrier and alter the pH and should not be overemphasised. Although antifungal powder does not eradicate infection, it may be used to prevent reinfection. It should be applied to the feet, not to the shoes, to prevent tinea pedis. Here, it is important to note that *T. interdigitale* which is the commonest species in some centres is preferentially harboured in the soles (Page 85).

Antifungal shampoos used in dermatophytosis are selenium sulfide (1% and 2.5%), zinc pyrithione (1% and 2%), povidone iodine (2.5%) and ketoconazole (2%). These are to be applied to the scalp and hair for 5 minutes, 2 to 4 times a week for 2 to 4 weeks or three times a week until the patient is clinically and mycologically cured. Neither of these adjunctive shampoos eradicates the disease, therefore they should be used in conjunction with systemic antifungals to eradicate tinea capitis. Adjunctive shampoo is recommended for all patients in order to decrease the viability and shedding of fungal spores present on the hair, hence preventing transmission to close contacts. It may also shorten the cure rate with oral antifungals. Antifungal shampoo is also recommended for all household contacts to prevent infection or eliminate the carrier state.

Thus most of the measures are adjunctive and not curative and may be just good to fill up 'patient handouts' which is the case in India.

8

Systemic Agents for Treatment of Dermatophytoses

Madhu Rengasamy, C Janaki, G Sentamilselvi

Systemic antifungal drugs used in the treatment of dermatophytosis are griseofulvin, terbinafine and triazoles such as fluconazole and itraconazole. Ketoconazole, an imidazole, introduced in the 1970s is no longer FDA approved for the treatment of superficial fungal infections.[1] There has been an increase in the prevalence of chronic, recurrent, extensive and difficult to treat dermatophytosis in India over the last 4–5 years, with a concomitant increase in the treatment failure.[2] Treatment regimens mentioned in the western and Indian standard textbooks have been found to be non-effective to result in clinical cure. Hence, an attempt has been made to provide the experience based dose and duration recommendations that are currently in vogue in addition to the standard textbook recommendations.

Indications for systemic antifungal therapy in the treatment of dermatophytosis are as follows:[3]

1. Failure of topical antifungal therapy
2. Extensive tinea corporis
3. Multiple sites involvement
4. Tinea pedis/tinea manuum
5. Chronic/recurrent dermatophytosis
6. Tinea of vellus hair
7. Hair infection by dermatophytes
8. Nail infection by dermatophytes
9. Steroid modified tinea/tinea incognito
10. Special forms—Majocchi granuloma, tinea imbricata

GRISEOFULVIN

Griseofulvin, a fungistatic drug isolated from *Penicillium griseofulvum* by Oxford, Raistrick and Simonart in 1939 was found to be effective in the treatment of dermatophytosis by JC Gentles in 1958.[4,5]

Mechanism of action: Griseofulvin causes disruption of microtubule spindle formation resulting in inhibition of nucleic acid synthesis, arrest of mitosis at the metaphase and inhibition of fungal cell wall synthesis.[5]

Spectrum of activity: It has a narrow spectrum of antimycotic activity and is indicated for the treatment of dermatophytosis of skin, hair and nail. It is effective against *Trichophyton, Microsporum* and *Epidermophyton* species. Griseofulvin does not act against *Malassezia, Candida* or other fungi causing deep mycoses.[6]

Pharmacokinetics

Half life: 9.5 to 22 hours[6]

Peak-post dosing levels: 2 to 4 hours[6]

Metabolism: Griseofulvin is best absorbed after a fatty meal and in micronised and ultra-micronized formulations. After oral administration, the drug reaches the stratum corneum (SC) within 4–8 hours. Sweat potentiates entry of the drug in the SC. It is tightly bound to the keratin during cell differentiation and persists in the keratin. It is mainly metabolized in the liver, with 6-demethyl griseofulvin and its glucuronide conjugate being the metabolites. Renal excretion is 50%, while 1% and 36% are excreted unchanged in urine and faeces respectively. It is also excreted in sweat.[6,7]

Indications: Griseofulvin is *US FDA approved* for the treatment of tinea corporis, tinea cruris, tinea pedis, tinea capitis and tinea unguium.[6]

It is used to treat tinea imbricata as an *off-label* indication.[6]

Dose and duration of treatment are given in Table 8.1.

Recommended Dose and Duration

Tinea corporis: 250 mg twice daily after a fatty meal for 6–8 weeks/until cure

Tinea pedis: 250 mg twice daily after a fatty meal for 8–10 weeks/until cure

Tablet strength of ultramicronised form is 330/375 mg.

Contraindications[5]

- Hypersensitivity to griseofulvin
- Pregnancy (category C drug)
- Patients with porphyria or hepatocellular failure
- Renal failure
- Systemic lupus erythematosus
- Acute intermittent porphyria

Side Effects[5,7]

Headache and nausea are the most common complaints. Incidence of headache is about 15% but it may disappear with continuation of drug.

Gastrointestinal: Vomiting, diarrhea, flatulence, dry mouth, angular stomatitis, heartburn.

Hematological: Leukopenia, neutropenia and punctate basophilia, which disappear despite continuation of therapy.

Hepatotoxicity

Skin: Photosensitivity (patient may be warned against exposure to intense sunlight).

Lupus erythematosus (LE), lupus-like syndromes or exacerbation of existing LE cold and warm urticaria, lichen planus, EMF-like rash, morbilliform eruption.

Renal: Albuminuria and cylindruria without evidence of renal insufficiency.

Table 8.1: Standard textbook regimen of griseofulvin (microsize) for tinea corporis and tinea pedis[6, 8–10]

Textbook	Tinea corporis		Tinea pedis	
	Dose/day	Weeks	Dose/day	Weeks
IADVL Textbook of Dermatology, 4th edition 2015[8]	500 mg OD	4–8	500 mg BD	4–8
Rook's Dermatology, 9th edition, 2016[9]	1 Gram	4	—	—
Fitzpatrick's Dermatology, 8th edition, 2012[10]	500 mg	2–4	—	—
Wolverton Comprehensive Dermatologic Drug Therapy, 3rd edition, 2013[6]	250 mg BD	Until cure	750 mg	4–8
Bolognia Dermatology, 3rd edition, 2012[11]	500–1000 mg (Microsize) 375–500 mg (Ultramicrosize)	2–4	750–1000 mg (Microsize) 500–750 mg (Ultramicrosize)	4

Menstrual Irregularity

Neurological symptoms—lethargy, vertigo, syncope, blurred vision, transient macular edema, peripheral neuritis, impairment of performance of routine tasks.

Rarely serum sickness syndromes and severe angioedema.

Drug Interactions[5,7]

- *Griseofulvin level is decreased* by barbiturates
- *Griseofulvin potentiates* the action of alcohol, resulting in disulfiram-like reaction
- Griseofulvin decreases levels of
  - Warfarin
    - Estrogen, oral contraceptives containing estrogen
    - Cyclosporin
  - Salicylates

FLUCONAZOLE

Fluconazole, a bis-triazole fungistatic drug, was approved for use in 1988 in United Kingdom and France and in the United States in 1990.[6]

Mechanism of action: Fluconazole inhibits the cytochrome P450 dependent lanosterol 14α-demethylase, which aids in the conversion of lanosterol to 14α-demethyl lanosterol and subsequently ergosterol, most important component in the fungal cell membrane. As a result, there is impaired biosynthesis of ergosterol along with the accumulation of 14α-methyl sterols which impair the functions of enzymes such as ATPases and other oxidative/peroxidase enzymes resulting in inhibition of growth of the fungi.[7]

Spectrum of activity: Fluconazole is active against dermatophytes, *Malassezia*, *Candida* species except *C. krusei*, *Cryptococcus neoformans*, *Histoplasma capsulatum*, *Coccidoides immitis* and *Blastomyces dermatidis*.[7]

Pharmacokinetics

Half life: 30 hours.[6]
Peak-post dosing levels: 1 to 2 hours.[6]

Metabolism: Fluconazole, a relatively hydrophilic molecule, is rapidly and almost completely absorbed after oral administration. Bioavailability is >90% and is unaltered by food or gastric acidity. After oral administration, drug accumulates in eccrine sweat and diffuses rapidly and extensively through the dermis and stratum corneum (SC). Much higher concentration is achieved in SC than in serum or plasma. Cerebrospinal fluid (CSF) concentration is 50–90% of the plasma level and it is hence useful in the treatment of fungal meningitis. Plasma protein binding of fluconazole is only 11–12% compared to the other azoles and terbinafine which have high affinity for plasma proteins. It undergoes little first-pass hepatic metabolism and is mainly eliminated through the renal system as 80% unchanged parent drug, 11% as metabolites and 2% in faeces.[6,7,12]

Indications[6]

- Fluconazole is *FDA approved* for the treatment of
  - Onychomycosis caused by dermatophytes,
  - Vaginal, oropharyngeal and esophageal candidiasis.
- It is used *off-label* in the treatment of
- Onychomycosis caused by *Candida* and non-dermatophyte molds
  - Tinea corporis/cruris, tinea capitis, tinea pedis
  - Pityriasis versicolor
  - Cutaneous and chronic mucocutaneous candidiasis

Dose and duration of treatment are given in Table 8.2.

Recommended Dose and Duration

Tinea corporis: Tab fluconazole 150 mg biweekly for 6–8 weeks or until cure.

Tinea pedis: Tab fluconazole 150 mg biweekly for 8 weeks or until cure.

Table 8.2: Standard regimens of fluconazole for tinea corporis and tinea pedis[3,6,8–12]

Textbook	Tinea corporis		Tinea pedis	
	Dose/day	Weeks	Dose/day	Weeks
IADVL Textbook of Dermatology, 4th edition 2015[8]	150–300 mg once/week	4–6	150–300 mg/ 1 dose/week	4–6
Rook's Dermatology, 9th edition 2016[9]	—	—	—	—
Fitzpatrick's Dermatology, 8th edition, 2012[10]	150–300 mg/ week	4–6	150 mg/week	3–4
Wolverton Comprehensive Dermatologic Drug Therapy 3rd edition, 2013[6]	150–300 mg once/week	2–4	150 mg once/ week	2–6
Sentamilselvi G, Handbook of Dermatomycology, 1st edition, 2006[3]	3 mg/kg biweekly	6	—	—
Bolognia Dermatology, 3rd edition, 2012[11]	150–200 mg/ week	2–4	150–200 mg/ week	4–6
Olafsson JH, Hay RJ, Antibiotic and Antifungal Therapies in Dermatology, 2017[13]	100 mg daily 150 mg/week	2–4 2–3	Longer duration	

Contraindications[6]

- Known hypersensitivity to fluconazole/ hypersensitivity to other azoles.
- Coadministration with terfenadine/aste- mizole likely to cause VT-torsades de pointes.
- Concomitant administration with quini- dine, pimozide.
- Pregnancy (category C drug)

Adverse Effects[6,7] (Table 8.3)

Cutaneous: Skin rash; Uncommon: Fixed drug eruption, Stevens-Johnson syndrome/TEN, acute generalised exanthematous pustulosis, increased sweating, alopecia.

Gastrointestinal: Nausea, vomiting, diarrhea, dyspepsia, constipation, abdominal pain

Neurological: Headache; Uncommon—dizziness, seizures, insomnia, paraesthesia, vertigo.

Hepatic: Elevated liver enzymes; Rarely: Hepatitis, hepatic failure, cholestasis.

Haematological: Uncommon—leukopenia, neutro- penia, thrombocytopenia, agranulocytosis.

Miscellaneous: Uncommon or rare anaphy- laxis (angioedema), oliguria, hypokalemia, hypertriglyceridemia, dysgeusia, fatigue, fever, malaise.

Drug Interactions[6,13–15] (Table 8.4)

- Fluconazole is a potent CYP2C9 inhibitor, moderate CYP3A4 inhibitor
- *Fluconazole level is decreased by* rifampin
- *Fluconazole level is increased by* hydro- chlorthiazide and possibly other thiazide diuretics
- *Fluconazole decreases levels of* oral contraceptives
- *Fluconazole increases levels of the following coadministered drugs:*
  - Anti-diabetic: Sulfonylurea
  - Anti-hypertensive: Nifedepine, losartan
  - Proton pump inhibitor omeprazole
  - NSAID: Diclofenac, ibubrufen, celecoxib, naproxen
  - Bronchodilator: Theophylline
  - Anti-convulsant: Phenytoin, carbamaze- pine

Table 8.3: Adverse effects of terbinafine, fluconazole and itraconazole[6,7,13]

Terbinafine	Fluconazole	Itraconazole
Cutaneous: Skin rash, pruritus. Rarely Stevens-Johnson syndrome/ TEN, angioedema, psoriasiform eruption or exacerbation of psoriasis, acute generalised exanthematous pustulosis, exfoliative dermatitis, exacerbation of cutaneous and systemic LE, alopecia	**Cutaneous:** Skin rash; Uncommon: Fixed drug eruption, Stevens-Johnson syndrome/TEN, acute generalised exanthematous pustulosis, increased sweating, alopecia	**Cutaneous:** Skin rash, pruritus, diaphoresis. Rarely Stevens-Johnson syndrome/TEN, acute generalised exanthematous pustulosis, exfoliative dermatitis, leukocytoclastic vasculitis, photosensitivity, alopecia
Gastrointestinal: Diarrhea, dyspepsia, abdominal pain, nausea, flatulence. Uncommon: Vomiting, pancreatitis	**Gastrointestinal:** Nausea, vomiting, diarrhea, dyspepsia, constipation, abdominal pain	**Gastrointestinal:** Nausea, vomiting, diarrhea, abdominal pain. Uncommon: Dyspepsia, pancreatitis, dysgeusia, constipation
Neurological: Headache, Uncommon: Depressive symptoms	**Neurological:** Headache, Uncommon: Dizziness, seizures, insomnia, paraesthesia, vertigo	**Neurological:** Headache, Uncommon: Dizziness, peripheral neuropathy, paraesthesia
Hepatic: Raised liver enzymes—LFT >2 times to upper limit of normal (reversible). Rarely: Idiosyncratic hepatic injury, hepatic failure	**Hepatic:** Elevated liver enzymes (reversible); Rarely: Hepatitis, hepatic failure, cholestasis	**Hepatic:** Raised liver enzymes (reversible); Rarely: Hepatitis, hepatic failure
Renal—Safe	**Renal**—Safe	**Renal**—Urinary tract infection
Haematological: Uncommon—severe neutropenia, thrombocytopenia, agranulocytosis, pancytopenia, anemia, altered prothrombin time with warfarin	**Hematological:** Uncommon—leukopenia, neutropenia, thrombocytopenia, agranulocytosis	**Hematological:** Uncommon—leukopenia, neutropenia, thrombocytopenia
Cardiac: Uncommon vasculitis	**Cardiac:** Uncommon—QT prolongation, torsades depointes	**Cardiac:** Uncommon congestive cardiac failure
Miscellaneous: Uncommon or rare—taste and smell disturbance, reduced visual acuity, visual field defect, hearing loss, anaphylaxis (angioedema), serum sickness like reaction, increased creatine phosphokinase, myalgia, arthralgia, photosensitivity, tinnitus, vertigo	**Miscellaneous:** Uncommon or Rare–anaphylaxis (angioedema), oliguria, hypokalemia, hypertriglyceridemia, dysgeusia, fatigue, fever, malaise	**Miscellaneous:** Uncommon or rare– peripheral edema, pulmonary edema, taste disturbance, dyspnea, transient or permanent hearing loss, anaphylaxis (angioedema), oliguria, hypertriglyceridemia, hypokalemia, myalgia, arthralgia, menstrual, disorders, erectlie dysfunction

Table 8.4: Drug interactions[6,13–15]		
	Fluconazole	*Itraconazole*
Antifungal level is decreased by	**Fluconazole is a potent CYP2C9 inhibitor, moderate CYP3A4 inhibitor** Rifampin	**Itraconazole is a potent CYP3A4 inhibitor** *Decreased absorption:* Antacids, H_2 receptor antagonists, proton pump inhibitors, *Increased metabolism:* Rifampicin, rifabutin phenytoin phenobarbitone, carbamazepine, INH, nevirapine
Antifungal level is increased by	Hydrochlorthiazide and possibly other thiazide diuretics	Erythromycin, clarithromycin, ciprofloxacin indinavir, ritonavir
Azole decreases levels of	Oral contraceptives	Oral contraceptives Amphotericin B (pretreatment with itraconazole may reduce activity)
Azole increases levels of co-administered drugs:		
Antidiabetic: Antihypertensive	Sulfonylurea	Sulfonylurea; nifedipine, verapamil
Gastric acid suppressors—proton pump inhibitor	Nifedipine, losartan Omeprazole, diclofenac,	Omeprazole, H_2 receptor antagonists
NSAID	Ibubrufen, celecoxib,	—
Bronchodilator	Naproxen, theophylline	—
Anticonvulsant	Phenytoin, carbamzepine	Phenytoin
Antiretroviral	Zidovudine, saquinavir	Zidovudine, saquinavir, indinavir
Benzodiazepines	Diazepam, midazolam,	Alprazolam, diazepam, midazolam,
Immunosuppressants	Triazolam, alprazolam,	triazolam
Anticoagulant	Cyclophosphamide	Cyclophosphamide
Antimycobacterial	Warfarin	Warfarin
HMG CoA inhibitor	Rifabutin	Rifabutin
Immunosuppressants	Atorvastatin, fluvastatin	Atorvastatin, fluvastatin
Antiarrhythmic	Cyclosporin, tacrolimus,	Cyclosporin, tacrolimus,
Antibiotic	Sirolimus—sufomethoxazole	Sirolimus
Narcotics	Fentanyl, alfentanil, methadone	Digoxin, verapamil, fentanyl
Tricyclic antidepressants	Amitryptiline, nortryptiline	Alfentanil, methadone
Glucocorticosteroids	—	Dexamenthasone, budesonide, Methylprednisolne, fluticasone

- Anti-retroviral: Zidovudine, saquinavir
- Benzodiazepines: Diazepam, midazolam, triazolam, alprazolam
- Cyclophosphamide
- Warfarin, rifabutin

- Atorvastatin, fluvastatin
- Cyclosporin, tacrolimus, sirolimus
- Sulfamethoxazole
- Fentanyl, alfentanil, methadone
- Amitryptiline, nortryptiline

ITRACONAZOLE

Itraconazole, a broad spectrum triazole fungistatic drug, synthesised in 1987 was approved in the United States for treatment of onychomycosis of finger and toe nails in 1995.[6]

Mechanism of action: Itraconazole inhibits 14α-demethylase like the other azoles and interferes with the formation of ergosterol, thus inhibiting the growth of the fungi.

Spectrum of activity: Itraconazole is effective against dermatophytes, *Malassezia* and *Candida* in addition to a wide range of fungi causing subcutaneous and systemic mycoses.[6]

Pharmacokinetics

Half-life: 21 hours.[6]

Peak-post dosing levels: 3 to 5 hours.[6]

Metabolism: Itraconazole is highly keratinophilic and lipophilic with increased drug specificity for fungal enzymes and a little effect on the mammalian cytochrome P450 enzymes. Oral absorption of itraconazole is variable and is enhanced by food and gastric acid. Bioavailability is 55% and it has been found to be maximal with itraconazole capsule form being taken immediately after meals and the oral solution in a fasting state. Capsule could also be taken in a fasting state along with cola beverage. Oral solution has increased bioavailability. Most of the absorbed drugs is strongly bound to plasma proteins (99.8 %). It is highly lipid soluble and is well distributed to sebum, sputum, adipose tissue. However, CSF penetration is poor. Skin concentration is four times higher and in the sebum, it is tenfold higher than in the plasma. Itraconazole accumulates in the plasma during multiple dosing by virtue of its non-linear pharmacokinetics. It is delivered to the skin by passive diffusion from the plasma. Although the drug is detectable in sweat within 24 hours after intake, there is minimal excretion in sweat unlike griseofulvin, ketoconazole and fluconazole. The drug persists in the SC for 3 to 4 weeks after cessation of therapy. In case of nail, drug reaches the free end of the nail plate via nail matrix and nail bed. It does not distribute back to the plasma, but remains in the nail until it is shed through normal growth. Hence it does not have to be given continuously. Studies state that the drug has been detected in the finger nails, 9 months after 2 pulses and in the toe nails 11 months after 3 pulse administration. It is metabolized in liver extensively by cytochrome CYP3A4 and is eliminated through the renal system as 40% inactive metabolites and in the feces as 3–18% of the parent drug.[6,16]

Indications[6]

Itraconazole is *FDA approved* for the treatment of

- Tinea unguium, oropharyngeal and esophageal candidiasis
- Deep mycoses: Histoplasmosis, blastomycosis and aspergillosis

It is used *off-label* in the treatment of:

- Onychomycosis caused by *Candida* and nondermatophyte molds
- Tinea corporis/cruris, tinea capitis, tinea pedis
- Majocchi's granuloma, tinea imbricata
- Pityriasis versicolor, pityriasporum folliculitis, seborrheic dermatitis
- Vaginal, cutaneous and chronic mucocutaneous candidiasis.

Dose and duration of treatment are given in Table 8.5.

Recommended Dose and Duration

Tinea corporis:

- Itraconazole 100 mg OD for 4 weeks
- Itraconazole 100 mg BD for 3–4 weeks

In the recent times, most often used dose is itraconazole 200 mg OD for 3–4 weeks, but based on PK/PD studies and skin levels a dose of 100 mg BD is better than 200 mg OD as this is a time dependent drug.

Table 8.5: Standard regimens of itraconazole for tinea corporis and tinea pedis[3,6,8–11]

Textbook	Tinea corporis		Tinea pedis	
	Dose/day	Weeks	Dose/day	Weeks
IADVL Textbook of Dermatology, 4th edition, 2015[8]	200–400 mg	1 1	400 mg OD 200 mg OD	1 2
Rook's Dermatology, 9th edition, 2016[9]	100 mg	2–4	400 mg	1–2
Fitzpatrick's Dermatology, 8th edition, 2012[10]	200 mg	1	200 mg BD	1
Wolverton Comprehensive Dermatologic Drug Therapy, 3rd edition, 2013[6]	200 mg 100 mg	1 2	400 mg 200 mg 100 mg	1 2–4 4
Bolognia Dermatology, 3rd edition, 2012[11]	200 mg	1	200–400 mg	1
Sentamilselvi G, Handbook of Dermatomycology, 1st edition, 2006[3]	200 mg 100 mg	1 2	—	—

Tinea pedis:
- Itraconazole 200 mg BD for 2 weeks
- Itraconazole 200 mg OD for 4 weeks

Contraindications[6,7]

- Known hypersensitivity to itraconazole
- Ventricular dysfunction, cardiac failure
- Terfenadine, astemizole, cisapride can cause ventricular tachycardia—torsades de pointes
- Pregnancy (category C): Effective contraception throughout therapy and until 2 months after cessation of drug should be adopted.

Adverse Effects[6,7] (Table 8.3)

- *Cutaneous*: Skin rash, pruritus, diaphoresis. Rarely Stevens-Johnson syndrome/TEN, acute generalised exanthematous pustulosis, exfoliative dermatitis, leukocytoclastic vasculitis, photosensitivity, alopecia.
- *Gastrointestinal:* Nausea, vomiting, diarrhea, abdominal pain. Uncommon: Dyspepsia, pancreatitis, dysgeusia, constipation
- *Neurological*: Headache; Uncommon— dizziness, peripheral neuropathy, paraesthesia
- *Hepatic*: Raised liver enzymes (reversible); rarely—hepatitis, hepatic failure
- *Renal*: Urinary tract infection
- *Hematological*: Uncommon—leukopenia, neutropenia, thrombocytopenia
- *Cardiac*: Uncommon—congestive cardiac failure.
- *Miscellaneous*: Uncommon or rare—peripheral edema, pulmonary edema, taste disturbance, dyspnea, transient or permanent hearing loss, anaphylaxis (angioedema), oliguria, hypertriglyceridemia, hypokalemia, myalgia, arthralgia, menstrual disorders, erectlie dysfunction.

Drug Interactions[6,13–15] (Table 8.4)

- Itraconazole is a potent CYP3A4 inhibitor
- *Itraconazole level is decreased by*
  - Drugs decreasing its absorption: Antacids, H_2 receptor antagonists, proton pump inhibitors
  - Drugs increasing its metabolism: Rifampicin, rifabutin phenytoin
  - Phenobarbitone, carbamazepine
  - INH, nevirapine

- Itraconazole level is increased by
  - Erythromycin, clarithromycin, ciprofloxacin, indinavir, ritonavir
- *Itraconazole decreases levels of* oral contraceptives
- *Itraconazole increases levels of the following coadministered drugs*:
  - Antidiabetic: Sulfonylurea
  - Antihypertensive: Nifedepine, verapamil
  - Proton pump inhibitor: Omeprazole, H2 receptor antagonists
  - Anticonvulsant: Phenytoin
  - Antiretroviral: Zidovudine, saquinavir, indinavir
  - Benzodiazepines: Alprazolam, diazepam, midazolam, triazolam
  - Cyclophosphamide
  - Warfarin, digoxin, rifabutin
  - Atorvastatin, fluvastatin
  - Cyclosporin, tacrolimus, sirolimus
  - Fentanyl, alfentanil, methadone

TERBINAFINE

Terbinafine, a fungicidal drug, was approved for use in the United States in 1996.[6]

Mechanism of action: Terbinafine acts by inhibition of squalene epoxidase enyme which results in accumulation of squalene and depletion of ergosterol. While the fungicidal activity of terbinafine is associated with accumulation of squalene, fungistatic activity is due to the depletion of ergosterol.[7]

Spectrum of activity: Terbinafine is effective against dermatophytes and fungi causing mycetoma, sporotrichosis, chromoblastomycosis and histoplasmosis.[6]

Pharmacokinetics

Half-life: 36 hours.[6]
Peak-post dosing levels: 2 hours.[6]

Metabolism: Terbinafine is a broad spectrum antifungal drug with keratinophilic and lipophilic properties. It is well absorbed after oral intake and its absorption is not affected by food. Though it is well absorbed, bioavailability is only 40% possibly due to the first pass metabolism. While it reaches high concentration in the sebum, it is not detectable in the sweat. Terbinafine is delivered by passive diffusion through sebum and basal keratinocytes to the sratum corneum. It is well distributed in the adipose tissue, skin and nails. The drug has been detected in stratum corneum, at a concentration above the mean inhibitory concentration for dermatophytes, 2–3 weeks, after the oral therapy is discontinued. Drug concentration in the SC is 70 times more than that achieved in the plasma. Plasma protein binding is >99%. Elimination by renal route is 70%.[6,17,18]

Indications[6]

Terbinafine is *FDA approved* for the treatment of:
- Tinea unguium and tinea capitis

It is used *off-label* in the treatment of
- Onychomycosis caused by *Candida* and nondermatophyte molds
- Tinea corporis/cruris, tinea pedis
- Majocchi's granuloma, tinea imbricata
- Seborrheic dermatitis
- Deep mycoses: Chromoblastomycosis, sporotrichosis, aspergillosis and black piedra.

Dose and duration of treatment are given in Table 8.6.

Recommended Dose and Duration

Tinea corporis: Terbinafine 250 mg OD for 4–6 weeks.
Tinea pedis: Terbinafine 250 mg OD for 6–8 weeks

Contraindications[6]

- Allergic reaction to terbinafine
- Pregnancy—first trimester (category B drug)

Warning: Not recommended in chronic active liver disease:
- To be avoided if creatinine clearance is <50 ml/mt

Table 8.6: Standard regimens of terbinafine for tinea corporis and tinea pedis[3,6, 8-11]

Textbook	Tinea corporis		Tinea pedis	
	Dose/day	Weeks	Dose/day	Weeks
IADVL Textbook of Dermatology, 4th edition, 2015[8]	250 mg	2	250 mg	2
Rook's Dermatology, 9th edition, 2016[9]	250 mg	2–3	250 mg	2
Fitzpatrick's Dermatology, 8th edition, 2012[10]	250 mg	2–4	250 mg	2
Wolverton Comprehensive Dermatologic Drug Therapy, 3rd edition, 2013[6]	250 mg	2–4	250 mg	2–6
Sentamilselvi G, Handbook of Dermatomycology, 1st edition, 2006	5 mg/kg 250 mg	2 1	5 mg/kg 250 mg	2 2
Bolognia Dermatology, 3rd edition, 2012[11]				

- To be discontinued if skin rash, neutropenia <1000 cells/cu mm, signs of LE,
- Taste and smell disturbance

Adverse Effects[6,7,13] (Table 8.5)

Though uncommon, the most common side effects were from gastrointestinal system and skin.

Cutaneous: Skin rash, pruritus. Rarely Stevens-Johnson syndrome/TEN, angioedema, psoriasiform eruption or exacerbation of psoriasis, acute generalised exanthematous pustulosis, exfoliative dermatitis, exacerbation of cutaneous and systemic LE, alopecia

Gastrointestinal: Diarrhea, dyspepsia, abdominal pain, nausea, flatulence. Uncommon: Vomiting, pancreatitis

Neurological: Headache; Uncommon—depressive symptoms

Hepatic: Raised liver enzymes—LFT > 2 times to upper limit of normal (reversible), rarely—idiosyncratic hepatic injury, hepatic failure

Hematological: Uncommon—severe neutropenia, thrombocytopenia, agranulocytosis, pancytopenia, anemia, altered prothrombin time with warfarin

Cardiac: Uncommon—vasculitis

Miscellaneous: Uncommon or rare—taste and smell disturbance, reduced visual acuity, visual field defect, hearing loss, anaphylaxis (angioedema), serum sickness like reaction, increased creatine phosphokinase, myalgia, arthralgia, photosensitivity, tinnitus, vertigo.

Drug Interactions[6,13-15]

Terbinafine does not interfere with the mammalian cytochrome P-450 enzymes and hence drug interactions are not common. However, there could be a few interactions as it inhibits CYP2D6.

- *Terbinafine level is decreased by* rifampicin
- *Terbinafine level is increased by* fluconazole, cyclosporine
- *Terbinafine increases levels of the following coadministered drugs*:
  - Tricyclic antidepressants, selective serotonin reuptake inhibitors
  - Beta-blockers
- Antiarrhythmics: Class 1c flecainide, propafenone
- MAO inhibitors type B
- Anticoagulants (increased prothrombin time with warfarin).

KETOCONAZOLE

Ketoconazole, an imidazole, was the first broad spectrum, fungistatic antifungal drug introduced in the United States in 1981. It is no longer approved by the FDA for use in superficial fungal infections due to the idiosyncratic hepatic toxicity.[1,6]

Mechanism of action: Similar to the other azoles.

Spectrum of activity: Ketoconazole is effective against dermatophytes, *Malassezia*, *Candida*, dimorphic and dematiceous fungi.[19]

Pharmacokinetics[19]

Ketoconazole is known for its time-dependent pharmacokinetics and sustained post-treatment antifungal effect.

Half-life: 2 hours during the first 10 hours and 8 hours thereafter. The half-life of ketoconazole increases with dose and duration of treatment.

Peak-post dosing levels: 1–2 hours

Metabolism: Ketoconazole is well-absorbed in an acidic milieu. Approximately 99% is bound to proteins and only a negligible proportion reaches the CSF. It is extensively metabolised in the liver and is converted into several inactive metabolites. The major route of excretion is through the bile into the intestinal tract. Approximately 13% of dose is excreted in urine, while 2 to 4% is unchanged in feces.

Indications[1,19]

Systemic ketoconazole was used in the treatment of dermatophytosis, extensive and recurrent pityriasis versicolor and candidiasis. In 2013, FDA warned against the use of ketoconazole tablets to treat skin and nail fungal infections and stated that it could be used to treat serious fungal infections when no other antifungal therapies are available.

Hence only topical ketoconazole cream/ lotion and shampoo are in use to treat dermatophytosis (glabrous skin infection and tinea capitis), pityriasis versicolor and muco-cutaneous candidiasis.

Contraindications[19]

Hypersensitivity to ketoconazole pregnancy/ lactation congenital or documented acquired QTc prolongation.

Concomitant administration with quinidine, methadone, disopyramide, quinidine, pimozide, saquinavir, simvastatin.

Adverse Effects[19]

Gastrointestinal: Nausea, vomiting, constipation.

Hepatic: Severe hepatitis can occur in 1:10,000 patients and it is because of this dreaded side effect, that in spite of being an effective broad spectrum antifungal agent, it has ceased to be in use.

Neurological: Headache, dizziness

Endocrinological: Adrenal insufficiency, decreased cortisol/testosterone
- Gynecomastia, impotence, alopecia
- Cutaneous: Urticaria

Drug Interactions[19–21]

- *Ketoconazole level is decreased by* rifampin, isoniazid, phenytoin, H_2 antagonists, antacids
- *Ketoconazole decreases levels of* oral contraceptives
- *Ketoconazole increases levels of the following coadministered drugs*:
  - Antidiabetic: Sulfonylurea
  - Anticonvulsant: Phenytoin, carbamazepine
  - Warfarin, rifabutin
  - Cyclosporin

Comparison of Efficacy and Adverse Effects of Systemic Antifungal Agents

All the five antifungal agents discussed so far, have dermatophytes in their spectrum of activity. However, there are a few facts for consideration. Ketoconazole is no longer indicated in the treatment of superficial dermatophytosis because of the hepatotoxicity. It is known that griseofulvin and fluconazole diffuse into the stratum corneum through sweat.[5,12] Hence it would be worthwhile to treat highly sweat prone patients with dermatophytosis or patients with tinea corporis in the submammary regions/axillae and tinea cruris with one of these drugs. Terbinafine is detected in the skin up to 2–3 weeks and itraconazole up to 3–4 weeks after the last dose.[6] This virtue of these drugs makes them the treatment of choice in case of chronic hyperkeratotic tinea pedis. Savin et al found that terbinafine was superior to griseofulvin in the treatment of moccasin type of tinea pedis.[22] In the case of intertriginous tinea pedis, an azole antifungal agent is preferred. Studies have shown that terbinafine was less effective in tinea capitis caused by *Microsporum* species compared to *Trichophyton* species.

Griseofulvin, fluconazole, itraconazole and terbinafine can cause hepatic dysfunction and raise liver enzymes. Among these, fluconazole may be given, monitoring the liver enzymes. In patients with renal dysfunction, terbinafine has to be reduced based on the creatinine clearance and hence itraconazole is preferred. Itraconazole has a negative ionotropic effect and is hence contraindicated in patients with cardiac failure. Itraconazole can cause pedal edema, hypertriglyceridemia and trigger hypertension, because of which it is best avoided in patients with metabolic syndrome. Itraconazole has a little effect on the mammalian cytochrome P450 enzymes compared to fluconazole. Terbinafine has less drug interactions than itraconazole, but has more propensity for the risk of SJS/TEN.

References

1. US Food and Drug Administration. FDA Drug Safety Communication: FDA Limits Usage of Nizoral (ketoconazole) Oral Tablets Due to Potentially Fatal Liver Injury and Risk of Drug Interactions and Adrenal Gland Problems. 2013. Available online: http://www.fda.gov/Drugs/Drug Safety/ucm362415.htm (accessed on 25 January 2017).

2. Verma S, Madhu R. The great Indian epidemic of superficial dermatophytosis: An appraisal. Indian J Dermatol 2017;62:227–36.

3. Sentamilselvi G. Dermatophytosis. In: Sentamilselvi G, Janaki VR, Janaki C, editors. The handbook of Dermatomycology and Colour atlas. 1st ed. India: Dr.G.Sentamilselvi; 2006.p.9–15.

4. JC Gentles. The Treatment of Ringworm with Griseofulvin. Br J Dermatol 1959; 71: 427–33.

5. Finkelstein E, Amichai B, Grunwald MH. Griseofulvin and its uses. International Journal of Antimicrobial Agents 1996;6: 189–94.

6. Gupta AK. Systemic antifungal agents. In: Wolverton SE, editor. Comprehensive dermatologic drug therapy. 3rd ed. China: Elsevier Saunders; 2013. p. 98–120.

7. Bennett. Antifungal drugs. In: Brunton L, Chabner B, Knollman, editors. Goodman and Gillmans. 12th ed. New York: McGraw-Hill Medical; 2011. p 1571 –92.

8. Manjunath Shenoy M, Suchitra Shenoy M. Superficial fungal infections. In: Sacchidanand S, Oberoi C, Inamdar AC, editors. IADVL Textbook of Dermatology. 4th ed., Vol. I. Mumbai: Bhalani Publishing House; 2015. p. 459–516

9. Hay RJ, Ashbee HR. Fungal infections. In: Griffiths CE, Barker J, Bleiker T, Chalmers R, Creamer D, editors. Rook's Textbook of Dermatology. 9th ed., Vol. II. West Sussex: Wiley Blackwell; 2016. p. 923–1018.

10. Schieke SM, Garg A. Superficial fungal infection. In: Goldsmith LA, Katz SI, Gilchrest BA, Paller AS, Leffel DJ, Wolff K, editors. Fitzpatrick's Dermatology in General Medicine. 8th ed., Vol. II. New York: The McGraw-Hill Companies; 2012. p. 2277–97.

11. Elewski BE, Hughey LC, Sobera JO, Hay R. Fungal diseases. In: Bolognia JL, Jorizzo JL, Schaffer JV, editors. Dermatology. 3rd ed., Vol II. China: Elsevier Saunders; 2012. p.1267.

12. Faergemann J1, Laufen H. Levels of fluconazole in serum, stratum corneum, epidermis-dermis (without stratum corneum) and eccrine sweat. Clin Exp Dermatol. 1993.;18:102–6.

13. Sigurgeirsson B and Hay RJ. The antifungal drugs used in skin disease. In: Olafsson JH, Hay RJ,

editors. Antibiotic and Antifungal therapies in dermatology. 1st Indian reprint, New Delhi: Springer (India) private Ltd; 2017. p. 141–156.

14. Bruggemann RJM, Jan-Willem C, Alffenaar Nicole MA Blijlevens Eliane M, Billaud Jos GW, Kosterink Paul E, Verweij David M, Burger Louis D, Saravolatz Clinical relevance of the pharma-cokinetic interactions of azole antifungal drugs with other coadministered agents. CID 2009;48: 1441–58.

15. Gubbins PO, Heldenbrand. Clinically relevant drug interactions of current antifungal agents. Mycoses 2009;53:95–113.

16. Hans Christian Korting, Claudia Schöllmann. The significance of itraconazole for treatment of fungal infections of skin, nails and mucous membranes. J Dtsch Dermatol Ges 2009; 7:11–19.

17. Jason G Newland, Rahman SMA.Update on terbinafine with a focus on dermatophytoses. Clinical, Cosmetic and Investigational Dermatology 2009; 2:49–63.

18. Faergemann J, Zehender H, Denouel J, Millerioux L. Levels of terbinafine in plasma, stratum corneum, dermis-epidermis (without stratum corneum), sebum, hair, and nails during and after 250 mg terbinafine orally once per day for four weeks. Acta Derm Venereol (Stockh) 1993; 73: 305–9.

19. Jeanne Hawkins Van Tyle. Ketoconazole; Mechanism of Action, Spectrum of Activity, Pharmacokinetics, Drug Interactions, Adverse Reactions and Therapeutic Use. Pharmacotherapy: The Journal of Human Pharmacology and Drug Therapy 1984;4:343–73.

20. David R. Bickers. Antifungal therapy: Potential interactions with other classes of drugs. J Am Acad Dermatol 1994;31:S87–S90.

21. Brodell RT, Elewski BE. Clinical pearl: systemic antifungal drugs and drug interactions. J Am Acad Dermatol 1995;33:259–60.

22. Savin RC. Oral terbinafine versus griseofulvin in the treatment of moccasin-type tinea pedis. J Am Acad Dermatol 1990; 23: 807–9.

CHAPTER

9

Rationale of use of Antifungal Drugs Based on Skin Pharmacokinetics

Pooja Arora Mrig, Kabir Sardana

INTRODUCTION

The menace of dermatophytosis in India in the form of increasing incidence of chronic and relapsing infections has led the clinicians to use higher doses of antifungal agents and their combinations without any evidence. Various studies are being carried out in this direction that mainly focus on laboratory evaluation of the susceptibility of the fungus to various antifungals. It is important to understand that *in vitro* susceptibility of an organism to an antifungal agent does not directly correlate with the therapeutic outcome. There are several factors related to the host (immune response, site of infection, underlying illness, reinfection from other sources), infecting organism (virulence potential of the infecting strain) and the antifungal agent (dose, quality of the drug and compliance, pharmacokinetics [PK], pharmacodynamics [PD], drug interactions) that are more important than susceptibility tests in determining the clinical outcome.

This chapter focuses on the role of pharmacokinetics in selection and dosing of oral antifungals to optimise therapy against dermatophytes. Not only will this help the clinician in choosing the most potent drug in the appropriate dose and interval of administration but will also help in planning clinical trials and formulating laboratory guidelines.

Pharmacokinetics and Pharmacodynamics

Study of pharmacokinetics involves understanding the interaction of a drug with the host that includes absorption, distribution, protein binding, metabolism and elimination. The goal is to achieve adequate drug concentration at the site of infection, which in the case of dermatophytosis is the skin or more appropriately the stratum corneum. The levels of various antifungals in the skin depend on the route of delivery of antifungals to the stratum corneum, which can be via sweat, sebum, keratin or via diffusion through the dermis. These vary for different classes of antifungals and relate with clinical efficacy.

Plasma or serum levels of antifungals are not an indicator of the concentration in target organ. The concentration in all skin tissue compartments exceeds that of plasma one week after stopping treatment and the elimination of the drugs is much faster in plasma than in the skin. In fact it has been shown that terbinafine (TER) and (ITR) persist in the skin for 3 weeks after stopping therapy.

Pharmacodynamics describes the relationship between pharmacokinetics and the outcome. It provides insight into the link between antifungal pharmacokinetics, *in vitro* susceptibility and treatment outcome. The relationship of drug and dosage has been described by *three* pharmacodynamic parameters. These include the peak concentration in relation to the MIC (C_{max}/MIC), the area under the concentration curve in relation to the MIC [24 hours area under the concentration curve (AUC)/MIC], and the time that drug concentrations exceed the MIC expressed as a percentage of the dosing interval (%T > MIC).[1,2] These are depicted in Fig. 9.1.

PD studies integrate drug PKs, including drug concentration over time, *in vitro* potency (MIC), and treatment efficacy. There are 3 major PK/PD questions that are critical for optimizing therapy.

1. Which PK/PD measure (index) is most closely linked to efficacy?

The predictive efficacy of a drug is largely dependent on the impact of drug concentration on organism survival over time. There are two patterns of activity, concentration dependent or concentration independent (also known as time dependent). Following exposure to concentration-dependent drugs, both the rate and extent of organism killing increase as the drug concentration is escalated.

The PD index associated with concentration-dependent action is the C_{max}/MIC. Here the ideal dosing strategy is administration of large doses infrequently to take advantage of the concentration-dependent action. Concentration-independent agents are characterized by a threshold of maximal activity that occurs at drug concentrations close to the MIC. The PD index most commonly associated with time-dependent action is %T > MIC. The dosing strategy associated with maximal efficacy, in this situation, is administration of lower doses more frequently to increase the duration of exposure at levels just above the MIC. Azoles are classically time-dependent drugs, hence giving a BD dose is better than a higher OD dose. This is the rationale of a 100 mg BD being better and more logical than 200 mg OD.

As in India, numerous pharmacological up-dosing regimens are followed, with a little logic we will dwell on this aspect. The impact of dosing interval on treatment efficacy is an important measure (Fig. 9.2). If one increases the dose administered from say terbinafine 250 mg BD to 500 mg OD, all three PD indices will increase proportionally. However, if the total dose over the dosing period is kept constant (as in a fractionation experiment), the interdependence is reduced. In this case, as the interval is increased (e.g. from once daily [q24h] to eight times daily [q3h]), each dose is appropriately decreased to keep the daily (or

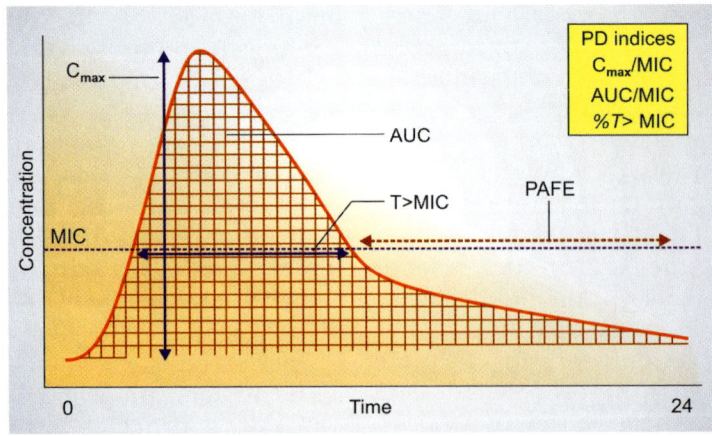

Fig. 9.1: Diagrammatic representation of pharmacokinetics/pharmacodynamics of oral antifungal drugs. Pharmacokinetic/pharmacodynamic relationship of antimicrobial dosing over time relative to organism MIC. The three PD indices are also listed, including C_{max}/MIC, AUC/MIC, and %T > MIC. PAFE: Post-antifungal effect

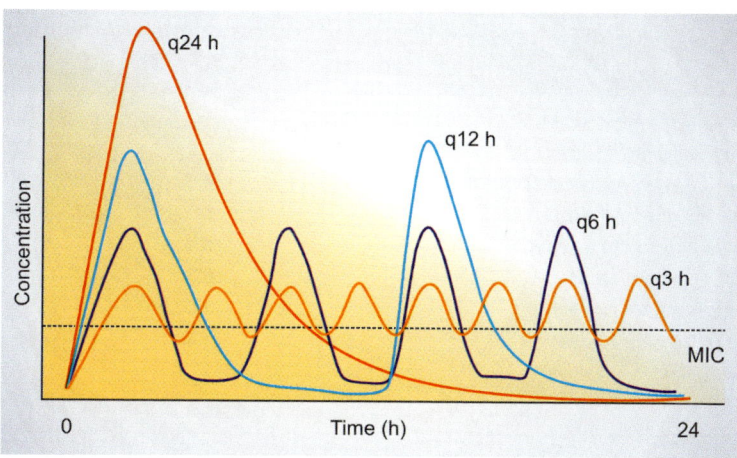

Fig. 9.2: Concentration and time profile showing the effect of fractionating a total daily dose into once-, twice-, four-, and eight-times daily fractions. AUC will remain the same because the total daily dose administered is the same in all four regimens; however, C_{max} will progressively decline and % T > MIC will progressively increase as the dose is fractionated into increasing fractions

total dose) the same (Fig. 9.2). Therefore, the AUC is approximately the same for each regimen as the same total daily dose is administered (i.e. the same drug exposure is occurring over the time period). However, as the interval is increased, and therefore the individual drug dose is decreased, the C_{max} will proportionally decrease as the fractionation is increased. Conversely, time above MIC will increase as the fractionation is increased (Fig. 9.2) with terbinafine a 250 BD >500 mg as the C_{max} is needed for a longer time.

When efficacy is enhanced with shorter dosing intervals, the %T > MIC is most closely linked to efficacy. Conversely, when treatment effect is optimal when larger doses are administered infrequently, the C_{max}/MIC is the predictive index. When outcome is similar among various dosing intervals, typically the AUC/MIC measure is predictive of efficacy. This aspect will be discussed further in relation to the drugs prescribed.

2. A *second* exposure-response factor, the post-antifungal effect (PAFE), can also influence PD relationships. The PAFE is the drug effect following drug exposures above the MIC. The C_{max}/MIC and %T > MIC are associated with prolonged antifungal effects (Fig. 9.1). For example, triazoles exhibit prolonged PAFE, and it has been shown that AUC/MIC is the optimal predictive index. Hence, *again for ITR giving the drug for a long time is not logical as it has a long PAFE.*

3. The *last aspect* is the levels of the drug in the skin. Here it must be appreciated that different drugs have different routes of secretion and the skin levels usually exceed the plasma levels (Fig. 9.3). Thus, in most cases, there is a little logic of increasing the doses of drugs.

This can be appreciated in Table 9.1. Also voriconazole has a very low skin secretion level and hence is inferior to the existing drugs for dermatophytoses.

There are other principles but for the practising clinician, knowledge of the above concepts should suffice. An understanding of the above principles of PK/PD of antifungals is important for selection of appropriate agent in the proper dosage to achieve maximal therapeutic outcome.

The relevant PK/PD parameters of the commonly used oral antifungals for dermatophytosis are mentioned in Fig. 9.3.

	Serum/plasma (μg/ml)	Epidermis–dermis (μg/g)	Stratum corneum (μg/g)
Griseofulvin 500 mg for 2 weeks	2.0	ND	20.6
Fluconazole 50 mg for 12 days	1.81	2.93	66.4
Fluconazole 150 mg once a week for 2 weeks	2.12	4.62	23.4
Itraconazole 200 mg for 7 days	0.5	ND	0.79
Ketoconazole 200 mg for 14 days	7.9	ND	5.18
Terbinafine 250 mg for 12 days	1.0	0.3	9.1
Terbinafine 250 mg for 28 days	1.39	1.03	14.40
Terbinafine 250 mg for 7 days	1.56	1.44	3.54
Terbinafine 250 mg for 14 days	1.46	2.00	7.63
Levels in the skin are XX higher than the serum			

Fig. 9.3: The levels of almost all antifungals except ketoconazole have a higher skin level than plasma. Note that the levels of FLU (50 mg × 12 days) are the highest. But it must be also noted (Table 9.1) that it has a low keratin adherence

Table 9.1: Comparison of the skin kinetics of orally active antifungal agents[2]				
	Sweat	Sebum	S. corneum	Keratin adherence
Terbinafine	ND	High	High	Strong
Itraconazole	Low	High	Low	Strong
Fluconazole	High	ND	Very high	Low
Griseofulvin	Very high	ND	High	Weak
Ketoconazole	High	Low	Low	Strong

ND: Not detectable.

Terbinafine (TER)

The route of distribution of terbinafine is dependent on sebum, whereas its concentration in sweat is nil. Also being lipophilic and having a strong keratin adherence, it is slowly eliminated from the skin and the cutaneous levels remain high even after stopping the treatment. The comparison of the skin kinetics of oral antifungal agents is depicted in Table 9.1.

For terbinafine, it is believed %T > MIC is the cardinal parameter that correlates with activity of the drug. Hence, twice a day dose is better than increasing the single dose as practiced by a few clinicians. Studies have shown that the T1/2 for TER range from 11.35 to 16.4 hours making twice daily dose more pharmacologically logical than once daily dose in cases where dose is escalated to 500 mg daily.[3–5]

A study by Sakai et al[6] has examined this aspect. A elaborate study depicts the MIC values % T > MIC and AUC/MIC values, as well as recommended terbinafine dosing interval for fungal pathogens (Table 9.2). Dosing intervals recommended herein are made on the basis of maintaining plasma concentration greater than the MIC for 100% of the dosing interval. Here the % T > MIC for dermatophytes seems to suggest appropriate use of terbinafine for superficial dermatophyte infections.

A higher dose as is prescribed in India (500 mg OD or 250 mg BD) can be justified if it is shown that the TER skin levels are not enough at a 250 mg OD dose to surmount the MIC 90. Also TER can cause asymptomatic liver damage in approved doses and such high doses can put the clinician open to medicolegal scrutiny.[7]

Table 9.2: Pathogen-specific terbinafine pharmacokinetic analysis and proposed dosing intervals (30–35 mg/kg)

Organism	Reported MIC (µg/ml)	T > MIC (h)*	AUC/MIC[†] (µg h/ml)	Proposed dosing interval
Blastomyces dermatitidis	0.06	18.8	13	Twice daily
Histoplasma capsulatum	0.06	17.6	13	Twice daily
Sporothrix schenckii	0.25–0.5	9.5	9	Three times daily
Coccidioides immitis	0.6	11	9	Three times daily
Pythium insidiosum	32	0	Not assessed	Not recommended
Microsporum spp.	0.01	17.6	13	Twice daily[‡]
Trichophyton mentagrophytes	0.01	17.6	13	Twice daily[‡]

*T > MIC data exhibited approximately 5% intersubject variability.
[†]AUC/MIC data exhibited approximately 10% intersubject variability.
[‡]For deep dermatophyte infections.

AZOLES

Itraconazole (ITR)

Sebum plays a major role in the delivery of itraconazole to the stratum corneum. The levels remain high up to 7 days after the end of therapy. Excretion via sweat is very low and does not play a significant role in delivery to the stratum corneum. Sweat levels follow the same kinetics as the plasma levels. Similar is the case with incorporation into the basal layer. However, this route of delivery continues to give itraconazole levels even when plasma, sweat and sebum levels are undetectable.[8, 9]

The difference in drug levels in the stratum corneum of different body areas can be explained by the difference in importance of these routes delivery to the skin.[2,10] Palms have a thick stratum corneum with no sebum and sweat excretion. Thus, ITR levels in palms are relatively low but persist at least 3 weeks after the end of therapy due to the thickness of stratum corneum.[2,10] The back has a rather thin stratum corneum with an even distribution of sebum and sweat glands. This results in levels higher than the corresponding plasma levels but in the disappearance of drug within 2 weeks after the end of therapy (parallel with disappearance of detectable sebum and sweat levels).[2,10] The beard region has a much higher level of sebum excretion. As a result,

ITR levels are extremely high and remain measurable unto 4 weeks after discontinuation of therapy.[10]

Studies that have evaluated the relation between dose and antifungal activity have found that TER in a dose of 250 mg daily was comparable to 200 mg/day ITR. However, ITR of dose 200 mg twice a day had a faster onset of action than TER and was found to have the closest to a complete fungicidal effect against *Trichophyton mentagrophytes*.[11]

It is important to note that ITR has a nonlinear PK (mentioned below) and increasing the dose would lead to a disproportionate increase in serum level. This is because the liver enzymes are saturable and as higher doses are given, the clearance goes down and thus the levels may rise to cause toxicity (Fig. 9.4).

Fluconazole (FLU)

FLU is found in high concentrations in the stratum corneum, eccrine sweat and dermis–epidermis. It directly diffuses from into the epidermis–dermis from capillary blood vessels, and a major portion of it exists in an unbound form (because of its small extent of binding to corneous keratin). It might be effective not only in the treatment to dermatomycoses localised to the stratum corneum but also in the treatment of fungal

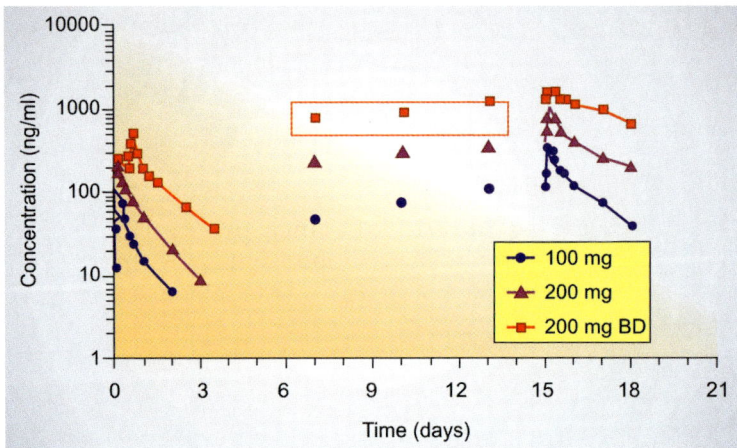

Fig. 9.4: Serum levels of ITR at day 1 and day 15 after 3 different doses. Note that the difference between 100 mg BD and 200 mg BD is not significant. This coupled with the high skin levels achieved is a sound logic for avoiding updosing

infections in deeper part of epidermis and dermis. But the drug levels decrease rapidly due to lack of keratin binding (Table 9.1), hence it has a little reservoir effect.

Ketoconazole

Ketoconazole reaches the stratum corneum by direct diffusion and sweat. Also it has a high binding capacity to corneocytes. Excretion in sebum and incorporation in basal layer are less important. Some clinicians are using this molecule and its efficacy might be related to its lower MIC than other drugs. Also there are a few brands hence the quality variation is minimal. But unlike other drugs it does not achieve high levels in the skin.

Griseofulvin

Sweat is the major route of delivery to the stratum corneum. The levels in stratum corneum are high but it does not have a tight binding to stratum corneum. Clinicians should use this drug only when a patient has profuse sweating as that is the major route of secretion. Its use across the board just based on a low MIC report[12] is not a logical concept.

CONCLUSIONS

The value of PK/PD studies is enormous as it helps us to choose drugs and their therapy rationally. Also it helps to scientifically approach the various practices being adopted in India and can help to understand what is wrong with these regimens (Table 9.3).

References

1. Andes D. Pharmacokinetics and pharmacodynamics of antifungals. Infect Dis Clin North Am. 2006; 20:679–97.

2. Sardana K, Arora P, Mahajan K. Intracutaneous pharmacokinetics of oral antifungals and their relevance in recalcitrant cutaneous dermatophytosis: Time to revisit basics. Indian J Dermatol Venereol Leprol 2017;83:730–732.

3. Jensen JC. Clinical pharmacokinetics of terbinafine (Lamisil) Clin Exp Dermatol 1989;14:110–3.

4. Sardana K, Gupta A. Rational for drug dosimetry and duration of terbinafine in the context of recalcitrant dermatophytosis: Is 500 mg better than 250 mg OD or BD. Indian J Dermatol 2017;62: 665–67.

5. Faergemann J, Zehender H, Denouël J, Millerioux L. Levels of terbinafine in plasma, stratum corneum, dermis-epidermis (without stratum corneum), sebum, hair and nails during and after 250 mg terbinafine orally once per day for four weeks. Acta Derm Venereol 1993;73:305–9.

Table 9.3: Strategies being practiced to enhance antifungal effect and their PK/PD rationale[2, 4, 5, 8–13]

Strategy	Rationale
Terbinafine 500 mg once daily	Higher dose is not needed as terbinafine, even at conventional doses, achieves skin levels that exceed plasma levels by a factor of 75
	An updosing is justified only if the minimum fungicidal concentration of the species prevalent in India is higher than the skin levels achieved by 250 mg daily
Terbinafine 250 mg twice daily	If a higher dose is given, divided dose has more rationale
Itraconazole 200 mg daily	It is the ideal dose and ideally fractionation of dose is better than a single dose (100 mg BD >200 mg OD)
Itraconazole 200 mg twice daily	Higher dose (200 mg BD) does not translate into higher antifungal effect but has a faster onset of action
	Also there is quality variation of the 105 brands and the topography and number of the pellets is crucial for efficacy. A good quality 100 mg capsule is better than an inferior 200 mg capsule
Use of griseofulvin	This drug has a little role in cutaneous dermatophytoses as it is fungistatic and its skin levels are lower and dependent on eccrine glands with a little keratin adherence to be of any value. Few studies have found high MIC value for this drug
Use of isotretinoin with itraconazole or terbinafine	*As both TER and ITR are primarily lipophilic and ISO reduces the sebum secretion they are perfectly antagonistic. Also the potential for side effects are high
Use of FLU	FLU attains very high levels in stratum corneum in a daily dose of 50 mg for 12 days and may be logical to administer in cases of clinical failure with TER/ITR, specially in patients with decreased lipid secretion
Use of voriconazole	Voriconazole is not to be used for the very simple fact that resistance in the lab has not been demonstrated in a large number of studies to existing AF. The complex pathogenesis of the disorder makes this a very minor component. The other drawbacks are:
	a. The cost
	b. Serum levels of voriconazole may vary widely among patients, primarily due to differences in metabolism. Voriconazole is extensively metabolized by the CYP450 enzymes and polymorphisms are common in the primary enzyme CYP2C19. Patients can possess polymorphisms that lead to either slow or rapid metabolism, placing them at risk for toxicity or therapeutic failure, respectively. Higher voriconazole concentrations, those exceeding 6 mg/ml, have been linked to adverse drug events, including hepatitis and delirium.
	c. Given the variability in metabolism of voriconazole amongst patients its use has to be monitored
	d. No comparison with ITR/TER or FLU in the skin exist to show it to be superior
	e. Most importantly its secretion in the skin is less than in the plasma. Thus, it is useless *in vivo* for dermatophytosis

*Pediatr Allergy Immunol. 2014 Jun;25(4):405–7. doi: 10.1111/pai.12181. Epub 2014 Jan 3. Systemic treatment with isotretinoin suppresses itraconazole blood level in chronic granulomatous disease. von Bernuth H, Wahn V.

6. Sakai MR, May ER, Imerman PM et al. Terbinafine pharmacokinetics after single dose administration in the dog. Vet Dermatol 2011;22:528–34.

7. Kramer ON, Albrecht J. Clinical presentation of terbinafine induced severe liver injury and the value of Laboratory monitoring: a critically appraised topic. Br J Dermatol 2017;177:1279–1284.

8. Andes D. Clinical utility of antifungal pharmacokinetics and pharmacodynamics. Curr Opin Infect Dis. 2004;17:533–40.

9. De Doncker P. Pharmacokinetics of oral antifungal agents. Dermatol Ther 1997;3:46–57.

10. Cauwenbergh G, Degreef H, Heykants J, Woestenborghs R, Van Rooy P, Haeverans K. Pharmacokinetic profile of orally administered itraconazole in human skin. J Am Acad Dermatol 1988;18:263–8.

11. Piérard G, Arrese J, De Doncker P. Antifungal activity of itraconazole and terbinafine in human stratum corneum: a comparative study. J Am Acad Dermatol 1995;32:429–35.

12. Miskeen AK, Uppuluri P. Laboratory diagnosis of fungal infections: A primer. In: Sardana K, Mahajan K, Arora P, editors. Fungal infections: Diagnosis and management. Delhi: CBS, 2017. p 23–39.

13. von Bernuth H, Wahn V. Systemic treatment with isotretinoin blood level in chronic granulomatous disease. Pediatr Allergy Immunol. 2014; 25;405–7.

10

Steroid Modified Tinea

Yogesh S Marfatia, Devi S Menon

INTRODUCTION

Tinea has assumed epidemic proportions in India. Tinea incognito is a dermatophyte infection of the skin where clinical presentation has been modified by the misuse of topical or systemic corticosteroids.[1] Tinea incognito is like an 'epidemic within an epidemic'.

The Indian market is flooded with preparations containing potent topical corticosteroids (TCS) in combination with antifungal, antimicrobial, and other ingredients because of their potent anti-inflammatory property. Clobetasol containing topical preparations are available over-the-counter and are used as self-medication without a definite diagnosis. Potent TCS containing skin lightening preparations enjoy huge market. They are also rampantly prescribed by family physicians, practitioners of alternate medicine and chemist, considering TCS as a "panacea" or "cure-all drug".

The most common cause of tinea incognito is TCS/TCS containing combinations. Nowadays, cases of tinea incognito with topical tacrolimus and pimecrolimus have also been described. These drugs suppress the normal cutaneous immune response to dermatophytes, thus enhancing the development of atypical superficial fungal infections.

Thus, topical and systemic corticosteroids, topical immunomodulators, and systemic immunosuppressives can modify clinical features of dermatophytosis making it difficult to diagnose and treat. This has also resulted in chronicity and recalcitrance. Persistence of fungus is responsible for contiguous spread, facilitating intrafamilial cases. High index of suspicion and careful enquiry about use of such medications can clinch the diagnosis of tinea incognito.

PHARMACOLOGIC ACTIONS OF TOPICAL CORTICOSTEROIDS

TCS acts through glucocorticoid receptor (GCR) which can be found in almost all types of human cells accounting for the long list of glucocorticoid receptor mediated effects and adverse effects (Table 10.1).

STEROID MODIFIED TINEA

Topical corticosteroids have a more profound disease modifying ability than systemic steroids and suppress the fungus-induced local immune response. Potent topical steroids can also increase the numbers of hyphae present on the surface of the skin in fungal infections and change the appearance of the lesions. Tinea incognito is more commonly caused by potent fluorinated steroids, like clobetasol and betamethasone, more so if applied under occlusion.[2]

In tinea incognito, the classical well-defined lesions become modified (Table 10.2). They become ill-defined with reduced itching and inflammation with spread of lesion. In many dermatoses like melasma, psoriasis, pemphigus, etc. which are steroid responsive, there can be superimposed tinea especially at occlusive sites. Therefore, before initiation of steroid, any occult foci of fungal infection like onychomycosis or tinea pedis must be ruled out.

Most common manifestation of dermatophyte is tinea cruris because the site provides an occlusive environment favorable for the growth of fungi. Due to its micro-environment, drug penetration in genito-crural region is highest in the body and hence, the site is more susceptible to the adverse effects of topical corticosteroids. The absorption quotient of scrotum is found to be 40 times that of the forearm. Anatomic, physiologic and mechanical factors as well as exposure to physiologic contact irritants like urine, vaginal secretions, etc. increases vulnerability of female genitalia to the infection. Steroid modified tinea is likely to be missed at this site. Absorption of topical steroids is found to be seven times higher in vulvar skin than forearm skin, thus making it more vulnerable to TCS adverse effects.[3]

When potent topical steroid-containing antifungal combinations are applied, there is temporary resolution of inflammation with alleviation of itching and redness but without effectively eliminating the dermatophyte. This, combined with other factors like tight-fitting clothing, high humidity, and daily commuting for work or studies causes the dermatophyte to spread. Because of the dramatic symptomatic improvement initially, patient may discontinue the treatment and present with a flare up. Self-medication and prolonged use is also very common.

Table 10.1: Pharmacologic effects vs adverse effects of topical corticosteroids	
Pharmacologic effects	*Clinical effects/adverse effects*
• Anti-inflammatory • Vasoconstriction • Anti-proliferative • Hypopigmentation • Anti-allergic • Immunosuppression • Suppression of cellular, vascular and immunologic response	• Masking of skin infections like tinea • Precipitation of infections • Hypopigmentation • Skin atrophy and striae • Telangiectasia, purpura • Acneiform eruptions

Table 10.2: Clinical features: Typical tinea vs steroid modified tinea	
Typical tinea	*Tinea incognito*
Itching present but less irritation	Itching less but irritation is troublesome
Oval or circular patch with well defined elevated borders and central clearing Peripheral vesiculation may be present	Ill-defined lesions with scattered papules, pustules, and hyperpigmentation Follicular papules may be present Ring within ring appearance
Erythema and scaling is characteristic	Blanching erythema Less scaly
Chances of recurrence and dissemination are less if treated adequately	Chances of recurrence and dissemination are higher

TINEA INCOGNITO

Diverse presentations of tinea incognito have been reported in literature (Figs 10.1 to 10.3 and Table 10.3). A study of 58 patients of tinea facei was conducted out of whom 25 (43.1%) patients presented with complaints of photosensitivity and in 2 patients' lesions resembled discoid lupus erythematosus. They were all applying topical steroid.[4]

Starace et al[5] reported a case of a 17-year-old male with pustular psoriasis of nail bed of toe, treated with topical steroids and vitamin D_3 derivative, which gave rise to a tinea incognito on dorsum of foot.

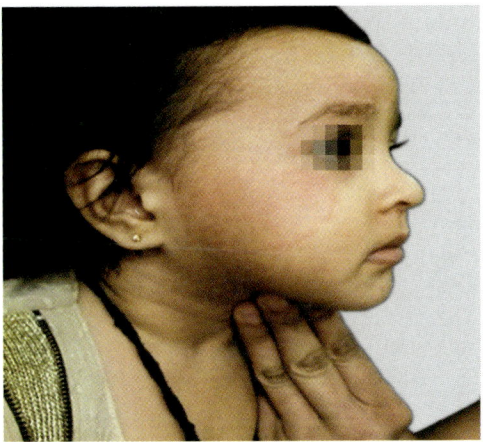
Fig. 10.3: Tinea incognito in a child

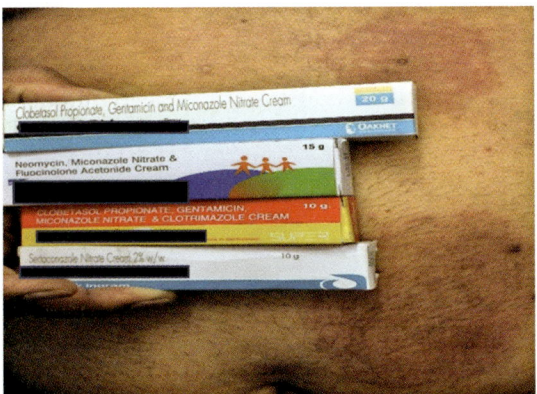
Fig. 10.1: Tinea incognito after applying topical antifungal steroid antibiotic combination

Table 10.3: Clinical characteristics of tinea incognito
1. Ill-defined skin lesion with diffuse scaling of long duration
2. Lesions occurring at sites like face, trunk, genitalia
3. Unresponsive to topical corticosteroids (including combination therapy)
4. Unresponsive to topical calcineurin Inhibitor
5. Presence of occult tinea like in the interdigital space, onychomycosis
6. Patient on immunosuppressive treatment for conditions like autoimmune dermatological and medical conditions

Lecamwasam et al[6] reported a case of 22-year-old pregnant woman with tinea incognito on face following application of an over-the-counter medication for skin lightening.

A 70-year-old hypothyroid, diabetic woman presented with huge patch of vitiligo over the trunk which showed an erythematous scaly plaque strictly limited within the depigmented patch. Scraping for fungus was positive and hence a diagnosis of tinea corporis limited to the patch of vitiligo was established.[7]

A case of Majocchi's granuloma of the face and the scalp has been described in a 55-year-old female who had been diagnosed with eczema and received systemic (intramuscular and oral) as well as TCS over a period of 7 months. Biopsy identified *Trichophyton*

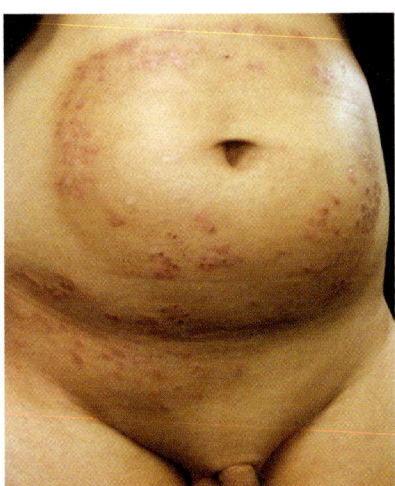
Fig. 10.2: Tinea incognito in a child

rubrum. The patient was treated with systemic itraconazole (200 mg once daily) and topical terbinafine (twice daily) for 8 weeks.[8]

Myriad Clinical Manifestations of Tinea Incognito

An immune-mediated phenomenon called "tinea pseudoimbricata" is a particular type of tinea incognito which has been described as "rings within the ring" and "double-edged tinea" appearance. *Trichophyton mentagrophytes,* instead of *Trichophyton concentricum,* is usually isolated from these lesions[9] (Figs 10.4 and 10.5).

Steroid Modified Tinea as a Koebnerizing Factor

Chronic nature of steroid modified tinea and persistent irritation facilitates koebnerization of co-existing dermatoses like psoriasis, lichen planus and vitiligo.

A case of lichen planus developing new lesions in a patch of steroid modified tinea presented in our outpatient department[7] (Figs 10.6 and 10.7).

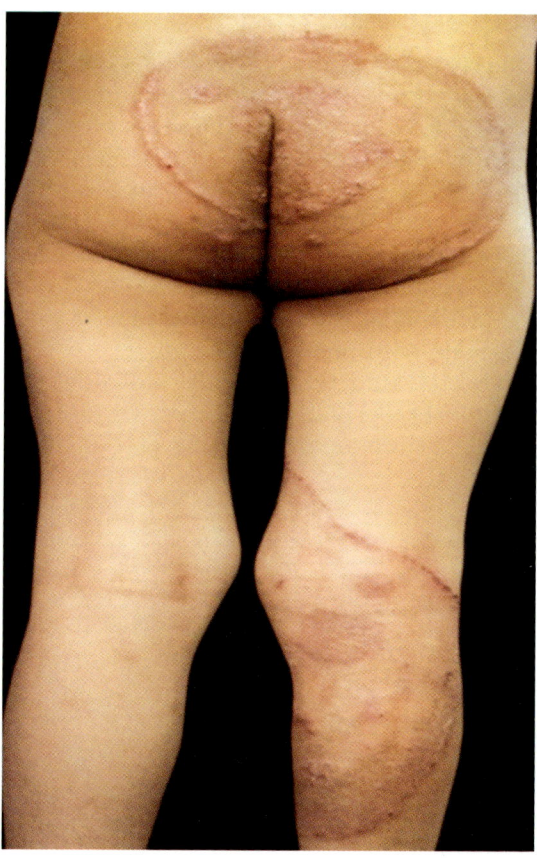

Fig. 10.5: Tinea pseudoimbricata

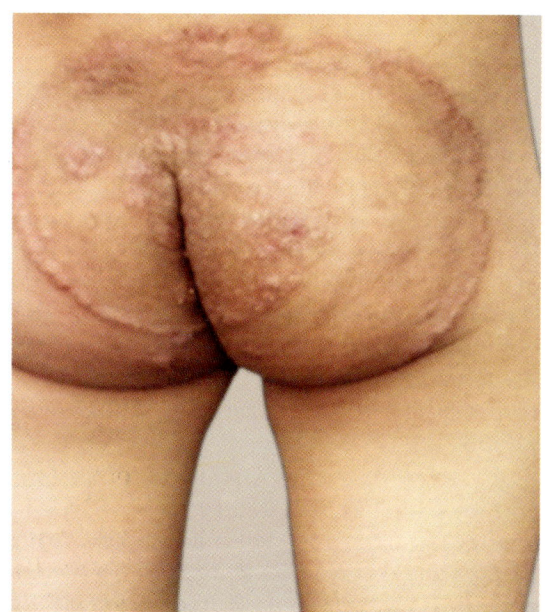

Fig. 10.4: Tinea pseudoimbricata

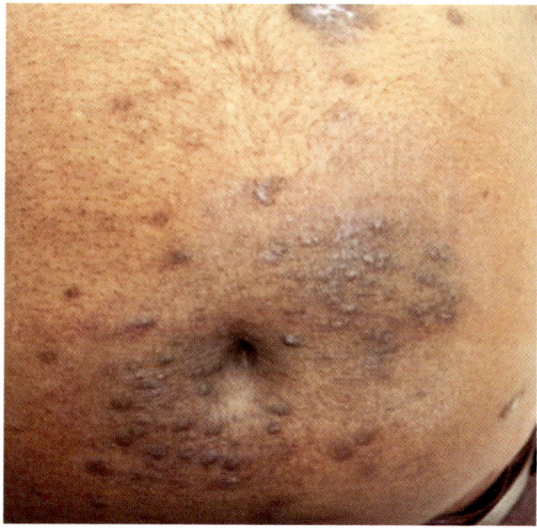

Fig. 10.6: Lichen planus

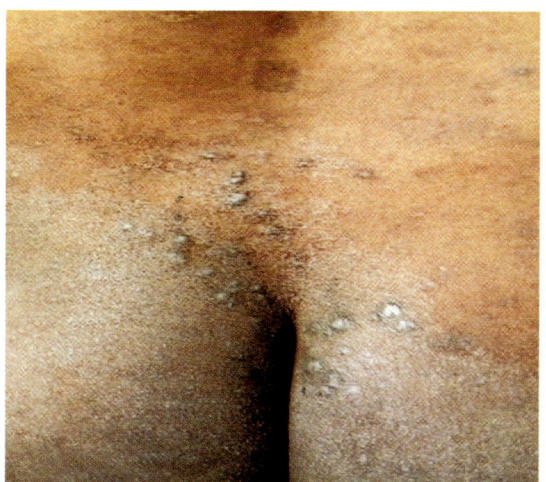

Fig. 10.7: Same patient with lichen planus developing new lesions in a patch of steroid modified tinea

Superimposed Tinea

Prolonged application of potent TCS in inflammatory dermatoses facilitates tinea superimposed on pre-existing dermatoses.

A case of eczema of feet (Fig. 10.8), scleroderma (Fig. 10.9), prurigo nodularis (Fig. 10.10) and papulonodular amyloidosis (Fig. 10.11) developed superimposed tinea after prolonged application of TCS.

Guenova et al[10] reported a case of 68-year-old female with pemphigus foliaceus for 13 years, on long-term oral and topical steroids with worsening of lesions mainly in facial, lower torso, and buttock areas. Periodic acid–Schiff (PAS) stain, fungal culture, and polymerase chain reaction analysis showed abundant *T. rubrum*.

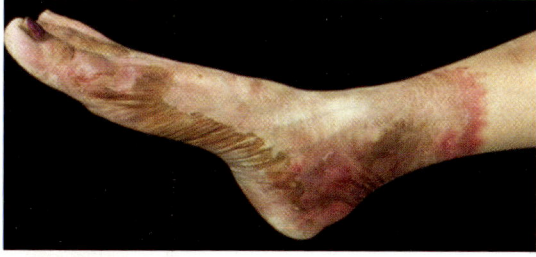

Fig. 10.8: Patient under treatment for eczema developed superimposed tinea incognito

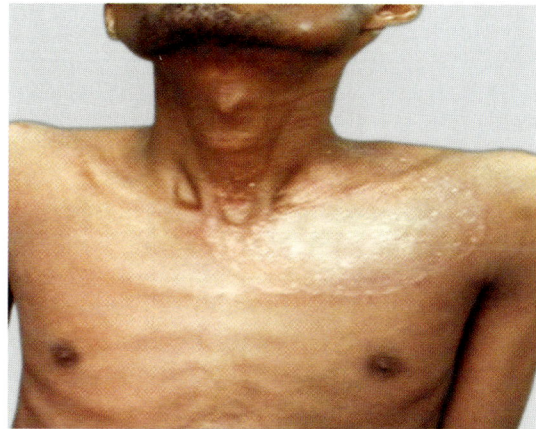

Fig. 10.9: Tinea corporis in patient with systemic sclerosis

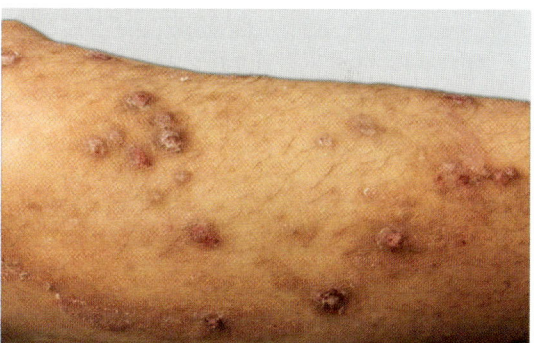

Fig. 10.10: Tinea corporis superimposed on prurigo nodularis

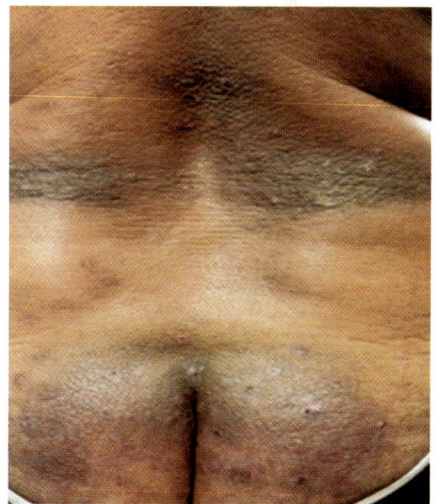

Fig. 10.11: Tinea corporis superimposed on papulonodular amyloidosis

Tinea and Atopic Dermatitis

Due to inherent pruritic and inflammatory nature of atopic dermatitis, TCS application is a preferred first line management. While TCS encourage tinea, pruritus disseminates the same.

A study of associated dermatoses was conducted in 97 atopic dermatitis patients. Superficial fungal infections were present in 23 cases. Tinea corporis and tinea cruris took 8 weeks to cure with oral fluconazole and topical antifungals instead of usual 4 weeks.[11]

Take home message
■ Before prescribing TCS for any dermatoses, rule out tinea. A careful look in webspace, groin fold and nail is essential.
■ On every follow up visit, such check for tinea is essential.
■ Meticulous history of self medication, use of over-the-counter products and other topical preparations as advised by chemist is essential.
■ Ask-your patient to bring fairness and skin lightening creams they are using to check whether it contains steroid or not. Infact, encourage patient to bring all the topical medications used for treatment of any other skin diseases.
■ When in doubt and when ill-defined scaly lesions are present in any dermatoses, potassium hydroxide scraping is essential to rule out superimposed tinea.
■ Control of itching in pruritic dermatoses is must in preventing development or dissemination of tinea.

CONCLUSION

Because of its potent antiallergic and anti-inflammatory effect, corticosteroids are prescribed for skin conditions of diverse etiology,often without establishing a definite cause. In tinea incognito, skin lesions become ill-defined with reduced itching and inflammation with spread of lesion. There is also more chances of recurrence and dissemination. Every patient attending dermatology clinic must be examined for evidence of fungal infection before initiation of oral and topical steroids.

In patients with chronic dermatoses, the potential for superimposed tinea remains high, as prolonged steroid application is the norm. Persistent itching and irritation in TCS modified tinea provides an opportunity for koebnerization of pre-existing chronic dermatoses.

Careful monitoring of cases using TCS, for occult foci of fungal infection like web spaces and nails is a necessity. Mycological examination like potassium hydroxide preparations and culture in Sabouraud's dextrose agar must be performed in suspicious lesions. Patients on systemic steroids must be evaluated periodically for aggravation of existing dermatosis or presence of atypical lesions if any.

Approximately half of the cases of tinea present as TCS modified tinea. Careful history, meticulous clinical and mycologic examination will go a long way in picking up tinea incognito.

Selection of topical and oral antifungals depends upon previous exposure and responsiveness to such medications. There is no substitute for elaborate patient education and counseling.

References

1. Marfatia, Jose. Tinea incognito and topical corticosteroid abuse in dermatology. World Clin Dermatol 2016;3(1):207–19.
2. Schaller M, Friedrich M, Papini M, Pujol RM, Veraldi S. Topical antifungal corticosteroid combination therapy for the treatment of superficial mycoses: conclusions of an expert panel meeting. Mycoses 2016;59:365–73.
3. Yogesh S Marfatia, Devi S Menon. Use and Misuse of topical corticosteroid in genital dermatosis. A Treatise on topical corticosteroids in dermatology 2017.
4. Mittal RR, Jain C, Gill SS, Jindal R. Atypical manifestations of tinea faciei. Indian J Dermatol Venereol Leprol 1996;62:98–9.
5. Starace M, Alessandrini A, Piraccini BM. Tinea incognito following the use of an antipsoriatic gel. Skin Appendage Disord 2016;1(3):123–5.

6. Lecamwasam KL, Lim TM, Fuller LC. Tinea incognito caused by skin-lightening products. J Eur Acad Dermatol Venereol 2016;30(3): 480–1.

7. Parimalam K, Dinesh DK, Thomas J. Vitiligo delimiting dermatophyte infection. Indian J Dermatol 2015;60:91–3.

8. Liu C, Landeck L, Cai SQ, Zheng M. Majocchi's granuloma over the face. Indian J Dermatol Venereol Leprol 2012;78:113–4.

9. Verma SB, Hay R. Topical steroid-induced tinea pseudoimbricata: a striking form of tinea incognito. Int J Dermatol 2015;54:192–3.

10. Guenova E, Hoetzenecker W, Schaller M, Röcken M, Fierlbeck G. Tinea incognito hidden under apparently treatment-resistant pemphigus foliaceus. Acta Derm Venereol 2007;88:276.

11. Mittal RR, Walia R, Gill AK, Bansal N. Dermatoses associated with atopic dermatitis (le). Indian J Dermatol Venereol Leprol 2000;66:218–9.

Overview of Causes and Treatment of Recalcitrant Dermatophytoses

Kabir Sardana, Ananta Khurana

INTRODUCTION

We have used the term "**recalcitrant**" as opposed to resistance as data from most centers have not found *in vitro* resistance commensurate with the number of patients failing treatment.[1,2] Hence recalcitrance can be an all encompassing term that can be used to describe the various scenarios that one sees in clinical practice (Fig. 11.1). Three important terms need elucidation here.

Relapse/Recurrence

This can be defined as a re-occurrence of the infection usually after 4 weeks of completion of approved systemic therapy. The duration of 4 weeks is based on concrete *in vitro* and *in vivo* data providing evidence that the two most commonly used drugs used in clinical practice, itraconazole (ITR) and terbinafine (TER), persist in levels higher than reported MICs of most dermatophytes for that much time.[3–5] However, whether the levels are sufficient in the wake of higher MICs (to TER) being reported now is a potential area for further research.

Recent Indian studies have demonstrated high rates of relapses with conventional treatment regimens. Majid et al reported relapses in 33.8% of the clinico-mycologically

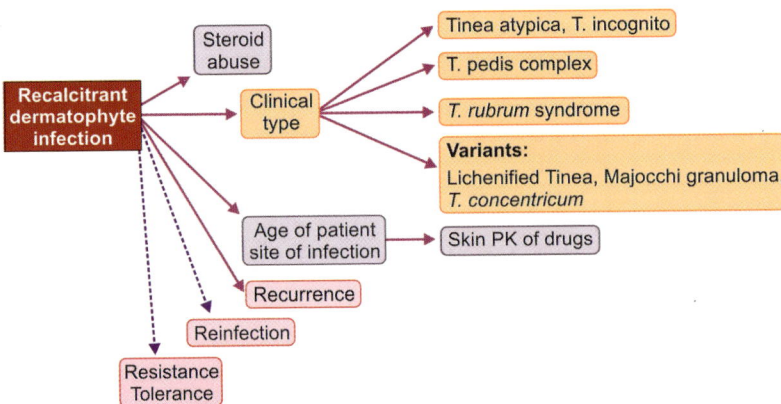

Fig. 11.1: An overview of the various factors that can lead to recalcitrant infection. *In vitro* resistance is not the overriding factor. These causes are to be considered once compliance, undertreatment and misdiagnosis and quality of brands are excluded

cured patients of tinea corporis/cruris, within the 12 weeks follow-up period.[6] Similarly, Sharma et al reported recurrence rates of 34.33% (26.92% in tinea corporis, 21.43% of tinea cruris and 80% in tinea pedis) patients.[7] Species-wise, the recurrence rates were 75% for *Trichophyton mentagrophytes* and 50% for *T. rubrum*.[1]

In India, recurrences are likely due to two major factors. One is possibly actual *resistance*[1,2] and second is the suppression of the *host immunity* due to steroid abuse.[8] Another possible cause is lack of *compliance*.[1,2]

Other causes may include humidity, sweating, clothing type, host immune response, barrier dysfunction and of course reinfection. A lack of adequate dose, or drug interactions may also play a role.[2]

Resistance

What we are seeing in India is *clinical* resistance, which is possibly a failure of therapy due to subtherapeutic drug levels at the site of the infection, caused by the pharmacokinetics of the drug, drug interactions or poor patient compliance. Other reasons for clinical failure include overwhelming infection, certain particular sites of infection and immune status of the host. Herein there is also the issue of the quality of the drug specially itraconazole (ITR).[2]

In vitro resistance: This is a microbiological term and is ideally to be used when the MIC of the organism isolated is more than a certain predefined level. For TER, it is >0.5 µg/ml (now 1 µg/ml).[9,10] Resistance to fluconazole is defined as MIC >64 µg/ml, and for ketoconazole and itraconazole as MIC >8 µg/ml.[11] Azoles, being static drugs, have a high potential for inducing resistance. The prevalence of azole resistance in dermatophytes has been reported to be as high as 19% in certain areas worldwide.[11] There are reports of resistance of *T. rubrum* to terbinafine due to alterations in the squalene epoxidase gene or a factor essential for its activity. In a report it was seen that usual MICs of 0.03 mg/ml are seen in susceptible strains of *T. rubrum*; while in these resistant strains, MICs were >1.0 µg/ml.[9,10] Importantly, resistance seen in dermatophytes, so far, is drug class specific and hence a strain resistant to one class *may* respond to another with a different mechanism of action.

Clinically a patient who has a persistent infection or relapses within 4 weeks of an adequate dose regimen and duration of an approved drug can possibly have resistance, if the immunological and extraneous factors (steroid suppression) have been *excluded*. Importantly, a documented *in vitro* resistance does not always translate into clinical failure. This is as the levels achieved by the antifungal drug in the skin, as opposed to the plasma, are much higher.[12,13] Hence the drug may exceed the *in vitro* MIC many times over.[12,13] This said, it is also known that in India the MIC to terbinafine is higher than itraconazole, but even then clinically ITR does not consistently show superior results. Griseofulvin (GRI) has low MIC, but by itself is a clinically ineffectual drug.[2] The low MIC reflects its lack of use in India since the last two decades.[2] It must be thus understood that the MIC levels reflect prescription practices and with a higher use of ITR, the MIC to it will also rise. With some drugs, e.g. fluconazole high MICs are seen, that does not mean a poor clinical outcome. Hence just a higher MIC is of a little value as the drug invariably achieves sufficiently high levels in the skin with a conventional dose. Further, the next step, after documenting high MICs, is to perform mutational analysis on these strains. This would finally confirm or discredit the resistance theory, as the case may be.

But here we may add that there is a simple tool to assess the efficacy of drugs based on *in vitro* data. If the MIC cut offs are close to the MFC (minimal fungicidal concentration), the organism is said to be sensitive. For example, butenafine, a drug not marketed in India, is 10–100 times more potent than the azoles and has 4 times greater activity than naftifine *in vitro* and this is based on a similar MIC and MFC data for this drug.[14]

Tolerance

This is when the organism apparently becomes clinically resistant to the drug in the tissues but is sensitive *in vitro*. This may also be important and may explain the scenario in some cases.

Chronic Dermatophytoses

Chronic dermatophytosis is defined as an infection that persists for 6 months to one year. This subset may have a unique immunological profile as discussed below.

AN OVERVIEW OF IMPORTANT FACTORS UNDERLYING RECALCITRANT INFECTIONS

Though there are several reasons propounded for recalcitrance, we will focus on the important factors and arrive at a logical assessment of what seems likely to be a plausible answer to the issues faced in India (Box 11.1). Issues like global warming, fungicide use in agriculture, clothing, weather, etc. are not discussed as they are not unique to India and are seen in the whole of South-East Asia (and they do not face this problem) which effectively discounts these theories.

1. Clinical Type of Tinea

It must be understood that apart from the common and classical form of tinea corporis, with an annular configuration and central clearing, many other variants are described. These other variants will *not* respond to conventional durations of therapy, without there being any *in vitro* resistance. The presentation depends on the species of *Trichophyton* (*see* below) and of course the host immunity, which is often compromised in India due to steroid abuse, and might explain some atypical variants. The extent of inflammation depends on the causative pathogen and the immune response of the host. Also, because hair follicles serve as reservoirs for infection, areas of the body with more hair follicles may be more resistant to treatment.

Tinea Corporis (Atypical Variants)

a. In case of topical corticosteroids abuse (tinea "incognito"), there is no scaling.[15] These cases are often diagnosed by pustules *within* the active border. A practical problem that we have faced is that in such cases the isolation and culture of fungi is

Box 11.1: Factors implicated in recalcitrant dermatophytoses	
Clinical type of tinea	Could there be certain *sites* and *types* that require a different management protocol without having *in vitro* resistance?
Fungal species (T. rubrum vs T. mentagrophytes and T. interdigitale) and type (zoophilic/anthropophilic)	Is there a species *shift* and does it matter?
Barrier integrity	How important is this in persistence or recurrence?
Host Immunity	Is there a reason for a depressed host immune response? Steroid abuse?
Drug: PK/PD and quality	What determines the secretion of drugs? Is there a quality issue?
Compliance	Does the patient take the desired therapy for the duration recommended?
Resistance	Is microbiological resistance in the lab in proportion to clinical failure? Is there a true *in vitro* resistance?

PK/PD = Pharmacokinetics/pharmacodynamics

also low. In studies from India, tinea incognito is the commonest presentation of topical steroid abuse.

b. Variants like *vesicular, granulomatous, or verrucous tinea* can be seen. *Deep or subcutaneous* dermatophytoses are very rare clinical entities, which have been reported under the names of disseminated trichophytic granuloma, dermatophyte mycetoma, tinea profunda cysticum and subcutaneous abscesses. These entities do not respond to conventionally recommended treatments and require prolonged therapy.

c. *Nodular perifolliculitis* (Majocchi granuloma), was originally described in women following shaving or waxing but is now often seen in many patients in India outside this narrow domain. Application of potent topical steroids and underlying immunosuppression are the contributory factors. Often there are only subtle follicular papules which become more prominent as the macular erythema around improves, with initiation of antifungal treatment. Their presence necessitates a much longer therapy.

d. Tinea imbricata is a dermatophytosis caused by the anthropophilic dermatophyte *T. concentricum*. In India, steroid misuse can lead to such a presentation.

Tinea Cruris

Tinea cruris is frequently associated with tinea pedis because clothing that is brought over the feet is contaminated and then comes in contact with skin in the groin region. Importantly, the lack of intervention for tinea pedis in such cases leads to frequent recurrences.

An increasing number of patients have chronic, leathery and lichenified lesions. This is a sign of Th1 depression and Th2 activation leading to the cycle of itching and lichenification.[16] In this case again a prolonged therapy is needed *without in vitro* resistance. Tinea genitalis, with severe inflammatory reaction necessitating prolonged high dose antifungals and often systemic steroids for initial anti-inflammatory effect, has been recently described and is thought to be sexually transmitted. [17]

Tinea Manuum/Pedis

Palms and soles are two sites where the infection is chronic and difficult to treat, with two predominant reasons, both of which discount the resistance theory and scientifically explain chronicity.

The *first* reason is related to the lack of sebaceous glands on the palms. In conjunction with this anatomical fact is the pharmacological fact that both of our first line oral drugs TER and ITR have a lipophilic secretion pattern (predominantly) which explains the *higher dose* and longer duration for infections of the palms and soles.[12,13] *Secondly*, there are many *nondermatophytes* implicated at these sites, which do not respond to conventional antifungals. Infections with *Neoscytalidium dimidiatum* and *N. hyalinum*, two nondermatophyte fungi, can have a tinea manuum-like appearance. Nondermatophyte pathogens that produce clinical findings identical with tinea pedis include *Neoscytalidium dimidiatum* and *N. hyalinum* (moccasin and interdigital types) and, occasionally, *Candida* spp. (interdigital type). Also the "dermatophytosis complex" (fungal infection followed by bacterial invasion) which again does not respond to antifungals alone. Prolonged administration of terbinafine, for 4–6 weeks, has been the standard recommendation for moccasin and hyperkeratotic tinea pedis and this does not mean "resistance".[18]

Other Sites

A large number of patients have tinea faciei and even scalp involvement with species that involve the skin. The type of species is not very important here, but the multiple unusual sites suggest a lowered immunity that allows rapid spread.

Invasive Dermatophytoses

Rarely, dermatophytes proliferate within the dermis. Invasion or dissemination of dermatophytes is most often seen in the setting of a chronic dermatophyte infection (most commonly *T. rubrum*) in an immuno-suppressed individual. Tinea profunda, Majocchi's granuloma and tinea genitalis have been described above in this regard. Hematogenous spread can lead to an acute onset of ulcerating or draining dermal and subcutaneous nodules. A more indolent process can also occur and most often presents as tender nodules on the extremities. In a pivotal study, all the patients with deep dermatophytoses had autosomal recessive CARD9 deficiency. Deep dermatophytoses appear to be an important clinical manifestation of CARD9 deficiency[19]

Currently, the recommended treatment is surgical excision (if localized) and systemic itraconazole or terbinafine but amphotericin B, griseofulvin and ketoconazole have also been used successfully.[20]

Implications

The basic underlying precept is that there are numerous atypical tinea presentations which are not consequent to resistance (*in vitro*). This should be borne in mind by the clinician:

1. Some sites have nondermatophytic infection and may require a different dosimetry.
2. Tinea pedis and manuum require higher doses, as ITR and TER are both lipophilic and may not achieve sufficient levels at these sites.
3. Certain clinical types may require longer therapy periods even in normal circumstances.

Two examples are the "leathery" variant of tinea corporis which is itchy due to an increased Th2 response and Majocchi granuloma, which has a follicular affliction. Hence recalcitrance does *not* necessarily mean resistance.

4. Invasive forms would of course require higher doses and prolonged treatment.

Here we may point out that there is definitely a rising MIC to TER, but not in all cases does it achieve resistance levels (>1 µg/ml). But conversely, there are cases of ITR failures even though ITR has a low MIC, which should make us think of other causes of recalcitrance (Fig. 11.1).

2. Fungal Species and Type (Zoophilic/Anthropophilic)

There are 3 major categories of dermatophyte causing human disease, of which zoophilic and anthropophilic ones are predominant (Box 11.2). Typically, a given dermatophyte induces a more severe inflammatory reaction in a host to which it is not adapted than it does in its natural host. In humans, anthropophilic species tend to cause chronic infections with minimal inflammation, while infections by zoophilic or geophilic species are generally highly inflammatory, acute and self-limiting.[21] The various clinical types are listed in Table 11.1.

Dermatophytes produce keratinases (enzymes that break down keratin), which allow invasion of the fungi into the stratum corneum. Mannans in the cell walls of dermatophytes have immuno-inhibitory effects. The mannans also *decrease* epidermal proliferation, thereby reducing the likelihood

Box 11.2: Types of dermatophytes based on mode of transmission		
Category	*Mode of transmission*	*Typical clinical features*
Anthropophilic	Human to human	Mild to non-inflammatory, chronic
Zoophilic	Animal to human	Intense inflammation (pustules and vesicles possible), acute
Geophilic	Soil to human or animal	Moderate inflammation

Table 11.1: Clinical presentations of various types of dermatophyte species	
Anthropophilic	*Clinical morphology*
Trichophyton rubrum	May produce concentric rings; can recur; causative organism in nodular perifolliculitis (Majocchi granuloma) and was the most common cause of tinea corporis at one time in India.
T. tonsurans	Commonly seen in adults who care for children with tinea capitis. In India, this is not common and most centres that identify this are probably incorrect as RFLP analysis of the PCR-amplified ITS1-5.8 s-ITS2 region helps to reclassify them as *T. interdigitale/mentagrophytes*.
Epidermophyton floccosum	Generally restricted to groin, feet; responsible for "eczema marginatum"
T. concentricum	Responsible for "tinea imbricata"; infections typically chronic. In India, steroid modified cases present with this morphology.
T. interdigitale (previously T. mentagrophytes var interdigitale)	Causes interdigital tinea pedis, tinea cruris, and onychomycosis.
Zoophilic	
T. mentagrophytes (previously T. mentagrophytes var. mentagrophytes)	May be associated with dermatophytid reaction; causes inflammatory tinea pedis and tinea barbae; associated with exposure to small mammals
Microsporum canis	Associated with pet exposure (cat or dog)
T. verrucosum	May mimic bacterial furunculosis; associated with exposure to cattle.

of the fungus being sloughed off prior to invasion.[16] This mechanism is thought to contribute to the chronicity of infections caused by *T. rubrum*, which produces this compound in higher amounts than others. Here it is relevant to note that the steroids (commonly abused in India) compound the immunosuppression and also reduce epidermal proliferation, thus inhibiting the host response.[15,16]

Host factors such as protease inhibitors may limit the extent of invasion. Other protective host factors include sebum, a functional skin barrier, pH, CO_2 levels, and transferrin.

Though most texts, before the epidemic we face in India, found *T. rubrum* to be the commonest cause, as per recent data, the proportions of *T. mentagrophytes* and *T. interdigitale* are increasing, though *T. rubrum* still predominates in most recently published reports except a recent one (Dabas et al)

which reported majority isolates (56%) to be *T. interdigitale* (Table 11.2).[22–24] Even though certain centers report *T. tonsurans* based on cultural characteristics or MALDI-TOF, molecular confirmation shows the species to be *T. mentagrophytes/interdigitale*. *T. mentagrophytes* spp is a term now only restricted to describe zoophilic species. The anthropophilic varieties of *T. mentagrophytes*, as well as several zoophilic strains previously classified as var *mentagrophytes* or var. *granulosum*, are not genetically distinguishable from *T. interdigitale* and are thus collectively known as *T. interdigitale* species. [25,26]

Implications

The various organisms that can cause tinea corporis and cruris are listed in Table 11.2. The important point here is that the source in many patients is probably the feet, as *T. interdigitale* affects the plantar skin and the chronicity is explained as anthropophilic species tend to subvert the immune system and cause recalcitrance.

Though no reason for the shift from *T. rubrum* to *T. interdigitale/mentagrophytes* has so far been proposed, the strains acquiring new virulence factors for subverting the host immune response, leading to improved host adaptability is a probable one. Thus the scenario may be an improved adaptation of these species to humans over the course of time, with the local immunosuppression by steroids making it easier to establish chronic infections. But the reasoning will remain conjectural till sound scientific data provides clear answers.

3. Barrier Defects

The first step in dermatophytes' pathogenicity is stratum corneum penetration. Thus, barrier can play a crucial role in host defense. The scratching and steroid abuse lead to compromised barrier integrity. Epidermal proliferation increases several fold in tinea affected skin and accordingly, proliferation and inflammation-associated keratins K6, K16, and K17 are expressed.[27,28] Expression of basal keratins K5 and K14 increases, whereas differentiation-associated K10 is reduced. Reduction of the cornified envelope proteins involucrin, loricrin, and the S100 protein filaggrin is also seen. Reduced filaggrin expression correlates with reduced skin hydration and thus tinea corporis patients have a compromised barrier. This was re-confirmed by another study, where dermatophytoses, except tinea pedis and tinea manuum, showed highly significant increase in transepidermal water loss (TEWL) compared with adjacent infection-free skin.[28]

It may be worthwhile to mention here that in individuals with an atopic background, in addition to the barrier function impairment, there further exists a selective or induced immune deficit for dermatophytic infections. Patients with allergic bronchial asthma or allergic rhinitis often develop chronic or recurrent fungal infections associated with high immediate-type hypersensitivity (high IgE levels) and low or waning delayed type hypersensitivity reaction to trichophytin.[29]

Implications

A concomitant or consequential barrier repair is of great use in preventing recurrences. A ceramide-based cream may be of use in preventing recurrences.

Here it must be pointed out that steroid abuse also leads to barrier compromise and is another pointer to the likely cause in India.

4. Immune Defects in Chronic Dermatophytoses

Waldman et al, in an experimental study involving patients with chronic dermatophytoses (>1 year; tinea corporis/pedis/manuum) demonstrated that patients with long-lasting dermatophytic infections exhibit a selective immune deficit, which had the following characteristics.[30]

(i) A significantly lower cytotoxic effect of T cells against dermatophytes when compared with normal controls. (ii) Suppression of lymphocyte proliferation response after incubation of peripheral blood mononuclear cells (PBMC) from chronic patients, with trichophytin or various dermatophyte homogenates. However, the culture of PBMC with nonspecific mitogens significantly enhanced the cell proliferation pointing to a selective defect. (iii) Incubation of PBMC with different dermatophytes homogenates (such as *T. rubrum*, *T. mentagrophytes*, or *M. gypseum*) resulted in the up regulation of HLA-DR and ICAM-1 expression by lymphocytes of normal population, but to a lesser degree of patients with chronic fungal infections, pointing to a defect in antigen presentation. (iv) Ultra-structure and histological evaluation of the culture of hyphae with CD4+ or CD8+ T cells showed more prominently destructive effects in the culture of cells that had been obtained from normal population, compared to those patients with long-lasting fungal infections.

Similarly, de Sousa et al[31] demonstrated that macrophages and neutrophils from patients with chronic widespread dermatophytoses presented with reduced phagocytic and killing abilities, and reduced H_2O_2 and NO release when compared with those of healthy donors. These macrophages secreted lower levels of the proinflammatory cytokines interleukin 1β (IL-1β), IL-6, IL-8, and tumor necrosis factor-α (TNF-α), but enhanced levels of the anti-inflammatory cytokine IL-10. Thus, the reduced levels of the cytokines with Th-1/Th-17-inducing properties, associated with the enhanced IL-10 release by macrophages, likely adversely affects the induction of an effective CMI response. On the same lines, McCarthy et al[32] reported that skin reactivity to trichophytin decreases with increasing disease chronicity. Further, treatment with terbinafine has been shown to improve trichophytin reactivity in those who achieved cure.[33]

However, an important point to consider here is that in these studies, *T. rubrum* was the predominant dermatophyte isolated, while what we are seeing presently is a high proportion of *T. mentagrophytes* and *T. interdigitale* as well.

There are a few reports in literature describing a "chronic trichophytosis" caused by anthropophilic strains of *T. interdigitale*.[34] A defective phagocytosis by neutrophils was reported in these patients, but subsequent literature, post the introduction of terbinafine, reported a good response (76%) to this drug with normalization of the phagocytic defect as well.

Thus, the propensity of the other species, which are being increasingly reported as causatives in our population, to produce chronic infections is not yet substantiated. It is an interesting proposition that these strains may also have acquired similar virulence mechanisms as *T. rubrum*, improving their ability to evade immune mechanisms.

a. The Cytokine Story

The primary production of the Th1 cell is the cytokine IFN-γ and the pro-inflammatory cytokine TNF-α, and that of the Th2/regulatory cell line is IL-10 (Fig. 11.2). In the early phase of the infection, IFN-γ levels are not changed and this is consequent to the high levels of IL-10 which down regulates the Th1 response. Over time, the response changes, and IL-10 production decreases, while the levels of IFN-γ increase. This correlates with clinical cure. The cytokine analysis in invasive dermatophytosis can shed more light on the immunological interplay (Fig. 11.3).

In the human disease, IFN-γ-positive cells were observed in the upper dermis in

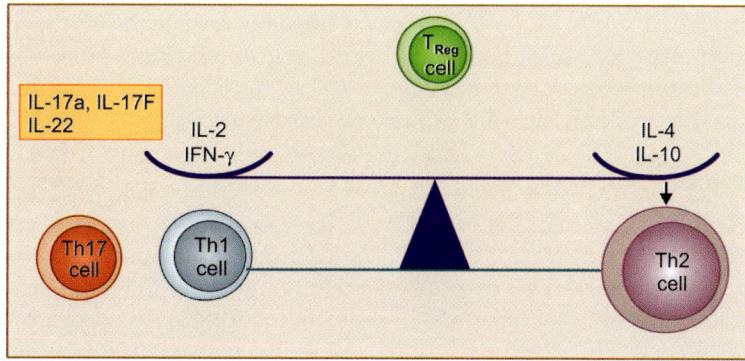

Fig. 11.2: Depiction of the balance between protective immunity (left) and the allergenic Th2 to response with T$_{Reg}$ cells balancing the immunity

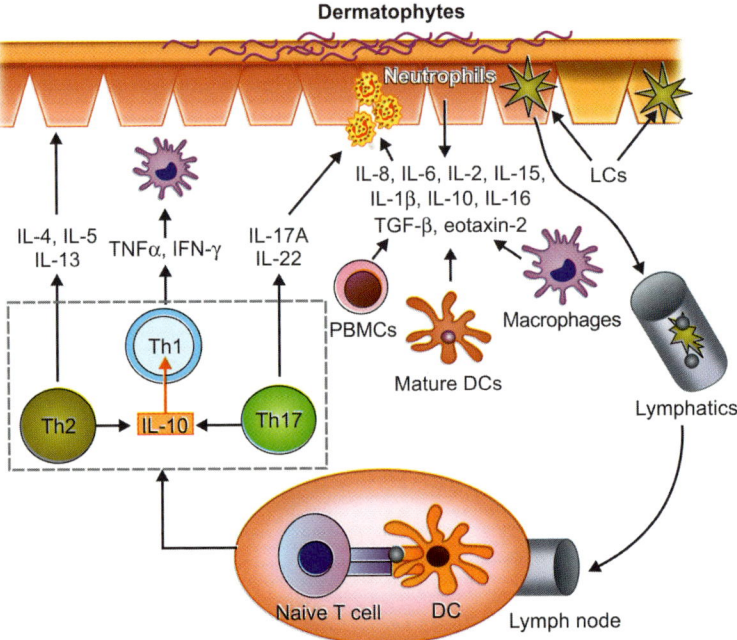

Fig. 11.3: Immune responses to dermatophytes. **Anthropophilic** dermatophytes such as *Trichophyton rubrum*, *Trichophyton schoenleinii* and *Trichophyton tonsurans* induce the production of interleukin-8, IL-6, IL-1β and eotaxin-2 in keratinocytes, peripheral blood mononuclear cells (PBMC), macrophages and dendritic cells (DC), while **zoophilic dermatophytes** such as *Arthroderma benhamiae* induce a wide range of cytokines including IL-1β, IL-6, IL-8, IL-10, IL-2, IL-15, IL-16, transforming growth factor-β (TGF-β), interferons (IFN-γ) (T-helper [Th]1), IL-17 (Th17), IL-4, IL-5 and IL-13 (Th2), leading to various pro-inflammatory processes such as neutrophil chemo-attraction as well as macrophage and DC activation resulting in fungal killing and clearance

lesions *in situ*[36] Campos et al.[37], also reported that the interaction of *Trichophyton rubrum* with phagocytic peritoneal cells induced production of IL-10. It must be remembered that there is a little humoral response in dermatophytosis.

The suppressive effect of steroids on Th1 cells does not need much elaboration and can succinctly explain the problem in India

b. Steroid Use and Dermatophytoses

There is a well-established role of cell- mediated immunity in the clearance of dermatophytes.[12] It is also amply clear that the Th1 response helps in clearing the infection, while what we are seeing is possibly a Th2 response that makes the disorder persistent much alike atopic dermatitis (AD).[12] Also, recent studies

suggest that the cutaneous acquired immune responses to dermatophytic infections involve Th1 and Th17 components, and this is in line with other studies involving *Trichophyton* spp (Fig. 11.3).[2]

Steroids reduce the Th1 response markedly and aggravate tinea. However, the effects of topical steroids on the established factors of the innate immune response to dermatophytes (Hspmolecules, pacC, hsf1) are not well documented.[35]

i. Rationale and consequences of steroid antifungal combinations: Not too long ago, such combinations were being prescribed by dermatologists as well. So, though now they are being restricted, let us take a look at the rationale of their use and continued approval in the West, so that a proper perspective is considered, and to understand how a "long lasting friend, suddenly become the enemy" situation.

The use of topical steroids is based on two unrelated but useful correlates which cannot be ignored as some of these products are still in vogue in the West.[20] In the USA, Lotrisone (Merck and Co, Inc, Whitehouse Station, New Jersey) and Mycolog-II (Bristol-Myers Squibb Co, New York), were in use. Lotrisone is a combination product composed of a high-potency topical steroid, betamethasone dipropionate 0.05% cream, and a topical antifungal agent, clotrimazole 1% cream. This combination drug is approved by the US Food and Drug Administration (FDA) for topical use. Mycolog-II is a combination of antifungal/steroid consisting of nystatin, an antiyeast agent, and triamcinolone, a medium-potency topical steroid. Interestingly while the former was approved for diaper dermatitis, Alston et al[39] showed that physicians frequently used Lotrisone for tinea corporis or tinea faciei in children younger than the then recommended age of 12 years and for longer than a 2-week period, resulting in recurrent and persistent infections.

Previous research, however, has shown that when combination antifungal/corticosteroid agents are used for fungal infections, they not only result in high rates of recurrence of fungal infections but also have greater side effect profiles. In these studies,[40] authors hypothesized that lack of clinical improvement was due to the immunosuppressive effects of the corticosteroid component in Lotrisone.[41] In the UK, guidelines from the National Institute for Health and Care Excellence currently recommend adding a mild to moderate steroid to a topical antifungal when the skin is particularly inflamed.[38] It has been surmised that patients who complain of intense pruritus in association with an infection-induced dermatitis are best treated by simultaneous application of a low- or medium-potency topical steroid for a limited period of 7–10 days, along with a topical antifungal agent that will be continued until clinical findings resolve (Fleischer AB).[42] Contrary to this, Rosen et al suggested that the steroid component may inhibit the effectiveness of the antifungal component when the latter has a limited or only fungistatic efficacy.[49] The scientific evidence on combination therapy is thus conflicting, with some older studies in favor of using combinations in the initial treatment period but more recent well-controlled studies[43–45] demonstrating that the combinations offer equal or lower mycological and clinical cure rates and that they may not be economically feasible as well[46] (although the situation related to the latter point is reverse in India). The inflammation would reduce with successful elimination of the fungi over time and furthermore some topical antifungals possess anti-inflammatory activity as well.

Topical steroids are well known to suppress local defense mechanisms favoring fungal growth, resulting in treatment failures. They have been demonstrated to stimulate fungal metabolism in low concentrations, while inhibiting fungal metabolism in high concentrations by their cytostatic effects.[47] However, in practice all steroid preparations might be considered as working at low concentrations since absorbed concentrations of steroids are expected to decrease after penetration through the skin layers.[48]

Possible interactions between steroid and antifungal components in a combination product may result from the following mechanisms: [47]

i. *chemical antagonism* (the combination of two substances in solution to form an inactive complex);

ii. *physicochemical antagonism* (reversible or irreversible competitive antagonism by receptor blockade);

iii. *biologic antagonism* (activation of the fungal metabolism by corticosteroids in low concentrations while inhibition of fungal metabolism by antifungal agent); and

iv. abolishing/diminishing of the antifungal *activity* through a cell membrane-protective activity of the corticosteroid component. The last effect may be especially important for azoles which act by inhibiting the production of fungal cell membrane component ergosterol.

The above data has major implications in India. It is important to note that all the above presented literature is with use of mild to moderate potency steroids, while the combinations with superpotent steroids as available in the Indian market are logically expected to fare worse with respect to clinical response rates and adverse effects. Further, no one adheres to the 14 days rule.

With the rampant use of these combinations in our patients, this factor can sufficiently explain the recurrences that we are seeing today and which have been reported before in the West (Reynolds RD). This may also answer the often heard question in certain forums, "why only now has this problem occurred in India". This is as there has been surreptitious change in the steroid compound of the available combination creams is a recent phenomenon due to the price regulations policy of the government.

Also it is relevant to point out that unlike the West,[39–41] we have been unable to restrict the use of such combinations. Sadly the numerous unenforceable dictates guiding the misuse of such creams in India target the wrong audience, and we should possibly look at the consumer and the GP, in that order.

ii. Cortisol suppression and steroid abuse— a surrogate marker of depressed immunity: Steroid suppression can be approximately equated with its suppression of cortisol levels. This can be roughly correlated with the suppression of the immune response. Herein it is important to understand that most of the

OTC combination creams contain clobetasol propionate and hence cause more suppression of immunity. The use of clobetasol propionate (0.05%) in a dose of 2 g/day can decrease morning cortisol level after a few days[50] and use over 100 g/week or 100–300 g/week can result in features of Cushing's syndrome and symptoms of adrenal insufficiency.[51]

Allenby et al. in their study found that adrenal suppression was to be expected with use of clobetasol propionate in a dose of more than 50 g/week.[52] In some studies, it has been shown that even a much less amount of topical steroid can induce systemic adverse effects; this may be due to the use of occlusion. A study of US FDA found that after at least 2 weeks of administration of topical glucocorticoids, about 40% of patients had abnormal adrenal responses.[52]

How to test it?

Levels of serum cortisol; taken at 0800 hrs, of less than 3 µg/dl (83 nmol/l) are diagnostic of adrenal suppression. Normal serum cortisol levels are 5–25 µg/dl (135–675 nmol/l).

How soon can it Happen?

Allenby et al found adrenal suppression in about 64% of adults applying **50 g** or more of a potent topical steroid for at least **2 weeks**.[53] Abnormal early morning, i.e. 8 am serum cortisol levels, have been reported in 29% of individuals in a retrospective study of children with vitiligo using moderate to potent topical steroid for a mean of 2 weeks. Kerner and workers found the frequency of cortisol suppression was 40% in patients using 0.05% clobetasol propionate for more than 3 weeks.[29] This steroid suppression *reverts* in about 2–3 weeks after stopping therapy.[52]

Implications

In India, patients often use steroid creams for months, much more than the 2 weeks shown to suppress the immunity.[53,54] Literature and

US FDA trial data have shown that the reversion of immune response takes about 3 weeks after stopping steroids.[52] This is only when it is used for 2–4 weeks. In India its months of misuse, and that includes IM steroids and oral betamethasone.

This can possibly explain the prolonged therapy and the lack of response in the first few weeks of antifungal drugs, as on an average it takes 3 weeks for the immune response to recover. Those of us who keep wondering why in India, must appreciate that combo creams available here contain the most potent steroids and India is the only country where steroid abuse is such a problem.

Now how can this be surmounted? One interesting observation is that *tacrolimus* may help preserve the barrier integrity and a comparative study has found this effect in AD.[55] Also, there is an interesting synergistic effect of tacrolimus and azoles on fungi including *T. mentagrophytes*, which is a causative prominent dermatophyte in India.[56] But it must be understood that there are also cases of tacrolimus causing persistence of infection and thus this issue is not yet clear. Probably a simple barrier cream would suffice.[57]

The above facts focussing on steroid modified cases, arguably the most common scenario in India, can explain the recalcitrance without resistance (*in vitro*).

5. Drug Factors (PK/PD and Quality)

There are a few important issues here that need to be looked at. How does the drug reach the skin, how long does it last and should we up dose (also *see* Chapter 9)?

Terbinafine (TER)

Terbinafine is delivered to the stratum corneum by passive dermo-epidermal diffusion, through sebum and through incorporation of drug from migrating basal keratinocytes.[3,4,10] High concentrations of drug (well above the MIC) are reached in the stratum corneum within hours of starting therapy.[3,4] Within 2 days of administering terbinafine 250 mg daily, the drug achieves high levels in the sebum.[3,4] TER has not however been detected in eccrine sweat. The elimination half-life of TER from the stratum corneum and sebum is 3–5 days. After administration of TER 250 mg daily for 12 days, drug concentrations above the previously reported MICs for most dermatophytes may be present for 2–3 weeks after oral therapy is discontinued.[3,4]

Itraconazole (ITR)[58–60]

Itraconazole is delivered to the skin mainly as a result of passive diffusion from the plasma to the keratinocytes, with strong drug adherence to keratin. Itraconazole becomes detectable in the sweat within 24 hours after the initial intake of drug. Despite the early detection in sweat, excretion of ITR by this route is minimal, in contrast to griseofulvin, ketoconazole, and fluconazole. There is extensive excretion of ITR into sebum. A negligible amount of ITR redistributes back from the skin and appendages to the plasma; therefore, ITR is eliminated as the stratum corneum renews itself, and when the hair and nails grow out. Itraconazole may persist in the stratum corneum for 3–4 weeks after discontinuation of therapy. In an *ex vivo* model, the therapeutic effect of ITR in the stratum corneum remained for 2–3 weeks after stopping therapy.

Fluconazole (FLU)[61–62]

When two doses of fluconazole (150 mg once weekly) are administered, the drug accumulates in the stratum corneum through sweat and by direct diffusion through the dermis and epidermis. Excretion in the sebum may be more limited. After discontinuation of therapy, there may be re-diffusion of FLU from the skin into the systemic circulation, but at a rate lower than elimination from the plasma. In healthy subjects, given a single FLU dose of 200 mg, the concentration in the plasma and stratum corneum was 3 µg/ml and 98 µg/g, respectively, 7 hours after administration. Faergemann J et al found that the maximum skin levels were achieved by FLU in a daily dose of 50 mg for 14 days. Over a 5-day FLU course (200 mg daily), the elimination of FLU from the stratum corneum occurred with a half-life of approximately 60–90 hours. This was 2–3 times slower than the elimination from plasma.

Combination of TER/ITR with Isotretinoin

Both terbinafine and itraconazole achieve high concentrations in sebum, which serves as a major route for transport of these drugs to their site of action (stratum corneum). Oral isotretinoin therapy reduces sebum produc-tion by up to 90%.[63] Hence, theoretically, it would block the secretion mechanism of both ITR and TER, markedly lowering their stratum corneum levels. Further, increased epidermal turnover is likely to adversely affect the "reservoir effect" of these drugs resulting in a shorter action span. Further, isotretinoin adversely affects ITR's pharmacokinetics. This has been documented in a case of chronic granulomatous disease, wherein co-adminis-tration of isotretinoin to a patient on long term ITR prophylaxis, made ITR's plasma levels undetectable.[64] These effects would have obvious implications on the expected thera-peutic outcome. Thus, to achieve a proposed advantage of improved epidermal turnover leading to faster fungal clearance from the stratum corneum, the combinations may compromise on achieving adequate drug levels in the skin. Hence, based on validated PK data for both ITR and TER, their combination with isotretinoin does not seem to be on a firm ground.

Implications

A plethora[3–5, 9, 10, 32–36] of concrete skin levels of antifungal (skinPK) data has shown that:
a. Most antifungal drugs achieve sufficiently high levels in the skin way beyond the MICs of the fungi.[3–5,12,13,58]

b. The drugs persist for about 3 weeks after stopping therapy[3-5]
c. Updosing beyond 250 mg BD of TER and 200 mg of ITR has a little pharmacological logic.[12,13,65,66] With the former there is also a risk of asymptomatic liver damage and the consequences of a "one way " medico-legal outcome.
d. The ideal drug will depend on the secretion profile and site. Hence on *oily skin* ITR and TER are good drugs but in *dry skin* FLU may be an ideal drug for sensitive strains. Again if *sweat* is the main route, GRI and ketaconazole are ideal drugs.[12]
e. Though FLU achieves the highest level in the skin (dose of 50 mg × 14 d), it has the least keratin adherence and hence is not the preferred choice in all care as it does not persist for sufficiently long time in the skin.
f. The proposed use of *voriconazole* is based on little science as the drug achieves only about 50% of the serum levels in the skin. Its use in tinea corporis and cruris is a cardinal error and its MIC is comparable to ITR, hence there is little justification of its use (Table 11.2).

Most importantly the *quality* is crucial with ITR and a brand with sufficient morphometric pellet characteristics achieves good results (Fig. 11.4). Considering the MIC levels, a topical drug achieves 100 × the MIC and a systemic drug achieves 10–30 × the MIC; hence we achieve 1000–3000 × MIC with combination of a systemic and topical and if even then the infections do not respond, this provides ample proof that the answer may lie elsewhere.

Here we draw the attention to a ethics cleared molecular work [67] (Table 11.2) where the low MIC of ITR and luliconazole makes these drugs a very efficient therapy. The high MIC 90 to TER explains its lowered efficacy. Here it may be pointed out that clinical experience suggest that even this combination (ITR +LULI) may not consistently work but

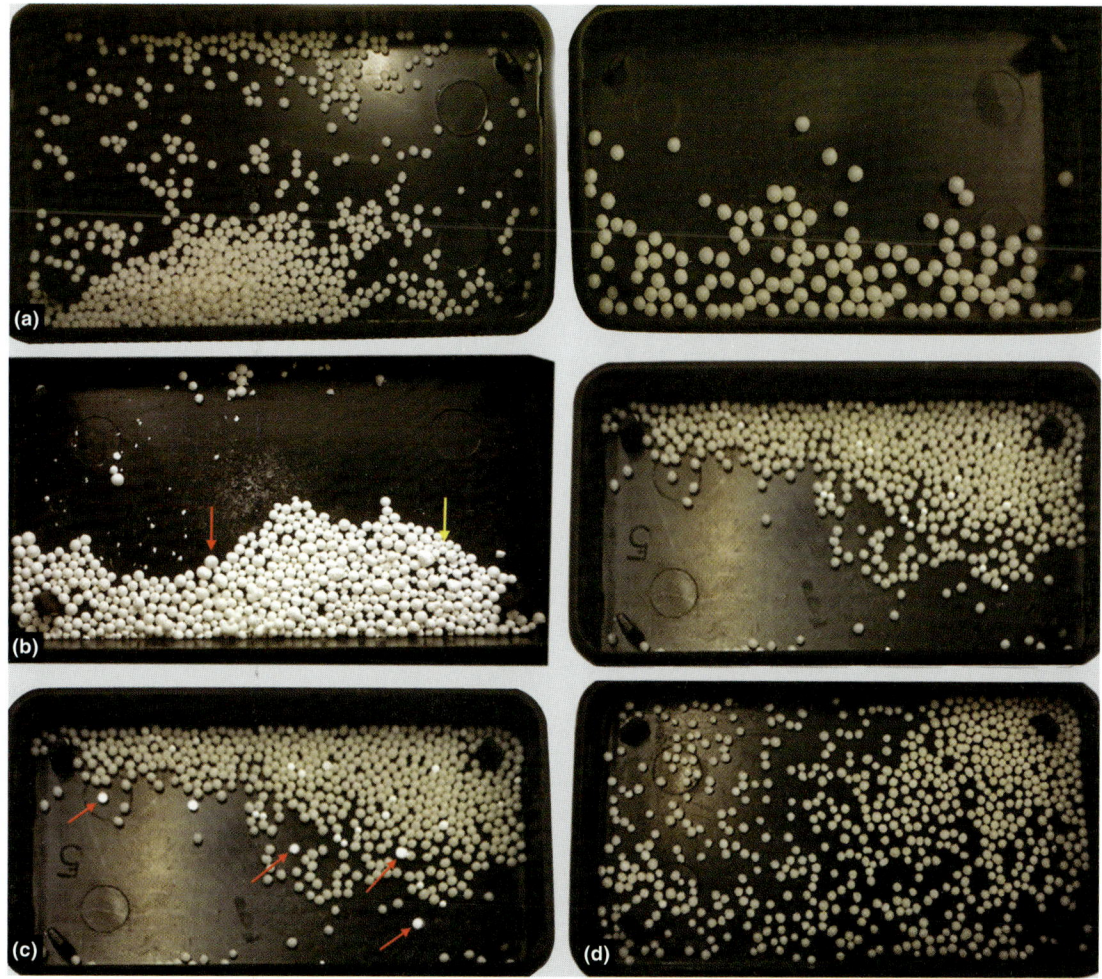

Fig. 11.4: Depiction of variable quality of pellets of itraconazole. (a) Shows on the left multiple uniform small pellets as compare to the brand on the right (left > right); (b) Variable pellets size red arrow (large pellets and yellow arrow small pellets); (c) Multiple dummy pellets (red arrow) use to increase the weight of the capsule; (d) Lower part of figure shows a reliable quality brand with multiple small pellets

based on mycology data, this seems the ideal combination. But here we may point out that synergism is based on *in vitro* "checkerboard studies" and not all combinations are additive.

Lastly it must be pointed that MIC data is not "the holy grail" and its interpretation depends on numerous other factors.[68,69] The reliance on MIC data has lead to ill conceived and unapproved updosing of drugs with 98 brands of ITR (ORG data) and still no "cure"

in sight; as the microbiology data is not the whole story.

6. Compliance

Though most clinicians recommend longer therapies of up to 8 weeks in all patients, in clinical practice this is rarely achievable as patients almost never take such long therapies consistently (Dr Asit Mittal, personal communication). It is also important

Table 11.2: Data on 8 recalcitrant cases of tinea confirmed by RFLP show high MIC to allylamine and low MIC to azoles

Clinical isolates	MIC range (μg/ml) (n = 3)									
	Fluconazole	Ketoconazole	Bifonazole	Clotrimazole	Itraconazole	Luliconazole	Posaconazole	Voriconazole	Terbinafine	Butenafine
T. mentagrophytes var. interdigitale KA-01	64	2	0.5	2	≤0.125	0.06–0.125	≤0.125	4	8	4
T. mentagrophytes var. interdigitale KA-02	64	0.25	≤0.125	≤0.125	≤0.125	≤0.004	≤0.125	0.5–0.25	8	2
T. mentagrophytes var. interdigitale KA-03	64	0.5–0.25	≤0.125	≤0.125	≤0.125	≤0.004	≤0.125	0.25≤0.125	≤0.015	≤0.125
T. mentagrophytes var. interdigitale KA-04	32–64	0.5	≤0.125	0.5–0.25	≤0.125	≤0.004	≤0.125	0.5	≤0.015	≤0.125
T. mentagrophytes var. interdigitale KA-05	64	0.25	≤0.125	≤0.125	≤0.125	≤0.004	≤0.125	0.25	8	2
T. mentagrophytes var. interdigitale KA-06	16–32	≤0.125	≤0.125	≤0.125	≤0.125	≤0.004	≤0.125	≤0.125	≤0.125.0.25	2
T. mentagrophytes var. interdigitale KA-07	32–64	≤0.125	≤0.125	≤0.125–0.25	≤0.125	≤0.004–0.008	≤0.125	≤0.125–0.25	2	2
T. rubrum ATCC28188	8	0.125	≤0.125	≤0.125	≤0.125	≤0.004	≤0.125	≤0.125	≤0.15	≤0.125

(Approved project on dermatophye resistance. PGIMER and Dr RML Hospital.) Among 8 dermatophyte isolates, 1 isolate has shown increased MIC to azoles and allylamine and 2 have shown increased MIC only to allylamine. Note that the azoles are generally better than allylamines.

Similar findings have been reported by a recent report from another Indian institute, which reported *T. interdigitale* to be the commonest isolated strain.

Dabas Y, Xess I, Singh G, Pandey M, Meena S. Molecular identification and antifungal susceptibility patterns of clinical dermatophytes following clsi and eucast guidelines. J. Fungi (Basel) 2017;32(2).

to note whether the patient is taking any potentially competitive drugs. Also the patient might fail to absorb the drug.

"Recurrence" may sometimes be caused by failure to eradicate the original infection rather than by reinfection. In India one of the most important cause for this is under treatment. That failure to clear the initial infection, rather than a reinfection, is a cause of many perceived "recurrences" is supported by the fact that culture frequently reveals the same organism that was found in the initial infection. Patients frequently stop the drugs altogether or start to use them on SOS basis after an initial improvement. Further our patients, especially the less educated ones, exercise their preferences in following prescriptions and often "choose" topical or systemic drugs as per their choice or the cost. Hence, it is essential that they understand the main focus of therapy and we should ensure that the prescription should have minimal essential drugs.

In a case of extensive tinea corporis, co-prescription of a topical antifungal may not be economically feasible, and it may be a good idea to co-prescribe a cheap emollient for barrier repair alongside a systemic antifungal, rather than burden a patient's limited resources with drugs from both routes and risking non-compliance and treatment failure. Another method we have adopted is to ask patients with extensive disease to use the topical agent only for the few most bothersome (there always are some) lesions.

We often encounter patients who complain of increased symptoms following starting of treatment. Some part of the problem may be related to stoppage of TCS which many would have been using, but this is also seen in those who have not used any TCS previously. This may be related to what the proponents of TCS combinations have described as "over treatment phenomenon", caused by the release of "fungal toxins".[70] Thus it is a good idea to inform the patients about this beforehand and prescribe antipruritics and

liberal use of emollients, at least during the initial part of the treatment, to ensure treatment long compliance.

Spending time with the distressed patients to educate them regarding drugs and fomite transmission goes a long way in achieving sustained cures. This also gives an important opportunity to emphasise the ill effects of TCS as a contributor to their condition and otherwise. A two-way interaction ensures long-term trust on the treating specialist and the patients are then less likely to fall back upon chemists and perform self medication.

Thus it is sensible to write an antifungal for 14 days and review. At that point it is a good practice to ask the patient to get the empty packs of the drug. This ensures compliance and can help to review and add or modify the therapy if needed.

7. Resistance (*in vivo*)

The argument of mycological resistance has sustained a boom in antifungal therapy but this has not correlated with any decrease in the incidence of infection/failures of treatment. This is when we have unapproved and supra pharmacological dosimetry of drugs (TER 500, ITR 400 mg) now. This in conjunction with some mycology studies where we have seen high MICs to TER. But at the same time inconsistent results with ITR in spite of low MICs to it makes the logic of "*in vitro* resistance" weak. Our own molecular (Table 11.3) work has shown that while ITR and other azoles have a low MIC, the patients do not consistently respond and this fact flies in the face of the "resistance story".

It must be noted that the MIC information provided by standard antifungal susceptibility test (AFST) methods may not always have clinical relevance. However, this issue (the "clinical utility" or "clinical relevance" of AFST) is rarely discussed. An important paper had articulated several important principles to consider when discussing the clinical utility of susceptibility test methods.[40,41] These principles include an understanding that the MIC is a construct that is largely defined by testing conditions, rather than a physical or chemical measurement.[40,41] This measure might correlate with clinical outcome, but a multitude of factors related to the host (immune response, underlying illness, site of infection), the infecting organism (virulence), and the antifungal agent (dose, pharmacokinetics, pharmacodynamics, drug interactions) may be more important than susceptibility test results in determining clinical outcomes for infected patients.[13] In particular, *in vitro* susceptibility of an organism to an antifungal agent does not consistently predict a successful therapeutic outcome.[12]

Hence, the existing data should be interpreted with caution as it discounts many other more important and relevant aspects of causation of dermatophytoses including the host immune response.

CLINICAL PRESCRIPTION WRITING

The plethora of hard scientific data suggests that the *in vitro* resistance theory does not "explain it all". The quantum of resistant strains seen in the laboratory does not correspond with the magnitude of treatment failures/recurrences we are seeing in the country today. In fact almost all the situations can be explained by steroid overuse except the species shift. It is important to use the evidence to give a rationale prescription. Though this is detailed in Fig. 11.5, it is important to remember that there are many scenarios where a longer therapy is needed for certain clinical types and sites of tinea without resistance being a cause. Also longer durations have been mentioned even in conventional texts and so 4–6 weeks therapy is *not long* as conventionally believed.

We are not covering nondermatophytes and will stick to conventional antifungals and how best to use them in India based on existing evidence. Also there is no concrete evidence for an immune booster, but this is a crucial and under-researched aspect. Without concrete evidence we cannot subscribe to the use of tacrolimus or any other oral drug at present as an immune booster.

Step 1: History and Examination

Assess steroid use, as if steroids have been used, a 3 weeks lack of response is expected. Also certain variants like lichenified tinea, Majocchi granuloma and steroid modified

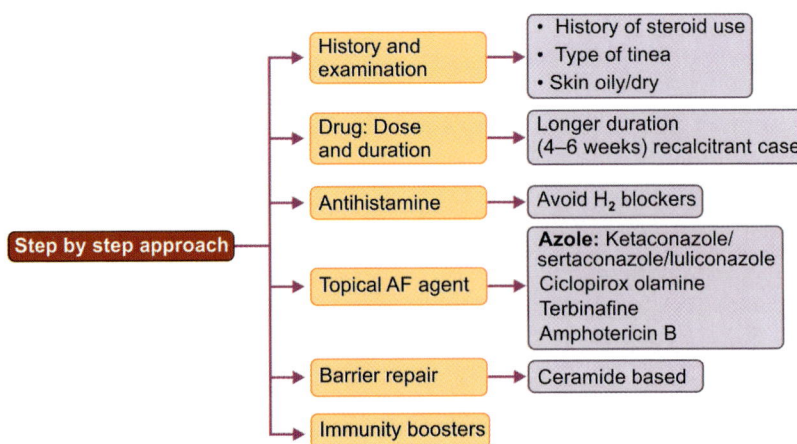

Fig. 11.5: Important points to consider while treating recalcitrant dermatophytosis

tinea are bound to take more time to respond *without* resistance. Hence not every prolonged therapy equates with *in vitro* resistance.

Also it is a good idea to assess whether the patient has a dry or oily skin as TER and ITR both are lipophilic and may not work in a patient with dry skin. Here fluconazole is a better option, if the strain is sensitive to it. For a patient with a predominant sweaty skin GRI and KET are good options.

Step 2: Drug: Dose and Duration

There is a form of persistent tinea infection usually caused by *T. rubrum* at sites in the groin or the trunk which, while responding initially to treatment with either terbinafine or itraconazole, relapses quickly. Different treatment regimens have been tried including combinations of oral azoles or allylamine plus topical azoles or allylamines. In contrast, tinea in immunosuppressed patients, including those with HIV/AIDS, usually respond to treatment although it is often necessary to double the normal dose.

A summary of the dose and duration is given below. The local mycological pattern is crucial and the preferred drugs today seem to be ITR or TER which should ideally be tailored based on *in vitro* data.

1. **Terbinafine:** The usual adult dose is 250 mg once daily. The duration of treatment depends on the site and severity of the infection. Standard dermatological therapy books have given a dose of 2–6 weeks in tinea pedis, 2–4 weeks in tinea cruris and 4 weeks in tinea corporis. [71]

   a. Tinea corporis and tinea cruris: **250 mg daily for 4 weeks**

   b. Tinea pedis and mannum: **250 mg daily for 2–6 weeks**

   c. Tinea imbricata: **250 mg PO daily for 4 weeks**

   d. Off-label double dose **(250 mg BD)**. This has been recommended only in immuno-suppressed patients including those with HIV/AIDS. [2]

We have been using 250 mg BD which makes a lot more pharmacological sense than 500 mg OD as this is a time dependent drug and not a concentration dependent drug (personal communication Dr David R Andes). The company that promoted 500 mg wrongly misinterpreted the quoted studies, as the promoted studies had actually used 250 mg BD (also *see* Chapter 9). [65]

2. **Itraconazole:** It is active against a wide range of dermatophytes and is effective in regimens of 100 mg for 15 days in tinea cruris and corporis or 30 days in dry-type tinea pedis. The currently preferred regimen by clinician uses 400 mg a day, given as two daily doses of 200 mg. [72,73] In tinea corporis, 1 week of therapy at this dosage is sufficient and in dry-type tinea pedis, 2 weeks. Occasionally, longer periods of treatment are needed.

   Here the dose of this drug is based on the AUC/MIC ratio and skin PK studies. Hence a higher dose is needed in palm and soles as these are not sebum rich sites while the drug is primarily *lipophilic*. [3–5,12,13] Studies have shown that 200 mg BD is not always needed as 100 mg BD achieves sufficiently high levels in the skin. But if used, this dose (200 mg BD) may achieve a faster response. [74]

   So the take home message is that 200 mg BD is ideally for lipid poor sites like palms and soles and using them for conventional lipophilic sites (corporis, cruris) is not required.

   a. Tinea corporis, tinea cruris

   > *Itraconazole:* **100 mg 7 to 14 days**
   > **200 mg BD 7 days**

   In India we often have to use a much longer duration. This may reflect two issues: One is the quality of the drug (98+ brands of ITR in India with variability in pellets) and also the local immune suppression due to steroids which takes time to recover. As 2–3 weeks is the time for the host immunity to recover after stopping steroids, during this period almost nothing would respond. This may account for the longer durations needed.

b. Tinea pedis and mannum

Itraconazole: **100 mg/day for 30 days**

200 mg daily for 2–4 weeks

200 mg BD for 7 days

c. Majocchi's granuloma: **Itraconazole 200 mg PO BD for 7 days, then off for 14 days (repeat 3 times total)**

d. Tinea imbricata: **Itraconazole 100 mg PO OD for 4 weeks**

3. **Fluconazole:** Though various regimens have been used, we feel that its use should be based on its secretion profile, and it is ideal for "dry" skin types and can achieve very high skin levels. But it must be noted that the levels do not last long enough after stopping therapy.[61,75]

Dose: **50–100 mg OD for 20 days.**

4. **Ketoconazole:** The suggested dosage is 200–400 mg daily for 4–8 weeks.

This drug has been found to have comparable efficacy, based on *in vitro* data, to ITR. But it requires frequent monitoring of liver functions. Some clinicians are using this drug as the abysmal quality of ITR brands have lead to a situation where patients are aware of the salt and its perceived "failure". With ketoconazole, quality is yet not an issue.

5. **Voriconazole:** The same has been discussed in a previous chapter. Without wasting time or breath it is sufficient to point out that the drug has a miniscule skin secretion. Thus except for side effects and cost and possible litigation, little extra will be achieved.

Its "perceived" use is possibly based on *in vitro* data, where it is found to be equipotent to ITR. But the incorrect use in dermatophytoses is inexplicable, more so when it does not reach the epidermis in sufficient amounts.

Considering the remarkably low MIC to ITR and luliconazole, there is no logic of combination or sequential therapy of oral antifungals. Extending this concept from deep fungal infection to tinea is scientifically ill conceived.

Overview of dosimetry is given in Fig. 11.6.

Step 3: Antihistamines

These are important to prevent skin damage consequent to incessant itching, which is one of the causes for penetration of the fungi (*see* barrier repair above). Most clinicians give hydroxyzine, while some administer doxepin which being a H_2 blocker may reduce the absorption of ITR. Hence an alternative drug should be used in case ITR is prescribed.

Step 4: Topical Drugs

(Luliconazole, ketoconazole, sertaconazole, terbinafine, ciclopirox-olamine, amphotericin B).

Topical drugs are useful as they reach higher skin levels than the systemic drugs. These should be continued for 2 weeks after resolution and ideally should be applied beyond the visible margins of the lesion.

A good adjuvant is *topical salicylic acid 6%,* which helps to increase the penetration of topical antifungals and desquamates the stratum corneum, the site of infection by dermatophytes. Whitfield ointment is another option.[76–78] These can be used in noninflamed tinea variants and are rapidly effective in combination with topical antifungal agents. However, irritancy may be an issue.

Our own experience is that luliconazole and ketoconazole are better than the other azoles. Butenafine is more efficacious than terbinafine and ciclopirox olamine is a potentially useful drug.

As far as *combination* of topical and oral is concerned, this is based on *in vitro* "checkerboard data".[79] Herein, varying levels of each drug are added to the culture plate and assessed. Such studies can show synergism or

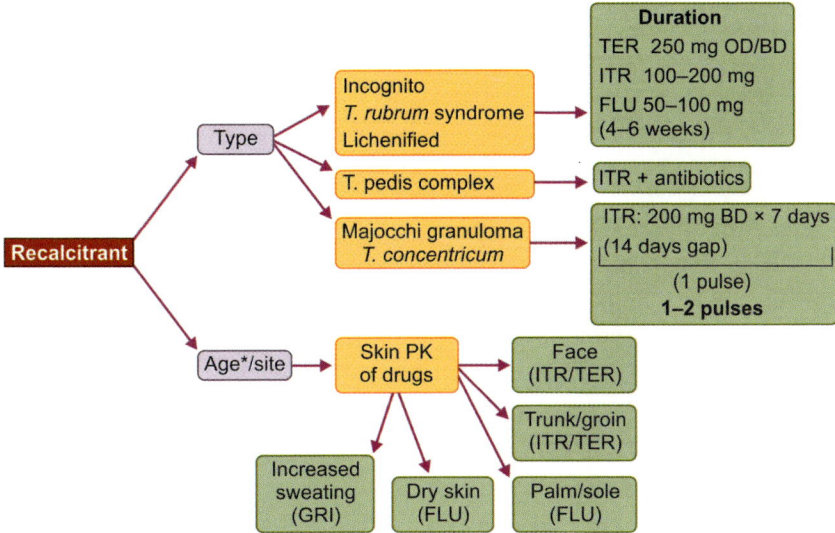

Fig. 11.6: A chart depicted the ideal drug based on site, age, skin type and morphology of tinea infection based on published *in vitro* and *in vivo* data gleaned from pubmed
*Ideal drug for children is fluconazole, based on its hydrophilic non-eccrine and non-lipophilic nature.
ITR: Itraconazole, FLU: Fluconazole, GRI: Grisefulvin, TER: Terbinafine

indifference. A classic example is *amphotericin B and azoles* which are antagonistic and thus should not be combined. *In vitro* susceptibility testing indicates that *ciclopirox* may have a broad antimicrobial profile including on dermatophytes, yeasts and other nondermatophytes. *In vitro* evaluation of activity of ciclopirox and terbinafine suggests many instances of synergy or additivism; for ciclopirox and itraconazole there may be indifference, synergy or additivism.

We have a two drug preference again based on mycological data. For those who cannot afford expensive drugs, topical ketaconazole is a good option (with low MIC values) while another good, but expensive, option is luliconazole which is plagued by the innumerable brands quality.

Step 5: Barrier Repair

This is a crucial step and should be added to the therapy with and after resolution. A good nonkeratolytic moisturiser with barrier repair will prevent recurrence too. And, at least in the initial phase of treatment, emollients have an adjunctive role in producing symptomatic relief as well. In fact, wherever the tinea eruption is inflamed, a simple barrier cream (ceramide) has salutary effects.

The use of barrier repair is based on studies that show that barrier repair helps both in upregulation of immunity and also helps to prevent relapses of dermatophyte infection. It also increases beta defensins.

CONCLUSIONS

We have detailed various plausible causes for the present epidemic of recalcitrant dermatophytoses in India in the text above. Apart from the most talked of and researched *in vitro* susceptibility testing, a plethora of factors related to the clinical presentation (lichenified tinea cruris, Majocchi's granuloma, tinea manuum/pedis, incognito tinea, etc.), organism (shift to *T. mentagrophytes* and *T. interdigitale*), host factors (steroid abuse, compliance, barrier defects) and drugs (ideal drug for a site, PK/PD characteristics, drug quality) are likely to play an important part (Fig. 11.7).

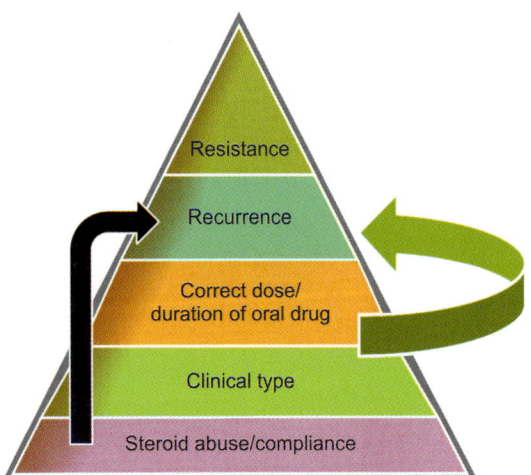

Fig. 11.7: Pyramid of causes of recalcitrant dermatophytosis. Most of the cases of recurrences can be explained by steroid abuse, lack of compliance, clinical type of infection and this in conjunction with the drug quality and doses can explain the situation. A thorough reading of *in vitro* data suggests that the issue of resistance is grossly overemphasized

Treatment should be guided by clinical response in conjunction with local *in vitro* sensitivity data. Updosing may be justified and offer pharmacokinetic and pharmacody-namic advantages but only till a certain point; more than 250 mg BD of terbinafine and more than 100 mg BD of ITR (except on plams and soles) is unlikely to produce any added effects (except probably the rapidity of response with higher dose ITR). Also some data shows that ketaconazole may be a better choice (mycolo-gically and economically) in certain cases.[83,84]

The need of the hour is to clinically correlate MIC sensitivity data and drug PK/PD studies. As the latter are not easy to do, we need to focus on clinical correlates of *in vitro* data. Also we need to see if virulence studies and data[51] would matter, though anthrophilic species have almost identical virulence secretors.[80] There is some recent data that has looked at genomic verifications of fungal proteins and enzymes regulated by multiple genes that are activated or repressed in response to the ambient environment of the host.[82] The HSP90, HSF1, and pacC genes are crucial and chemical inhibition of HSP90 results in increased susceptibility of *T. rubrum* to itraconazole.[82] These molecules provide arenas that may be potential therapeutic targets, as the presently available antifungal drugs are largely focused on a few limited metabolic pathways. Potential antifungal agents undergoing clinical investigation include: VT-1161, Drug 33525, LAS41003, ME-1111.[85]

We also need to focus on the pathogenesis of dermatophytoses and look beyond the drugs, towards the host immunity and its suppression. This will make us appreciate that sometimes the "truth is simpler than it seems". How the steroid abuse will be curtailed is luckily not in our purview, but needless to say most of this mess is due to a replication of our prescriptions by GPs and thus an emphatic dictate by us on our prescriptions may probably get the message across. As they say "imitation is the best form of flattery"; where legislation has failed this might succeed!

References

1. Odom R. Pathophysiology of dermatophyte infections. J Am Acad Dermatol. 1993;28:S2–S7.

2. Sardana K. Recalcitrant Dermatomycosis: Focus On Tinea corporis/cruris/pedis in Fungal Infections Diagnosis and Treatment. Sardana K, Mahajan K, Mrig PA. CBS Publishers, 2017, Delhi. 104–26.

3. Lever LR, Dykes PJ, Thomas R, et al. How orally administered terbinafine reaches the stratum corneum. J Dermatol Treat 1990;1:23–5.

4. Faergemann J, Zehender H, Denouël J, et al. Levels of terbinafine in plasma, stratum corneum, dermis-epidermis (without stratum corneum), sebum, hair and nails during and after 250 mg terbinafine orally once per day for four weeks. Acta Derm Venereol 1993;73:305–9.

5. Cauwenbergh G, Degreef H, Heykants J, et al. Pharmacokinetic profile of orally administered itraconazole in human skin. J Am Acad Dermatol 1988;18:263–8.

6. Majid I, Sheikh G, Kanth F, Hakak R. Relapse after Oral Terbinafine Therapy in Dermatophytosis: A

Clinical and Mycological Study. Indian J Dermatol. 2016;61:529–33. doi: 10.4103/0019-5154. 190120.

7. Sharma R, Adhikari L, Sharma RL. Recurrent dermatophytosis: A rising problem in Sikkim, a Himalayan state of India. Indian J Pathol Microbiol. 2017:541–45.

8. Mahar S, Mahajan K, Agarwal S, Kar HK, Bhattacharya SK.Topical Corticosteroid Misuse: The Scenario in Patients Attending a Tertiary Care Hospital in New Delhi. J Clin Diagn Res. 2016; 10:FC16–FC20.

9. CLSI document M38A-2 (2008a) Reference method for broth dilution antifungal susceptibility testing of lamentous fungi: approved standard, 2nd edn. Clinical and Laboratory Standards Institute, Wayne, PA.

10. Favre B, Ghannoum MA, Ryder NS (2004) Biochemical characterization of terbina fine-resistant *Trichophyton rubrum* isolates. Med Mycol 42:525–29.

11. Ghannoum M Azole. Resistance in Dermatophytes: Prevalence and Mechanism of Action. J Am Podiatr Med Assoc. 2016;106:79–86.

12. Khurana A, Sardana K. Reinterpreting minimum inhibitory concentration (MIC) data of itraconazole versus terbinafine for dermatophytosis-time to look beyond the MIC data? Indian J Dermatol Venereol Leprol. 2017 Dec 14.

13. Sardana K, Arora P, Mahajan K. Intracutaneous pharmacokinetics of oralanti fungals and their relevance in recalcitrant cutaneous dermatophytosis: Time to revisit basics. Indian J Dermatol Venereol Leprol. 2017;83:730–32.

14. Ghannoum M, Isham N, Verma A, Plaum S, Fleischer A Jr, Hardas B. *In vitro* antifungal activity of naftifine hydrochloride against dermatophytes. Antimicrob Agents Chemother. 2013;57: 4369–72.

15. Dutta B, Rasul ES, Boro B. Clinico-epidemiological study of tinea incognito with microbiological correlation. Indian J Dermatol Venereol Leprol. 2017;83:326–31.

16. Dahl MV. Dermatophytosis and the immune response. J Am Acad Dermatol 1994;31: S34–41.

17. Luchsinger I, Bosshard PP, Kasper RS, Reinhardt D, Lautenschlager S. Tinea genitalis: a new entity of sexually transmitted infection? Case series and review of the literature. Sex Transm Infect. 2015;91:493–6.

18. McClellan KJ, Wiseman LR, Markham A. Terbinafine. An update of its use in superficial mycoses. Drugs. 1999;58:179–202.

19. Lanternier F, Pathan S, Vincent QB, Liu L, Cypowyj S, Prando C, et al. Deep dermatophytosis and inherited CARD9 deficiency. N Engl J Med. 2013;369:1704–14.

20. Chastain MA, Reed RJ, Pankey GA. Deep dermatophytosis: report of 2 cases and review of the literature. Cutis. 2001:67:457–62.

21. Weitzman I, Summerbell RC. The dermatophytes. Clin Microbiol Rev. 1995;8:240–59.

22. Manjunath M, Mallikarjun K, Dadapeer, Sushma. Clinicomycological study of Dermatomycosis in a tertiary care hospital Indian J Microbiol Res 2016;3:190–3.

23. Ramaraj V, Vijayaraman RS, Rangarajan S, Kindo AJ. Incidence and prevalence of dermatophytosis in and around Chennai, Tamil Nadu, India. International Journal of Research in Medical Sciences. 2016, 4:695–700.

24. Bhatia VK, Sharma PC. Determination of minimum inhibitory concentrations of itraconazole, terbinafine and ketoconazole against dermatophyte species by broth microdilution method. Indian J Med Microbiol. 2015;33:533–7.

25. Nenoff P, Herrmann J, Gräser Y. *Trichophyton mentagrophytes sive interdigitale*? A dermatophyte in the course of time. J DtschDermatolGes. 2007;5:198–202.

26. Dhib I, Khammari I, Yaacoub A, HadjSlama F, Ben Saïd M, Zemni R, Fathallah A. Relationship Between Phenotypic and Genotypic Characteristics of *Trichophyton mentagrophytes* Strains Isolated from Patients with Dermatophytosis. Mycopathologia. 2017;182:487–93.

27. Jensen JM, Pfeiffer S, Akaki T, Schröder JM, Kleine M, Neumann C, Proksch E, Brasch J. Barrier function, epidermal differentiation, and human beta-defensin 2 expression in tinea corporis. J Invest Dermatol. 2007;127:1720–7.

28. Lee WJ, Kim JY, Song CH, Jung HD, Lee SH, Lee SJ, Kim do W. Disruption of barrier function in dermatophytosis and pityriasis versicolor. J Dermatol. 2011;38:1049–53.

29. Jones HE. Immune response and host resistance to human dermatophyte infection. *J Am Acad Dermatol* 1993; 28: S12–S18.

30. Waldman A, Segal R, Berdicevsky I, Gilhar A. CD4+ and CD8+ T cells mediated direct cytotoxic

effect against *Trichophyton rubrum* and *Trichophyton mentagrophytes*. Int J Dermatol. 2010;49:149–57.

31. de Sousa Mda G, Santana GB, Criado PR, Benard G. Chronic widespread dermatophytosis due to *Trichophyton rubrum*: A syndrome associated with a *Trichophyton* specific functional defect of phagocytes. Front Microbiol2015;6:801.

32. MacCarthy KG, Blake JS, Johnson KL, Dahl MV, Kalish RS. Human dermatophyte-responsive T-cell lines recognize cross-reactive antigens associated with mannose-rich glycoproteins. *Exp Dermatol* 1994;3:66–71.

33. Schmid-Wendtner MH[1], Korting HC. Effective treatment for dermatophytoses of the foot: effect on restoration of depressed cell-mediated immunity. J Eur Acad Dermatol Venereol. 2007;21:1013–8.

34. Gregurek-Novak T[1], Rabatiæ S, Silobrciæ V. Defective phagocytosis in chronic trichophytosis. J Med Vet Mycol. 1993;31:115–20.

35. Martinez-Rossi NM[1], Peres NT[2], Rossi A[3] Pathogenesis of Dermatophytosis: Sensing the Host Tissue. Mycopathologia. 2017;182(1–2): 215–227.

36. T. Koga, H. Duan, K. Urabe, M. Furue Immunohistochemical detection of interferon-gamma-producing cells in dermatophytosis. Eur. J. Dermatol., 11 (2001), pp. 105–7.

37. MRM Campos, M Russo, E Gomes, SR Almeida stimulation, inhibition and death of macrophage infected with *Trichophyton rubrum* Microbes Infect., 8 (2005), pp. 372–79.

38. National Institute for Health and Care Excellence. Fungal skin infection—body and groin. https:// cks.nice.org.uk/fungal-skin-infection-body-and-groin#!scenariorecommendation:1

39. Alston SJ, Cohen BA, Braun M. Persistent and recurrent tinea corporis in children treated with combination antifungal/ corticosteroid agents. Pediatrics 2003;111:201–3.

40. Barkey WF. Striae and persistent tinea corporis related to prolonged use of betamethasone dipropionate 0.05% cream/clotrimazole 1% cream (Lotrisone cream). J Am AcadDermatol 1987;17: 518–9.

41. Reynolds RD, Boiko S, Lucky AW. Exacerbation of tinea corporis during treatment with 1% clotrimazole/betamethasone dipropionate (Lotrisone). Am J Dis Child 1991;145:1224–5.

42. Fleischer AB, Feldman SR. Prescription of high-potency corticosteroid agents and clotrimazole-betamethasone diproprionate by pediatricians. ClinTher1999;21:1725–31.

43. Evans EG, James IG, Seaman RA, Richardson MD Does naftifine have anti-inflammatory properties? A double-blind comparative study with 1% clotrimazole/1% hydrocortisone in clinically diagnosed fungal infection of the skin. Br J Dermatol. 1993;129:437–42.

44. Nada M, Hanafi S, al-Omari H, Mokhtar M, el-Shamy S, Mühlbacher J. Naftifine versus miconazole/ hydrocortisone in inflammatory dermatophyte infections. Int J Dermatol. 1994;33:570–2.

45. Smith EB, Breneman DL, Griffith RF, Hebert AA, Hickman JG, Maloney JM, Millikan LE, Sulica VI, Dromgoole SH, Sefton J, et al. Double-blind comparison of naftifine cream and clotrimazole/ betamethasone dipropionate cream in the treatment of tinea pedis. J Am Acad Dermatol. 1992;26:125–7.

46. Greenberg HL, Shwayder TA, Bieszk N, Fivenson DP. Clotrimazole/betamethasone diproprionate: a review of costs and complications in the treatment of common cutaneous fungal infections. PediatrDermatol. 2002;19:78–81.

47. Högl F, Raab W. The influence of steroids on the antifungal and antibacterial activities of imidazole derivatives (author's transl)]. Mykosen. 1980; 23:426–39.

48. Erbagci Z. Topical therapy for dermatophytoses: Should corticosteroids be included? Am J ClinDermatol. 2004;5:375–84.

49. Rosen T, Elewski BE. Failure of clotrimazole-betamethasone dipropionate cream in treatment of *Microsporum Canis* infections. J Am Acad Dermatol. 1995;32:1050–1.

50. Kelly A, Nelson K, Goodwin M, McCluggage J. Adverse effects of topical corticosteroids. BMJ. 1972;14:114.

51. Allenby CF, Main RA, Marsden RA, Sparkes CG. Effect on adrenal function of topically applied clobetasol propionate (Dermovate) Br Med J. 1975;4:619–21.

52. Wolverton SE. 2nd ed. Philadelphia: Elsevier Inc; 2007. Comprehensive Dermatologic Drug Therapy; p. 144.

53. Kwinter J, Pelletier J, Khambalia A. High-potency steroid use in children with vitiligo: a retrospective

study. Epub 2006 Oct 20 ed :J Am AcadDermatol 2007; 56: 236–41.

54. Kerner M, Ishay A, Ziv M, Rozenman D, Luboshitzky R. Evaluation of the pituitary-adrenal axis function in patients on topical steroid therapy. J Am A cad Dermatol 2011; 65: 215–6.

55. Chittock J, Brown K, Cork MJ, Danby SG. Comparing the Effect of a Twice-weekly Tacrolimus and Betamethasone Valerate Dose on the Subclinical Epidermal Barrier Defect in Atopic Dermatitis. Acta DermVenereol. 2015 ;95:653–8.

56. Onyewu C, Eads E, Schell WA, Perfect JR, Ullmann Y, Kaufman G, Horwitz BA, Berdicevsky I, Heitman J. Targeting the calcineurin pathway enhances ergosterol biosynthesis inhibitors against *Trichophyton mentagrophytes in vitro* and in a human skin infection model. Antimicrob Agents Chemother. 2007;51:3743–6.

57. Bhari N, Saginatham H, Verma KK Tacrolimus induced dermatophyte infection overlying a plaque morphea. DermatolTher. 2017;30(1).

58. Cauwenbergh G, Degreef H, Heykants J, et al. Pharmacokinetic profile of orally administered itraconazole in human skin. J Am Acad Dermatol 1988;18:263–8.

59. Grant SM, Clissold SP. Itraconazole: a review of its pharmacodynamic and pharmacokinetic properties, and therapeutic use in superficial and systemic mycoses. Drugs 1989;37:310–44.

60. Piérard G, Arrese J, De Doncker P. Antifungal activity of itraconazole and terbinafine in human stratum corneum: a comparative study. J Am Acad Dermatol1995;32:429–35.

61. Faergemann J, Laufen H. Levels of fluconazole in serum, stratum corneum, epidermis-dermis (without stratum corneum) and eccrine sweat. ClinExpDermatol1993;18:102–6.

62. Wildfeuer A, Faergemann J, Laufen H, et al. Bioavailability of fluconazole in the skin after oral medication. Mycoses 1994;37:127–30.

63. Gollnick H[1], Cunliffe W, Berson D, Dreno B, Finlay A, Leyden JJ, Shalita AR, Thiboutot D; Global Alliance to Improve Outcomes in Acne. Management of acne: a report from a Global Alliance to Improve Outcomes in Acne. J Am Acad Dermatol. 2003;49:S1–37.

64. von Bernuth H, Wahn V. Systemic treatment with isotretinoin suppresses itraconazole blood level in chronic granulomatous disease. Pediatr Allergy Immunol. 2014;25:405–7.

65. Sardana K, Gupta A. Rational for Drug Dosimetry and Duration of Terbinafine in the Context of Recalcitrant Dermatophytosis: Is 500 mg Better than 250 mg OD or BD? Indian J Dermatol. 2017;62:665–667.

66. Khurana A, Sardana K, Bhardwaj V. Response to 'Clinical presentation of terbinafine-induced severe liver injury and the value of laboratory monitoring: a critically appraised topic'. Br J Dermatol. 2017 Nov 18. doi: 10.1111/bjd.16134.

67. Kabir Sardana. Aastha Gupta, RK Gautam, PK Sharma, Shamik Ghosh: Recalcitrant Dermatophyte Infections: A clinical mycological and mutational Study. Ethics Approval. PGIMER and RMLH. August 2017.

68. Rex JH, Pfaller MA. Has antifungal susceptibility testing come of age? Clin Infect Dis 2002;35:982–89.

69. Daniel J. Diekema and Michael A. Pfaller. Utility of Antifungal Susceptibility Testing and Clinical Correlations. In GS Hall (ed.), Interactions of Yeasts, Moulds, and Antifungal Agents: How to Detect Resistance, 131–58, 2012, Springer New York Dordrecht Heidelberg, London.

70. Havlickova B[1], Friedrich M.The advantages of topical combination therapy in the treatment of inflammatory dermatomycoses. Mycoses. 2008;51:16–26.

71. Gupta AK, Chaudhry M, Elewski B. Tinea corporis, tinea cruris, tine anigra and piedra. Dermatol Clin 2003;21:395–400.

72. Parent D, Decroix J, Heenen M. Clinical experience with short schedules of itraconazole in the treatment of tinea corporis and/or tinea cruris. Dermatology 1994;189:378–81.

73. Gupta AK, De Doncker P, Heremans A, et al. Itraconazole for the treatment of tinea pedis: a dose of 400 mg daily given for 1 week is similar in efficacy to 100 or 200 mg daily given for 2 to 4 weeks. J Am Acad Dermatol1997;36:789–92.

74. Piérard G, Arrese J, De Doncker P. Antifungal activity of itraconazole and terbinafine in human stratum corneum: a comparative study. J Am Acad Dermatol1995;32:429–35.

75. Stary A, Sarnow E. Fluconazole in the treatment of tinea corporis and tinea cruris. Dermatology 1998;196:237–41.

76. Russell D, Russell AD.Treatment of ringworm: old remedy vs. new. J Infect. 1992;24:333.

77. Logan RA, Hay RJ, Whitefield M. Antifungal efficacy of a combination of benzoic and salicylic

acids in a novel aqueous vanishing cream formulation. J Am Acad Dermatol. 1987;16:136–8.

78. Thaker SJ, Mehta DS, Shah HA, Dave JN, Kikani KM. A comparative study to evaluate efficacy, safety and cost-effectiveness between Whitfield's ointment + oral fluconazole versus topical 1% butenafine in tinea infections of skin. Indian J Pharmacol. 2013;45:622–4.

79. Gupta AK, Kohli Y. *In vitro* susceptibility testing of ciclopirox, terbinafine, ketoconazole and itraconazole against dermatophytes and nondermatophytes, and *in vitro* evaluation of combination antifungal activity. Br J Dermatol. 2003; 149:296–305.

80. Tran VD, De Coi N, Feuermann M, Schmid-Siegert E, Bãguþ ET, Mignon B, Waridel P, Peter C, Pradervand S, Pagni M, Monod M. RNA Sequencing-based Genome Reannotation of the Dermatophyte Arthrodermabenhamiae and Characterization of Its Secretome and Whole Gene Expression Profile during Infection. mSystems. 2016; pii: e00036–16.

81. Elavarashi E, Kindo AJ, Rangarajan S. Enzymatic and Non-Enzymatic Virulence Activities of Dermatophytes on Solid Media. J ClinDiagn Res. 2017;11:DC23-DC25.

82. Martinez-Rossi NM, Peres NT, Rossi A. Pathogenesis of Dermatophytosis: Sensing the Host Tissue. Mycopathologia. 2017;182:215–27.

83. Bhatia VK, Sharma PC. Determination of minimum inhibitory concentrations of itraconazole, terbinafine and ketoconazole against dermatophyte species by broth microdilution method. Indian J Med Microbiol. 2015;33:533–7.

84. Afshari MA, Shams-Ghahfarokhi M, Razzaghi-Abyaneh M. Antifungal susceptibility and virulence factors of clinically isolated dermatophytes in Tehran, Iran. Iran JMicrobiol. 2016;8:36–46.

85. Gupta AK[1,2], Foley KA[3], Versteeg SG. New Antifungal Agents and New Formulations Against Dermatophytes. Mycopathologia. 2017; 182:127–41.

12

Treatment of Dermatophytic Infection of Hair

Taru Garg, Sucheta Sharma, Sanjay Kr Rathi

INTRODUCTION

Tinea capitis is superficial fungal infection of the scalp caused by dermatophytes. It mainly affects children. However, it may also be seen in adults in certain circumstances as with immunodeficiency. Dermatophytes have the ability to invade the hair. This ability varies for different species, with some of the species like *M. audouinii, T. schoenleinii* and *T. violaceum* having more propensity for hair invasion. Tinea capitis can be caused by zoophilic or anthropophilic dermatophytes with predominance of later. Zoophilic species cause severe inflammation leading to inflammatory type of tinea capitis. Species of dermatophytes causing tinea capitis may differ in various geographical areas.[1] In India, *T. violaceum* has been most commonly reported to cause tinea capitis.[2,3]

CLINICAL FEATURES

Different types of dermatophytes invade the hair shaft in different manner causing diverse clinical manifestations.

Clinically all types of tinea capitis are characterized by partial, patchy/focal hair loss. Inflammation of varying degrees is seen depending upon causative organisms and host response. Broadly infection can be classified as inflammatory and non-inflammatory types (Tables 12.1 and 12.2).

Atypical presentation of tinea capitis: Tinea capitis is rare after puberty because of certain protective factors, namely the fungistatic property of the sebum, sweat, greater thickness of hair, and presence of *Pityrosporum ovale* as a competing agent in this age group.[4,5] It is rare in adults, but cases have been reported in immunocompromised as well as in immunocompetent adults. Tinea capitis in adults accounts for approximately less than 3% of all tinea capitis cases.[6,7] However, incidence as high as 11% has been reported in the literature.[8]

Mould-induced (other than dermatophytes) tinea capitis should be considered in clinically resistant and atypical cases.[9] In immunocompetent adults, the clinical features are often atypical.[5] The disease may resemble bacterial folliculitis, folliculitis decalvans, dissecting cellulitis, the scarring related to lupus erythematosus,[10] or annular scaly plaques of tinea corporis (Figs 12.5 and 12.6).

In some cases, alopecia is minimal or absent and infection presents as generalized, diffuse scaling of the scalp, resembling dandruff. It may present as concentric rings of papules and pustules with slight scaling on the scalp along with diffuse thinning of hair.[11] In any adult with a patchy, inflammatory scalp disorder, mycological samples should be sent for laboratory analysis. It has been suggested that adult family members of children with tinea

Table 12.1: Types of hair invasion		
Microsporum type		
Hair shaft is invaded at the level of mid follicle. Intrapilary hyphae grow inwards towards the bulb of the hair. Arthroconidia are present on the surface.		
Species	M. audouinii M. audouinii var. rivallieri M. canis M. canis var. distortum M. equinum M. ferrugineum	M. gypseum M. fulvum M. nanum
Size of arthroconidia	2–3 micrometer	5–8 micrometer
Type (based on spores)	Small-spored ectothrix	Small-spored ectothrix
Wood's lamp examination	Fluorescence is characteristic	Fluorescence in some cases
Clinical type	Grey patch	Grey patch
Trichophyton types		
Arrangement of hyphae and spores	Extrapilary hyphae form arthroconidia on external surface of the hair shaft	Intrapilary hyphae form arthroconidia within the hair shaft	Broad regular septate hyphae and air spaces are present within the hair shaft
Species	T. verrucosum T. mentagrophytes T. megninii T. rubrum (rarely)	T. tonsurans T. soudanense T. violaceum T. yaoundei T. gourvilii T. rubrum (rarely)	T. schoenleinii
Size of arthroconidia	10 micrometer	8 micrometer	—
Type	Large-spored ectothrix	Endothrix	No spores
Clinical type	Kerion	Black dot	Favus

Table 12.2: Clinical manifestations of tinea capitis			
Non-inflammatory		Inflammatory	
Grey patch	Black dot	Kerion	Favus
Patches of partial hair loss with numerous broken off dull grey hair due to presence of arthrospores on the surface. Well defined patches with minimal or no inflammation and fine white scales (Fig. 12.1)	Usually multiple patches of hair loss with minimal scaling, characteristically showing black dots, which are broken off hair caused by breakage of hair shaft close to the surface of the scalp (Fig. 12.2)	Painful, inflammatory boggy swelling covered with pustules and loose matted hair Lymphadenopathy is common. Superadded bacterial infection may occur (Figs 12.3 and 12.4)	Characterized by scutula, which are yellowish cup shaped crusts around hair shaft. Neighboring crusts may coalesce. Scarring and atrophy are features of this type of tinea capitis
Green fluorescence			Greenish grey fluorescence

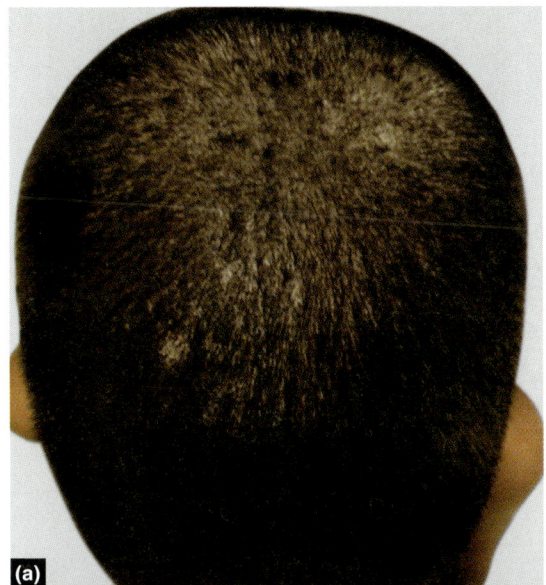

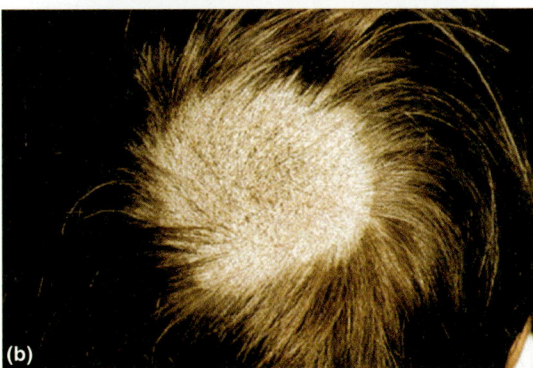

Figs 12.1a and b: Patchy hair loss with scalp scaling

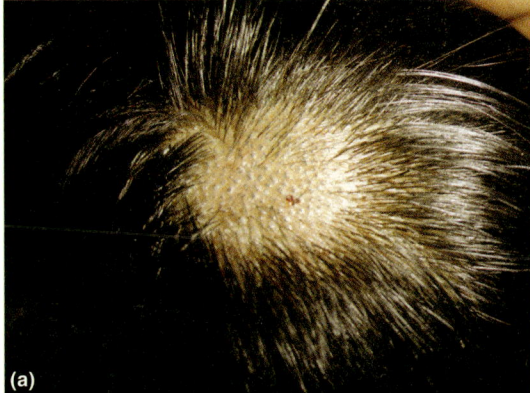

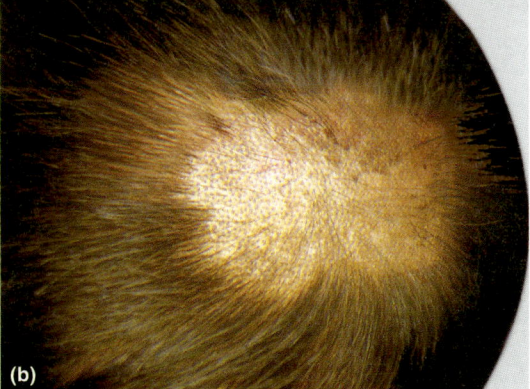

Figs 12.2a and b: 'Black dot' type of tinea capitis

capitis infection, should be treated prophylactically with antifungal shampoos as they may be asymptomatic carriers of the dermatophytes.[12]

DIFFERENTIAL DIAGNOSIS

It includes conditions characterized by focal and or patchy hair loss, with (lichen planopilaris, discoid lupus erythematosus) or without scarring (alopecia areata, trichotillomania, traumatic alopecia), or scalp scaling (seborrheic dermatitis, tinea amiantacea), or pustules (bacterial pyoderma, folliculitis decalvans, dissecting cellulitis of scalp).[1, 13]

INVESTIGATIONS

Microscopy, culture and Wood's lamp examination are the main methods for confirmation of diagnosis after clinical suspicion. Culture is gold standard for the diagnosis. Hair infected by certain dermatophytes produces a characteristic fluorescence (as mentioned in Table 12.1) in UV light filtered by Wood's glass. Trichoscopy is a rapid, non-invasive, inexpensive and reliable diagnostic tool.[14] Comma hair, corkscrew hair, pigtail hair and morse code-like hair are specific trichoscopic features, seen in tinea capitis (see Chapter 4).[14]

Future diagnostic tools which are being studied, are molecular ones (different types of PCR). However, large scale studies are required to compare the diagnostic sensitivity of microscopy, culture and PCR.[13, 15]

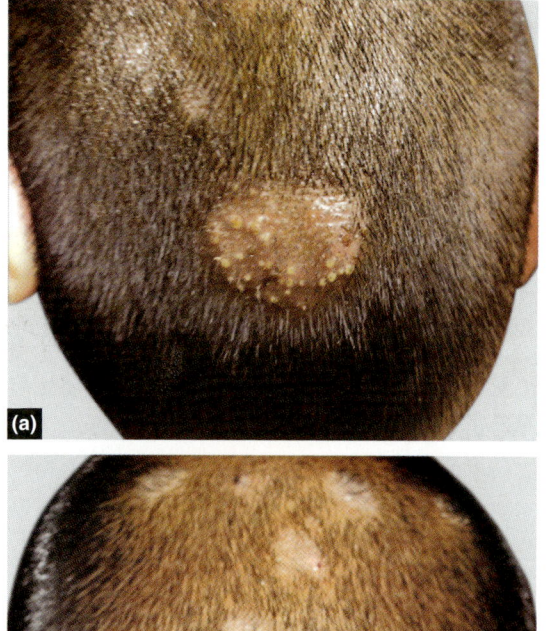

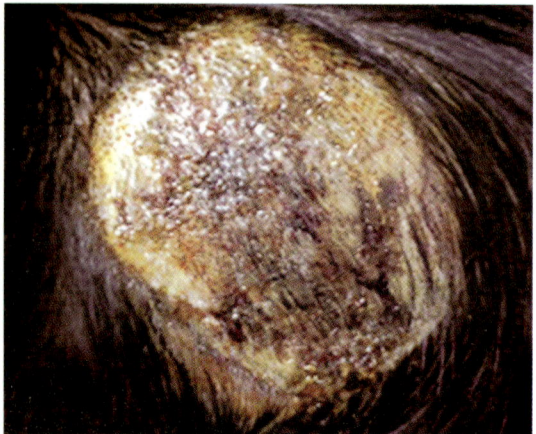

Figs 12.3a and b: Boggy swelling studded with pustules: Kerion

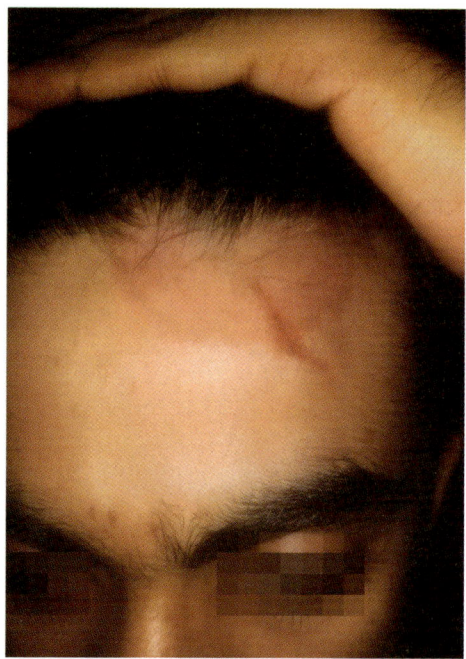

Fig. 12.5a: Annular scaly plaque extending onto the scalp

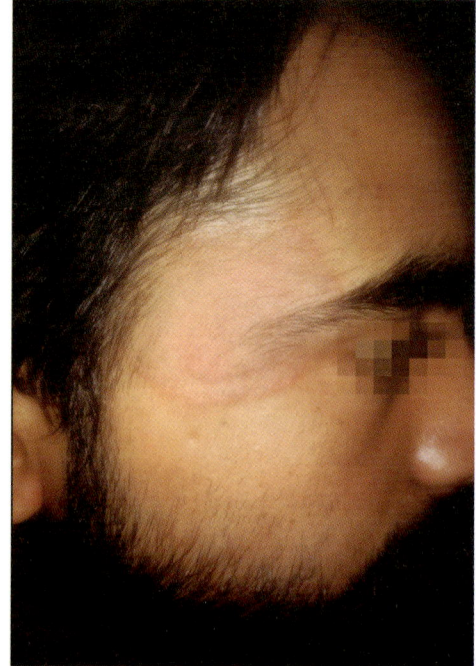

Fig. 12.4: Patchy hair loss with pus and crusting on the surface

Fig. 12.5b: Annular plaque on face with involvement of eyebrow

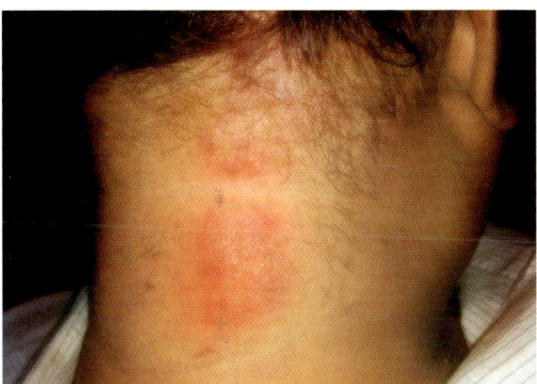

Fig. 12.6: Annular plaque on neck with involvement of scalp

Collection of Sample for Microscopy and Culture

Affected, easily pluckable loose and dull hairs are removed with help of forceps along with scalp scrapings with the help of surgical blade from the lesion. Brush samples may be taken for culture. Disposable toothbrush is brushed firmly through the hair and is then pressed against the culture medium in a Petri dish. This technique is helpful in screening large number of children. In cases of kerion, a transport swab is wiped after de-roofing the pustules and is sent for potassium hydroxide (KOH) smear, Gram's stain and for culture and sensitivity for bacteria (see Chapter 3).[1,16]

Microscopy

It should be carried out on scalp scrapings and plucked hair, by mounting in 10% KOH.[1] Infected hair are very delicate and tend to disintegrate if left for more than a few minutes in KOH, so the smear should be examined as soon as possible after mounting.[1] Presence of hyphae and/or arthroconidia should be reported. It is the most rapid method to establish fungal infection when culture report is awaited. However, false negative result range from 5 to 15% and depends on the skill of observer as well as quality of sampling. Calcofluor white may be added to facilitate the visualization of fungal structures, but

fluorescence microscope is required for this (see Chapter 3).[16]

Culture

Different media for culture are Sabouraud's dextrose agar (SDA), Emmon's modification of SDA, mycobiotic agar and dermatophyte test medium (DTM). Antibiotics and cycloheximide are added to reduce the bacterial contamination and to inhibit the growth of non-dermatophytic moulds respectively. Cultures are incubated at 20–30°C for 3–4 weeks and examined macroscopically twice a week. Usually signs of growth are seen at 7–10 days. Patients are asked to collect the culture report at 4th week after sample collection (see Chapter 3).[16]

TREATMENT

Oral antifungal therapy is the mainstay of treatment in tinea capitis. Topical antifungals are used as an adjuvant to prevent the transmission to other people. Topical agents include: Povidone–iodine, ketoconazole 2% and selenium sulfide 1% shampoos.[15] Asymptomatic carriers who harbor infection without any signs and symptoms of tinea capitis should be treated with antimycotic drugs.[16] Screening of all the family members is recommended.[15] General measures must be explained in detail, as not to share pillows, towels and combs.

Griseofulvin was the first effective oral drug used for the treatment of tinea capitis. Other drugs are terbinafine, itraconazole, fluconazole and ketoconazole. For the infections caused by *Trichophyton* species, *terbinafine* is superior to griseofulvin while for infection by *Microsporum* species, *griseofulvin* is superior to terbinafine.[15,17] We have seen good response to terbinafine even in grey patch type of tinea capitis, caused by *Microsporum* species without any treatment failure.

Griseofulvin

Griseofulvin is a fungistatic drug that inhibits nucleic acid synthesis, arrests cell division at metaphase and impairs synthesis of the cell wall. Currently it is available with us in micronized form. Earlier ultra-micronized form was also available. Suspension form is available in very few countries but not in India. Treatment duration with griseofulvin is longer as compared to terbinafine and itraconazole. It is given at the dose of 15–20 mg/kg for 6–8 weeks. Taking the drug with fatty food may increase the absorption and improve bioavailability. Higher dosage (25 mg/kg) for longer period may be required in resistant cases.[15]

Side-effects occur in 20% of cases, mostly gastrointestinal upset, particularly diarrhea, rashes and headache. The drug is contraindicated in pregnancy and men are cautioned against fathering a child for 6 months after the treatment.

Other contraindications: Lupus erythematosus, porphyria, severe liver disease.

Drug interactions: With warfarin, ciclosporin and oral contraceptive pills.

Terbinafine

Terbinafine is an allylamine that acts on the cell membrane and is fungicidal. It shows activity against all dermatophytes, but has higher efficacy against *Trichophyton* species than *Microsporum*. At higher dosage, terbinane is more effective against *M. canis* but confers no advantage over griseofulvin, and prolonging treatment duration does not improve efficacy. This is partly because the minimum inhibitory concentration of terbinafine (and to some extent for itraconazole) can exceed the maximum reported concentration of the drug in hair infected with *M. canis*, contributing to treatment failures. Additionally, terbinafine is not excreted in the sweat or sebum of prepubertal children, and cannot be incorporated into the hair shaft, thereby does not effectively reach the scalp surface where the arthroconidia are located in infections caused by *Microsporum* species, accounting for its relative inefficacy in such infections.[15]

The absorption characteristics of terbinafine are not altered when it is taken with food. The dose is given according to weight as: 62.5 kg for weight <20 kg, 125 mg for weight 20–40 kg and 250 mg for weight >40 kg/day. Duration of treatment is 4–6 weeks, shorter than griseofulvin.

Side-effects include gastrointestinal disturbances and rashes.[17]

Advantages: Fungicidal, shorter treatment regimens, better compliance and safety.

Drug interactions: Plasma concentration is decreased by rifampicin and is increased by cimetidine.

Itraconazole

Itraconazole exhibits both fungicidal and fungistatic activity depending on the tissue concentration of the drug. However, like other azoles, its primary mode of action is fungistatic, through depletion of cell-membrane ergosterols, which interferes with membrane permeability. Doses of 50–100 mg daily for 4 weeks or 5 mg/kg daily for 2–4 weeks have comparable efficacy with griseofulvin or terbinafine.[15,17] Absorption of itraconazole may be increased when it is administered with a cola beverage.

All these oral antifungals are available in tablet/capsule formulations. For griseofulvin and terbinafine scored tablet of 250 mg is available which can be divided/broken and can be given according to weight of the child. If children cannot take tablets or the dose is less than the available preparation then it can be dispensed in the form of powder or suspension by the pharmacist.

SUMMARY

To summarize investigations as detailed above, are carried out in clinically suspected cases of tinea capitis for confirmation of diagnosis and to exclude other differential diagnosis. Treatment is started based on clinical type, while awaiting culture report. Terbinafine is easily available, required for shorter duration and is primarily used for infection due to *Trichophyton* species. However, griseofulvin should be used wherever *Microsporum* species is suspected to be the cause. General measures and need for antifungal shampoos should be explained to prevent the transmission of infection. Ideally the endpoint of treatment is clinical and mycological cure.

Acknowledgment

Figures 12.1b, 12.2b and 12.4 are contributed by Dr Sanjay K Rathi, MD, Consultant Dermatologist Siliguri.

References

1. Hay RJ, Ashbee HR. Mycology. In: Burns DA, Breathnach SM, Cox N, Griffith CS (eds). Rook's Textbook of Dermatology. 8th ed. Oxford: Wiley Blackwell 2010; 25–8.

2. Kalla G, Begra B, Solanki A, Goyal A, Batra A. Clinicomycological study of tinea capitis in Desert District of Rajasthan. Indian J Dermatol Venereol Leprol 1995; 61:342–5.

3. Grover C, Arora P, Manchanda V. Tinea capitis in the pediatric population: A study from North India. Indian J Dermatol Venereol Leprol 2010; 76:527–32.

4. Lateur N, J Andre, J de Maubeuge, Poncin M, Song M. Tinea capitis in two Black African adults with HIV infection. Br J Dermatol 1999; 140:722–4.

5. Cremer G, Bournerias I, Vandemer Lerbroucke E, Houin R, Revuz J. Tinea capitis in adults: Misdiagnosis or reappearance? Dermatology 1997; 194:8–11.

6. Pursley TV, Raimer SS. Tinea capitis in the elderly. Int J Dermatol 1980; 12:220.

7. Terragni L, Lasagni A, Oriani A. Tinea capitis in adults. Mycoses 1989; 32:482–6.

8. Lee JY, Hsu ML. Tinea capitis in adults in Southern Taiwan. Int J Dermatol 1991; 30:572–5.

9. Chokoeva AA, Zisova L, Chorleva K, Tchernev G. *Aspergillus niger* — a possible new etiopathogenic agent in tinea capitis. Presentation of two cases. Braz J Infect Dis 2016; 20:303–7.

10. Sperling LC. Inflammatory tinea capitis (kerion) mimicking dissecting cellulitis. Occurrence in two adolescents. Int J Dermatol 1991; 30:190–192.

11. Narang K, Pahwa M, Ramesh V. Tinea capitis in the form of concentric rings in an HIV positive adult on antiretroviral treatment. Indian J Dermatol 2012; 57:288–90.

12. Management of scalp ringworm. Drug Therap Bull 1996; 34:5–6.

13. Hay RJ, Tinea Capitis: Current Status. Mycopathologia 2017; 182:87–93.

14. Elghblawi E. Idiosyncratic findings in trichoscopy of tinea capitis: Comma, zigzag hairs, corkscrew, and morse code-like hair. Int J Trichol 2016;8:180–3.

15. LC Fuller, RC Barton, MF Mohd Mustapa, LE Proudfoot, SP Punjabi, EM Higgins. British Association of Dermatologists' guidelines for the management of tinea capitis. Br J Dermatol 2014; 171:454–63.

16. Bennassar A, Grimalt R. Management of tinea capitis in childhood. Clin Cosmet Investig Dermatol 2010; 3: 89–98.

17. Chen X, Jiang X, Yang M, González U, Lin X, Hua X, et al. Systemic antifungal therapy for tinea capitis in children. Cochrane Database Syst Rev., 2016; 5.

13

Treatment of Dermatophytic Infection of Nail

Chander Grover, Prachi Kawthekar

INTRODUCTION

Among the various dermatological diseases, tinea unguium (dermatophyte infection of the nail) remains a formidable challenge. It is cosmetically distressing, causes a functional compromise, is a reservoir for dermatophyte skin infections and at the same time is very difficult to manage.[1] It is an important co-morbidity in patients with diabetes or immunosuppression.

CAUSATIVE FACTORS

Onychomycosis, a fungal infection of nails can be caused by many fungi; however, the majority of these are dermatophytes (68%).[2] Other fungi include yeasts (*Candida* species) and non-dermatophyte moulds. The most common dermatophyte implicated is *Trichophyton rubrum*.[2]

Clinical Features

Depending on the pattern of invasion, an individual nail can present with any of the following clinical types. More often however, a combination of different types exists:

1. **Distal and lateral subungual onychomycosis (most common):** The fungus infects the keratin of the hyponychium followed by proximal migration to involve the nailbed and plate (Fig. 13.1). It is most commonly caused by *Trichophyton rubrum*.

2. **Endonyx onychomycosis:** The fungus infects the nail plate, growing between its lamellae. It is most commonly caused by *T. soudanense* and presents as milky white discoloration of nail plate with no nail plate hyperkeratosis or onycholysis (Fig. 13.2).

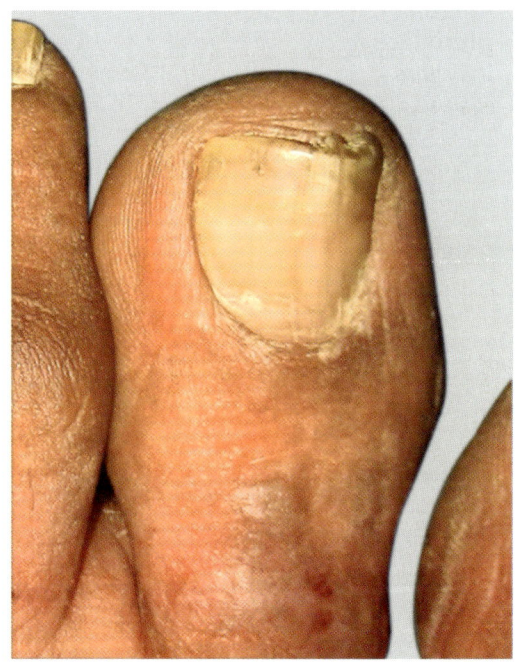

Fig. 13.1: Distal and lateral subungual onychomycosis

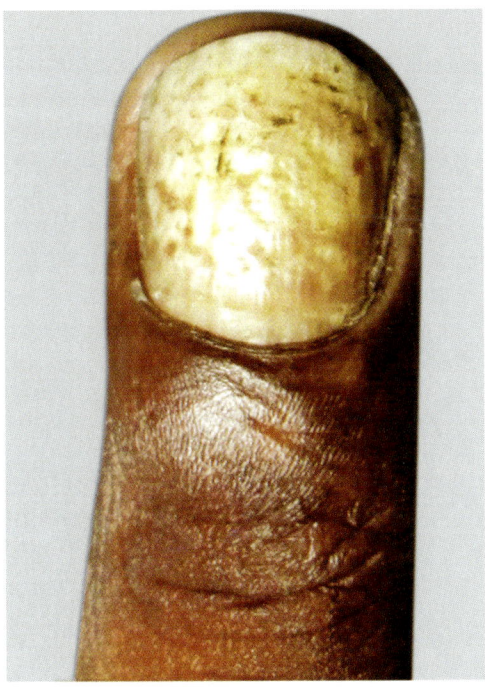

Fig. 13.2: Endonyx onychomycosis

3. **Superficial white onychomycosis:** The fungus infects the dorsal aspect of the nail plate followed by entire nail plate involvement (Fig. 13.3). It is most commonly caused by *T. mentagrophytes.*

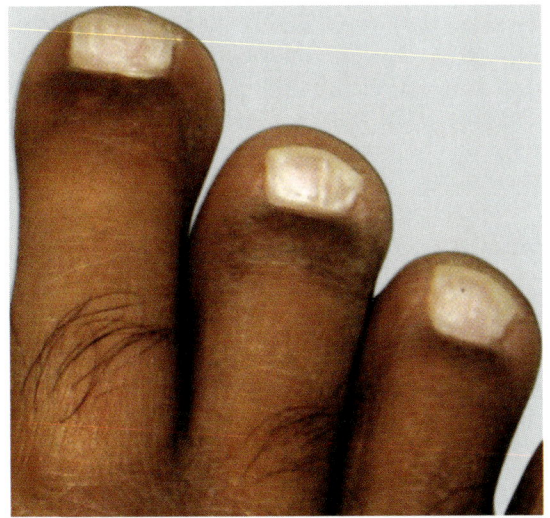

Fig. 13.3: Superficial white onychomycosis

4. **Proximal subungual onychomycosis:** The fungus first infects the proximal part of the nailbed followed by migration distally (Fig. 13.4). It is most commonly caused by *T. rubrum* and *T. megninii.*

5. **Total dystrophic onychomycosis:** This could be primary as seen with chronic mucocutaneous candidiasis or could be secondary to extensive involvement with any of the types identified above (Fig. 13.5).[2]

Dermatophytoma is a special type presenting as single or multiple white or yellow bands visible on the nail plate (Fig. 13.6). It is proposed that biofilm contributes to the development of the same, which further leads to decreased drug penetration and resistance to therapy. Usually a combination of different therapeutic approaches is required to manage a dermatophytoma.[3]

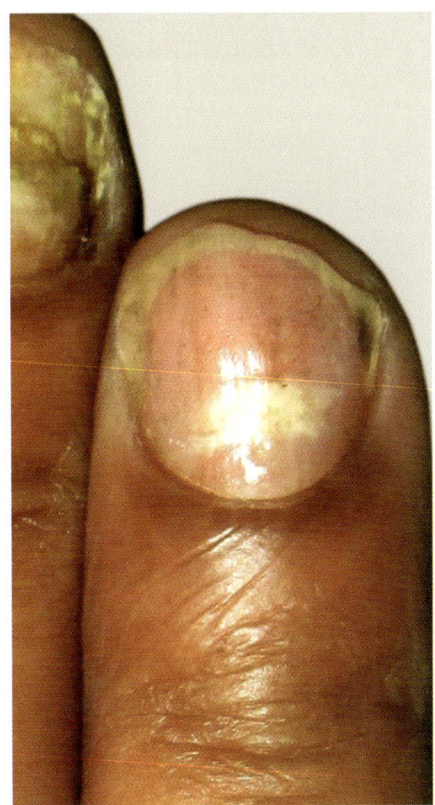

Fig. 13.4: Proximal subungual onychomycosis

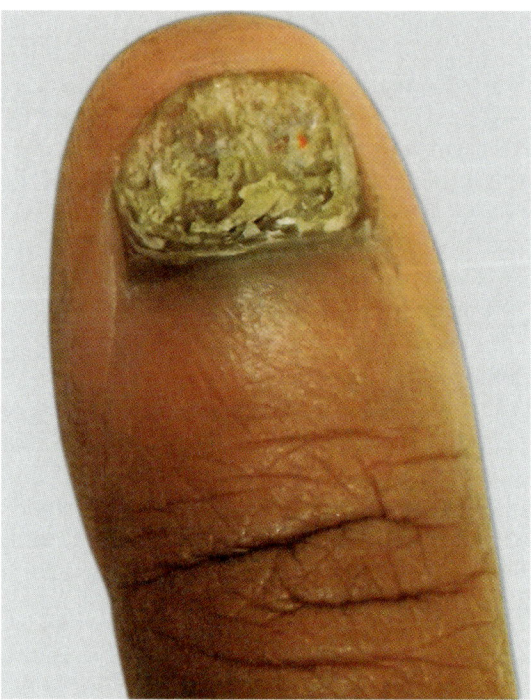

Fig. 13.5: Total dystrophic onychomycosis

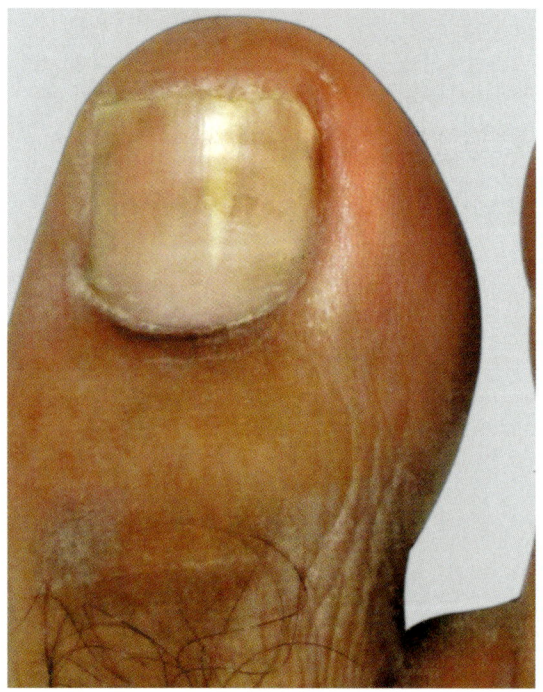

Fig. 13.6: Dermatophytoma

Differential Diagnosis

Roughly 50% of nail dystrophies are a result of onychomycosis; other mimickers could include traumatic damage, AGNUS (asymmetrical gait nail unit syndrome), nail psoriasis or chronic paronychia induced nail changes. It is especially important to rule out inflammatory and systemic causes of nail dystrophy, in case a large number of nails is involved.[4]

Diagnostic Considerations

It has been shown that onychomycosis cannot be reliably diagnosed based on clinical criteria alone. An isolated study from the US concluded that empirical treatment with terbinafine is more cost-effective than confirmatory tests done beforehand; however, this may be applicable to dermatophyte infections only. Also, economic considerations may be different for different countries, and the length of treatment along with potential medicolegal implications of prolonged therapy need to be kept in mind. Hence, it is recommended to confirm diagnosis before starting the treatment by direct microscopy, fungal culture and/or histopathology with PAS staining.[2, 5]

The diagnostic advantage offered by onychoscopy (dermatoscopy of nail) is being increasingly recognized. The characteristic reported changes include jagged proximal edge of onycholysis; characteristic color changes in an "Aurora Borealis" pattern; and whitish spikes within the onycholysed areas[6] (Fig. 13.7).

Management Considerations

In the past clinicians often faced the question, whether to treat onychomycosis or not, primarily because of limited treatment options. However, as of today, clinicians prefer to treat onychomycosis with the wider options available, especially because of the compromised quality of life, potential disabilities and limitations, risk of dissemination and secondary complications these patients encounter.[7]

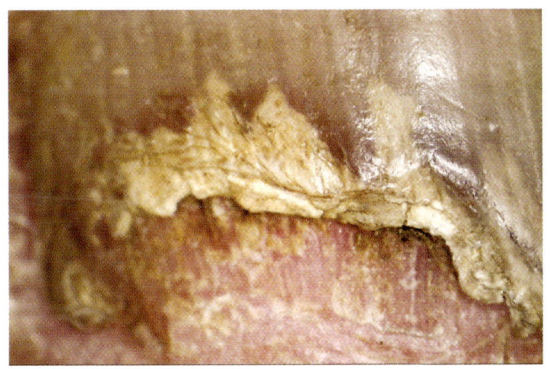

Fig. 13.7: Jagged proximal edge of distal onycholysis in a case of onychomycosis (Dinolite AM7915MZT with 50X)

Pre-treatment Considerations

The goal of treatment is to have clinically healthy nails free of fungus. Different studies have used different criteria for evaluating treatment efficacy in the form of clinical cure (defined as varied percentages of diseased free nail), mycological cure (defined as negative microscopy and culture) or complete cure (a combination of clinical and mycological cure).

A determination of baseline disease severity can be done with a numerical severity grading system known as the Onychomycosis Severity Score (OSI) devised by Carney et al (Table 13.1). It is a simple numerical score that could help in prognosticating and determining treatment outcomes. However, further research needs to be done in finding the correlation between the severity based on scores and the treatment outcomes. Other scoring systems include those by Sergeev et al and Baran et al, which were however not validated.[2, 8]

Poor prognostic factors for onychomycosis are detailed in Table 13.2.

General Measures

A number of general measures can help improve treatment outcomes. These need to be advised to the patients.

- Patients should be advised to wear loose shoes and to keep the nails short.
- Patients should be advised to avoid nail polish due to lack of data on the efficacy of topical formulations applied to polished but diseased nail plates.[9]
- Patients should also avoid walking barefoot, especially in public places, to avoid further dissemination.[10]
- Public swimming pools, spas, etc. are a common source of infection; so are unhygienic manicure and pedicure instruments.

Topical Therapy

Indications for topical therapy include:
1. Distal subungual onychomycosis affecting <50% area of the nail without:

Table 13.1: Onychomycosis severity index (OSI score)					
Area of involvement hyperkeratosis >2 mm		Proximity of disease to matrix		Presence of dermatophytoma or subungual	
Affected nail %	No. of points	Amount of involvement from distal edge	No. of points	Present	No. of points
0	0	< 1/4	1	No	0
1–10	1	1/4–1/2	2	Yes	10
11– 25	2	>1/2–3/4	3		
26–50	3	> 3/4	4		
51–75	4	Matrix involvement	5		
76–100	5				

OSI—score of area of involvement multiplied by the score of the proximity of disease to the matrix and 10 points added if dermatophytoma + or subungual hyperkeratosis >2 mm. 0—cured, 1–5—mild OM, 6–15—moderate OM, 16–35—severe OM.

Table 13.2: Poor prognostic factors for onychomycosis	
Morphological considerations	1. Total dystrophic variety 2. Lateral edge involvement 3. Thick nail involvement (subungual hyperkeratosis of >2 mm) 4. Dermatophytoma
Host factors	1. Old age 2. Immunosuppression 3. Poor peripheral circulation 4. Other dermatoses, e.g. nail psoriasis 5. Genetic predisposition
Agent factors	1. Drug resistance 2. Non-responsive organisms (e.g. non-dermatophyte moulds)
Environmental factors	1. Occupational factors 2. Occlusive footwear 3. Prolonged contact with water or sugary food

- Nail matrix involvement
- Presence of yellow streaks along the lateral margin of the nail
- Central yellow onycholytic area suggestive of dermatophytoma.
2. "Classical" superficial white onychomycosis.
3. Onychomycosis due to moulds (except *Aspergillus species*) as they usually do not respond well to systemic agents.
4. Unwilling patients or patients unable to tolerate systemic agents.
5. Maintenance therapy after a course of systemic antifungals.[1]

Various Topical Agents

1. Ciclopirox

Introduction: 8% ciclopirox solution is a synthetic antifungal available in a lacquer formulation indicated for mild to moderate onychomycosis in immunocompetent patients. It is the first FDA approved topical formulation for onychomycosis. If used as a monotherapy, cure rates are low (with complete cure in 25% cases). Therefore, it is commonly used as an adjunct therapy.

Mechanism of action: Although the mechanism of action is poorly understood, it is proposed to act on target proteins including metal-dependent enzymes affecting DNA replication and repair; cellular growth, metabolism and transport. It is fungicidal and has broad spectrum action on dermatophytes, NDM and yeasts.

Directions for use
- The patient is first advised to trim and file away the loose material under the nail.
- The lacquer is then applied evenly on the nail plate (including the undersurface), nail folds, and over the nailbed with an applicator brush.
- The lacquer is removed with alcohol every 7 days.
- It is used daily/twice daily for 48 weeks.

Side effects: These are few and include mild, transient irritation, burning and itching in the nailbed or neighboring skin.[1, 11, 12]

2. Amorolfine

Introduction: 5% amorolfine is a morpholine derivative that has a broad spectrum of action. It has fungistatic and fungicidal action on dermatophytes, NDM and yeasts.

Mechanism of action: It inhibits enzymes 14-reductase and δ-7, 8-isomerase, therefore, interfering with ergosterol biosynthesis.

Directions for use
- *Therapeutic:* Apart from the general instruction for using nail lacquer, patient

has to use it once or twice a week for 6–12 months.

- *Prophylactic:* It can be used once in two weeks.[1, 11, 12]

3. Tavaborole

Introduction: 5% tavaborole is an oxaborole derivative approved by FDA for treatment of onychomycosis in 2014.

Mechanism of action: It acts by inhibiting protein synthesis by inhibiting leucyl-transfer tRNA synthetase. Following this, there is an inhibition of fungal cell growth which ultimately leads to cell death.

Directions for use: Apart from basic instructions, it is to be applied once daily for 48 weeks. It does not require debridement of the affected toenail.

Side effects: Rare (1%) and include erythema, exfoliation and dermatitis.[1, 11–13]

4. Efinaconazole

Introduction: 10% Efinaconazole solution is a triazole antifungal and is FDA approved for onychomycosis.

Mechanism of action: It is similar to other triazole antifungals (inhibition of 14α-demethylase). Efinaconazole's fungicidal activity is comparable to that of amorolfine and superior to that of ciclopirox.

Directions for use: Similar to 5% tavaborole application.

Side effects: Dermatitis and vesicles at the application sites have been reported.[1,10, 11]

Systemic Therapy

Various agents used in this category are as follows:

1. Terbinafine

Introduction: It is an allylamine derivative and as of now, it is the first-line agent for onychomycosis.

Mechanism of action: It inhibits squalene epoxidase, resulting in depletion of ergosterol that in turn leads to cell death due to inhibition of cell membrane synthesis and intracellular accumulation of toxic squalene.

Dosage

- Continuous dosage: 250 mg daily for 6 weeks (fingernail infection) and 12 weeks (toenail infection)
- Pulsed dosage: 250 mg twice daily for one week a month—for 2 months (fingernails) and 3 months (toenails)
- Dosage in children is 125 mg (20–40 kg); and 62.5 mg (<20 kg)

Side effects: It is an overall well-tolerated drug with mild gastrointestinal side effects, asymptomatic liver enzyme abnormalities, skin rashes, pancytopenia and agranulocytosis. In patients with liver dysfunction, terbinafine should be avoided.[1, 11, 12]

2. Fluconazole

Introduction: It is a triazole introduced for management of *Candida albicans* infections. Although a very commonly used medicine, it is not FDA approved for onychomycosis.

Mechanism of action: It is similar to other triazoles and is hence, fungistatic.

Dosage schedule: 150 mg to 450 mg once a week, to be used for 6 months (fingernails) and 12 months (toenails). Despite moderate results, advantages of fluconazole use include once weekly dosing, few drug interactions and a relatively fewer side effects.[1,11, 12]

3. Itraconazole

Introduction: It is a triazole antifungal with a broad spectrum of action on dermatophytes, non-dermatophytes and yeasts. It is FDA approved for onychomycosis. It is a lipophilic compound, thus can persist in the nail plate for 6–9 months; enabling its use as pulse therapy.

Mechanism of action: Similar to triazoles.

Dosage

- Continuous regimen: 200 mg daily for 2 months (fingernails) and 3 months (toenails)

- Pulsed regimen: 200 mg BD for 1 week every month, 2 months (fingernails) and 3 months (toenails)

Side effects: It is generally tolerated well with adverse effects being seen in up to 3% of the patients. Headache and gastrointestinal upset are the most common adverse effects. Significant hepatic side effects (when continuous dosing beyond 4 weeks), or cutaneous symptoms (including pruritus, urticaria, acute generalized exanthematous pustulosis) have also been reported. It is contraindicated in patients with congestive heart failure (CHF) or history of CHF. Simultaneous use of medications that are metabolised by CYP 450 3A4 such as cisapride, quinidine should be done with precautions. Because of the greater risk of side effects with it, as compared to terbinafine, the latter is considered as the first line treatment.[1, 11, 12]

4. Other Drugs

Griseofulvin, ravuconazole, posaconazole have been tried but are not routinely used.

Surgical Therapy or Debridement

Thickened nail with subungual hyperkeratosis is one of the main reasons for the poor treatment response in patients with onychomycosis. Therefore, the following methods of debridement can be tried, with varied and slightly less satisfactory results:

1. Chemical removal: 40% urea in lacquer base, 50% potassium iodide
2. Mechanical (including surgical) removal: By aggressive debridement, partial or total nail plate avulsions, combined with chemical and mechanical matricectomy.

Partial nail plate avulsions are preferred due to lesser side effects as compared to total avulsions like shrinkage of nailbed, distal ingrowing edge and upward growth of bed, etc. However, all of these methods, act as adjunct treatments only, and need to be combined with systemic and topical treatments.[1, 11]

Newer Treatment Options/Device Based Therapies

These include the following given as follows.

1. Lasers

Introduction: Various types of lasers used for treatment of onychomycosis include 1064 nm Nd:YAG (Pinpointe laser and Genesis plus are FDA approved devices), CO_2 laser, femtosecond IR titanium sapphire laser.

Mechanism of action: Cellular photodamage in the absence of exogenous dyes or other photosensitising drugs is proposed as the mechanism of action of lasers. The exact chromophore targeted in the fungus is however not known.

Indications: Lasers are FDA approved for 'temporary enhancement of clear nail' in patients with onychomycosis. In the review by Bristow and colleagues, investigators concluded that the evidence for laser in onychomycosis was "limited and of poor methodological quality".[1,11, 14]

2. Photodynamic Therapy

Introduction: Potential use of PDT for management of onychomycosis has been studied in the literature.

Mechanism of action: The exogenous 5-aminolevulinic acid (ALA) is taken up directly by the organism, which then causes increased protoporphyrin (PPIX). Following light irradiation of the same, there is cellular damage and death.

Indications: Although it is not approved by FDA, PDT may be used for chronic recalcitrant nail infections, even the non-dermatophyte infections. However, detailed studies on efficacy of PDT including the treatment protocol need to be done.[1, 11]

3. Iontophoresis

Low level of electrical current may overcome the physical barrier and may help in increased transfer of topical antifungal agents, e.g.

topical terbinafine through the nail plate to reach nail bed and matrix.[11]

Special Considerations

- **Pregnancy:** In pregnant females with onychomycosis, treatment should be considered when benefits outweigh risks.
- **Children:** Although no medication is FDA approved for pediatric population, there are some differences in the management of the same. Due to thinner nail plate and faster nail growth, topical treatments work better and faster in children (as little as 4 months). A review by Feldstein and colleague also stated that systemic treatments have good efficacy with low incidence of side effects in the pediatric population.[14]
- **Diabetics:** Diabetic patients are much more prone to have onychomycosis than the normal population, especially with atypical organisms such as yeast. Presence of peripheral neuropathy further increases the risk. Furthermore, diabetics with onychomycosis are at higher risk of developing diabetic foot and its complications. Topical therapies, especially tavaborole and efinaconazole have showed good efficacy in this population.
- **Immunosuppression (including HIV):** Patients with immunosuppression have higher risk of infections including onychomycosis especially with atypical organisms. They may therefore benefit from preventive topical medications, although no agent is currently approved for the same.
- **Geriatric:** Onychomycosis is one of the most common infections in this age group. Due to multiple comorbidities, as well as other age related changes (locally and systemically), the management of onychomycosis in the elderly is tricky. It is crucial to analyze co-morbidities as well as the medications the patient is on to ensure a proper plan of management. Furthermore, for an assessment of cure, mycological cure should be the preferred criterion, as clinical cure may be difficult to achieve in view of age-related changes in the nail structure.[15]

CONCLUSION

Onychomycosis is one of the most common and resistant nail problems, and its management continues to be elusive. In this category, dermatophyte nail infections are the most common, even though more treatment responsive than non-dermatophytes. There are a variety of treatment modalities currently available including topical, systemic, mechanical and light based devices. However, because of low cure rates, a combination of various treatment approaches is usually preferred. The future lies in the advancement of device based therapies which can actually enhance penetration and availability of antifungal drugs in the difficult to reach areas of the distorted nail plates.

References

1. Grover C, Khurana A. An update on treatment of onychomycosis. Mycoses. 2012;55:541–51.
2. Grover C, Khurana A. Onychomycosis: newer insights in pathogenesis and diagnosis. Indian J Dermatol Venereol Leprol 2012;78:263–70.
3. Leeyaphan C, Bunyaratavej S, Prasertworanun N, Muanprasart C, Matthapan L, Rujutharanawong C. Dermatophytoma: An unrecognised condition. Indian J Dermatol Venerol Leprol 2016;82:188–9.
4. Richert B, Cappelletti ML, André J. [Differential diagnosis of onychomycosis].Rev Med Brux. 2011;32:219–23.
5. Mikailov A, Cohen J, Joyce C, Mostaghimi A.Cost-effectiveness of confirmatory testing before treatment of onychomycosis. JAMA Dermatol 2016;152:276–81.
6. Grover C, Jakhar D. Onychoscopy: A practical guide. Indian J Dermatol Venereol Leprol 2017;83:536–49.
7. Queller JN, Bhatia N. The dermatologist's approach to onychomycosis. J. Fungi 2015; 1: 173–84.
8. Carney C, Tosti A, Daniel R. A new classification system for grading the severity of onychomycosis: Onychomycosis severity index. Arch Dermatol 2011; 147: 1277–82.

9. Del Rosso JQ. Application of nail polish during topical management of onychomycosis: Are data available to guide the clinician about what to tell their patients? J Clin Aesthet Dermatol 2016;9: 29–36.

10. Vasudevan B. Clinical Correlation with diagnostic implications in dermatology. Jaypee Brothers. 1st ed., 2017.

11. Paiser DM, Jellinek NJ, Rich P. Efficacy and safety of onychomycosis treatments: An evidence-based overview. Semin Cutan Med Surg 2015; 34: S46–50.

12. Jellinek NJ, Rich P, Paiser DM. Understanding onychomycosis treatment: mechanism of action and formulation. Semin Cutan Med Surg 2015; 34:S51–3.

13. Sharma N, Sharma D. An upcoming drug for onychomycosis: Tavaborole. J Pharmacol Pharmacother 2015;6:236–9.

14. Gupta AK, Foley KA, Versteeg SG. Lasers for Onychomycosis. J Cutan Med Surg 2017;21:114–6.

15. Rich P, Jellinek NJ, Paiser DM. Management strategies for onychomycosis in special patient population. Semin Cutan Med Surg 2015;34:S54–5.

14

Treatment of Fungal Infections in Special Conditions

Ananta Khurana

Details of the various topical and systemic modalities of treatment of dermatophytoses have been covered in the respective chapters. This chapter highlights the management considerations in certain special patient groups/conditions like pregnancy, pediatric, elderly patients, renal dysfunction and liver diseases. A summary for pregnancy, hepatic and renal dysfunction is provided in Box 14.1. Further details are given in individual sections.

PREGNANCY

Prescribing any drug during pregnancy requires careful assessment of maternal benefit and fetal risks, including fetal loss, congenital malformations, organ toxicity and prematurity.

In addition to the pharmacodynamics, pharmacokinetics and intrinsic antifungal activity of a given drug, specific parameters to be considered are the period of gestation, level of fetal drug exposure and maternal physiological pharmacokinetic changes.[1] The drug pharmacokinetics may be altered by many factors like vomiting—increased gastric pH, increased cardiac output and increased intestinal blood flow. Increased intra- and extravascular blood flow and reduced serum albumin concentration enhance the distribution of unbound drugs. Finally, increased renal filtration/elimination and increased (3A4, 2D6, 2C9, 2A6) or decreased (1A2, 2C19) cytochrome activities can modify drug clearance. Fetal exposure relies on the drug's ability to cross the placenta, depending on the

Box 14.1: Summary of preferred treatment for certain special patient groups	
Condition	*Preferred drug*
Pregnancy	Topicals preferred;
	First line: clotrimazole, miconazole
	Second line: terbinafine
	Systemic: Terbinafine cat B but scarce human data precludes routine use
Pediatric	Same drugs as adults; with weight based dosing
Hepatic dysfunction	Cautious use of fluconazole (safer than others)
Renal dysfunction	Fluconazole with dose adjustments
	Terbinafine with dose adjustments

stage of pregnancy (placental maturation with enhanced fetal exposure in later term) and on intrinsic drug parameters (liposolubility, molecular weight, protein binding).[2-4]

Information on drug safety during pregnancy can be accessed from certain online resources like Teratogen Information System (TERIS); the European Network of Teratology Information Services (ENTIS); an American equivalent of ENTIS, known as the Organization of Teratology Information Specialists (OTIS); the International Centre for Birth Defects Surveillance and Research (ICBDSR) and Reprotox.

The drug pregnancy classification systems widely used include US FDA, European *Farmaceutiska Specialiteter i Sverige* (FASS or Swedish Catalogue of Approved Drugs) and the Australian Drug Evaluation Committee (ADEC) systems (Table 14.1). However, following much criticism, the US FDA system was abolished in 2014 and is to be replaced gradually by a new system called Pregnancy and Lactation Labelling Rule (PLLR) with narrative-based labeling requirements. The same is stated to be completed by June 2018, and till then both systems may be used by providers.

We wish to highlight a few points which the reader must keep in mind while interpreting the following tables regarding pregnancy categorizations of US FDA (and other systems). According to the US FDA system, new drugs are readily classified as category B based on negative animal studies and lack of human data. Following an "innocent until proven guilty" policy, drugs remain in category B unless future data indicate risk in animal or human fetuses.[5] If, however, there are animal studies showing fetal risk, but no human studies to refute this conclusion, or if there is a paucity of both human and animal data, drugs are assigned to category C. When controlled studies are lacking, established medications may be labeled category C, despite decades of use in pregnant women with few or no reports of adverse effects. Therefore,

rating under pregnancy category B or C can be inaccurate and misleading. It is recommended to exercise caution when considering therapy for a pregnant patient with a newer medication labeled as category B, and alternatively, one may consider established category C medications with a little or no evidence of adverse effects as a therapeutic option.[6]

Topical Antifungals

The pregnancy safety evidence regarding the various topical antifungals is presented in Table 14.2.

Miconazole: Miconazole cream was evaluated in two studies from the Hungarian Case-control Surveillance of Congenital Abnormalities, which compiled 22843 newborns/fetuses with congenital abnormalities and 38151 control newborns, from 1980 to 1996. Treatment during the first trimester did not increase the risk of congenital abnormalities (Odd's ratio 0.9, range 0.6–1.6).[7] Further, data of 2236 women exposed in first trimester did not have an increased association with cardiovascular defects, oral clefts, and spina bifida.[8] Further data obtained from the same program (1985–1990) found no linkage with congenital defects among 7266 newborns exposed during the first trimester. Thus, miconazole is safe in pregnancy and may be used as first-line agent.

Clotrimazole: 0.5% of topically applied clotrimazole is absorbed systemically.[9] Animal studies with high doses did not cause teratogenicity.[9] Hungarian Case-control Surveillance of Congenital Abnormalities (1980–1992) dataset did not find any association between vaginal and topical clotrimazole use and congenital anomalies. A large surveillance study of 2624 exposed newborns and other smaller studies also reported no adverse fetal outcomes from clotrimazole use.[10-12] Thus, topical clotrimazole is safe in pregnancy, and some authors consider it a first-line topical medication for cutaneous mycoses in pregnancy.[13,14]

Table 14.1: Comparison of pregnancy labeling by US FDA, FASS and ADEC		
US FDA	FASS	ADEC
A: Clinical data show no evidence of risk to the fetus	A: Reliable clinical data indicate no evidence of disturbance of their productive process	A: Extensive clinical experience in pregnant women and women of childbearing age has shown no increase in the frequency of malformations or other harmful effects on the fetus
B: Clinical data are limited or not available, but animal studies show no evidence of risk to the fetus, or clinical data show no evidence of risk to the fetus, but animal studies show adverse effects to the fetus	B: Clinical experience of use in pregnant women is limited or insufficient. Classification is based on animal data, by allocation to 3 subgroups (B1, B2, and B3) B1—animal experiments have not given evidence of an increased incidence of fetal damage; similar to FDA category B B2—animal experiments are inadequate; similar to FDA category C B3—reproduction toxicity studies in animals have revealed an increased incidence of fetal damage, the significance of which is considered uncertain in humans; similar to FDA category C	B: Human data are lacking or inadequate. Limited use in pregnant women and women of childbearing age has shown no increase in the frequency of malformation or other harmful effects on the human fetus. Classification is based on available animal data into 3 subcategories (B1, B2, and B3). Note: Allocation to category B does not imply greater safety than category C B1—studies in animals have not shown evidence of an increased occurrence of fetal damage; similar to FDA category B B2—studies in animals are inadequate or lacking, but available data show no evidence of an increased occurrence of fetal damage; similar to FDA category C B3—studies in animals have shown evidence of an increased occurrence of fetal damage, the significance of which is considered uncertain in humans; similar to FDA category C
C: Clinical data are not available and animal studies are not available, or clinical data are not available, but animal studies show adverse effects to the fetus	C: Data suggest pharmacologic effects may have adverse effects on the reproductive process	C: Drugs which, owing to their pharmacologic effects, have caused or may be suspected of causing, harmful effects on the human fetus or neonate without causing malformations. These effects may be reversible
D: Positive evidence of risk to the fetus from clinical data	D: Data indicate an increased incidence of malformations in humans	D: Drugs which have caused, are suspected to have caused, or may be expected to cause, an increased incidence of human fetal malformations or irreversible damage. These drugs may also have adverse pharmacologic effects. Note: Drugs in category D are not absolutely contraindicated in pregnancy. In some cases, the D category has been assigned on the basis of suspicion
X: Contraindicated based on animal studies or clinical data		X: Contraindicated in pregnancy

FASS: Swedish catalogue of approved drugs; ADEC: Australian Drug Evaluation Committee

Table 14.2: Pregnancy categorization of topical antifungals			
Topical drug	US FDA	FASS	ADEC
Clotrimazole	B	A	A
Miconazole	C		
Nystatin	C: Topical A: Vaginal	A	A
Terbinafine	B	B1	B1
Ciclopirox	B	A	—
Selenium sulfide	C	A, B3	—
Luliconazole	C	—	—
Amphotericin B	B	—	—
Ketoconazole	C	—	—
Oxiconazole	B	—	—
Naftifine	B	—	—

FASS: Swedish catalogue of approved drugs; ADEC: Australian Drug Evaluation Committee

Oxiconazole: Animal studies using doses up to 57 times the typical human doses based on mg/m^2 did not report fetal harm.[15] No studies or reports of oxiconazole in human pregnancies have been published. The use of topical oxiconazole is permitted after other safer alternatives, such as clotrimazole and miconazole.

Luliconazole: Pregnancy safety data in humans is lacking. No embryofetal toxicity or malformations were noted in animal studies except increased incidence of skeletal variation in rats at 3 times the maximum recommended human dose (MRHD).[16]

Ketoconazole: Animal studies using doses 10 times the oral MRHD reported fetal syndactylia and oligodactyly.[17] Studies or reports of topical ketoconazole use in human pregnancies are lacking. Oral ketoconazole use has however been associated with decreased androgen production and reports of limb malformation and hydrops fetalis.[18] Thus, in presence of safer alternatives, topical ketoconazole should not be used in pregnancy.

Terbinafine: Topical terbinafine demonstrates minimal absorption after topical use. Data on human exposures is still sparse. A prospective follow up study of 23 pregnant women exposed to topical terbinafine did not report teratogenic potential above the baseline risk of 1–3%.[19] Due to limited human data, topical terbinafine may be used after safer alternatives such as miconazole and clotrimazole.

Naftifine: 6% of the topical 1% cream is absorbed systemically. Animal studies using 12–150 times the recommended topical dose demonstrated no fetal harm.[20] Although human studies are lacking, no problems have been reported from topical use.[21] Limited application is likely safe.

Ciclopirox: Animal studies have not demonstrated any fetotoxicity or teratogenicity. Human studies are lacking but the drug is likely safe for topical use during pregnancy.[21]

Amorolfine: The drug has poor systemic absorption and has not shown deleterious effects in animals. It may hence be used during pregnancy.[22]

Nystatin: Nystatin is poorly absorbed orally, if at all and has long been categorized as category A by US FDA. A surveillance study reported 489 newborns exposed to nystatin during the 1st trimester and 1881 newborns at any time in pregnancy, and found no association with congenital malformations such as oral clefts, cardiovascular defects, spina bifida, polydactyly, limb reduction defects, and hypospadias.[23] Four other studies also concluded topical nystatin is safe in pregnancy.[24–27] However, a possible association between hypospadias and nystatin was reported in another case-control study.[13] Recent Hungarian data also raises the possibility of a slightly increased risk of hypospadias in exposed fetuses, although otherwise safe. Accordingly it may be prudent to avoid use during the critical period for this malformation (8–14 weeks of gestation).[22]

Selenium sulfide: No animal or human studies are available. However, short-term use over limited areas may be considered safe.[28]

Salicylic acid: Although not an antifungal, the drug is used to enhance fungal clearance along with the conventional anti-fungals and is hence mentioned here. Following topical application, about 9–25% of the dose is systemically absorbed.[29, 30] A large prospective study of 50,282 pregnant women did not report any adverse events.[31] But, when used in the 3rd trimester, salicylic acid can cause premature closure of ductus arteriosus and oligohydramnios.[32] Therefore, avoid widespread use in the 3rd trimester, application over large surface areas for prolonged time periods, or application under occlusive dressings at any time during pregnancy, as this may enhance systemic absorption.[33]

Systemic Antifungals (Table 14.3)

Terbinafine

Oral reproduction studies do not evidence any embryo—fetotoxicity in rabbits and rats administered up to 23 times the maximum recommended human dose.[34] It is not known whether terbinafine crosses the human placenta. There is limited data on human exposure. A follow-up on 54 women gestationally exposed to terbinafine (26 oral and 23 topical), with 24 exposures occurring during the first trimester and with a mean duration of exposure being 32 ± 9 days, reported no increased risk for major malformations above the baseline risk.[19] It has been classified as pregnancy category B, but oral prescription should preferably be postponed until after delivery.

Itraconazole

Itraconazole has been shown to be embryotoxic and teratogenic in rodents, inducing craniofacial and rib abnormalities.[34] However, a prospective study involving 229 women exposed to itraconazole, including 198 during the first trimester [daily doses ranged from 50 to 800 mg (median of 200 mg) for a median of 3 days (range 1–90)], failed to identify any increased risk of fetal malformations.[35] Another study on 206 women exposed during the first trimester also did not find an increased risk of malformations (mean daily dose of 182 + 63 mg for a mean of 6.9 + 6.4 days). An increase in early fetal loss was however reported.[36] Based on the present data, the drug should be avoided in pregnancy especially during the first trimester.

Fluconazole

Fluconazole readily crosses the placenta and has shown teratogenic and embryotoxic effects at high doses in animals.[37] Oral fluconazole treatment has been linked to a distinct pattern of birth defects in five infants of mothers who were treated for severe fungal infections with

Table 14.3: Pregnancy categorization of systemic antifungals			
Systemic drug	US FDA	FASS	ADEC
Griseofulvin	C	—	B3
Fluconazole	C/D	B3	D
Ketoconazole	C	B3	B3
Itraconazole	C	B3	B3
Terbinafine	B	B1	B1

FASS: Swedish catalogue of approved drugs; ADEC: Australian Drug Evaluation Committee

400 to 800 mg daily during most or all of the first trimester of pregnancy.[38–41] Similar defects have been observed in animals exposed to systemic azole antifungal agents.[42–44] In 2011, the US FDA issued a drug-safety announcement concerning the possible teratogenic risks conferred by long-term, high-dose fluconazole treatment. The FDA pregnancy category for fluconazole was consequently changed from C (adverse fetal effects in animals and no adequate human data) to D (evidence of human fetal risk, but benefits may warrant use), with the exception of the use of fluconazole at a single dose of 150 mg, for the treatment of vaginal candidiasis.[45]

Griseofulvin

Griseofulvin is carcinogenic, embryotoxic and teratogenic in rodents at 3–45 times the human dose.[34] A retrospective study compared 38151 normal pregnancies and 22843 pregnancies with birth defects in relation to their exposure to griseofulvin (reported in 7 and 21 cases, respectively) and did not find any association with any birth defect or with any excess of conjoined twins, as reported previously.[46,47] But human data are still limited to allow its use in pregnancy, especially in the first trimester.

Ketoconazole

It is unclear to what extent ketoconazole crosses the placenta; however, ketoconazole has been shown to be embryotoxic and teratogenic at high doses (80 mg/kg/day) in animals (2 times the human recommended dose).[48] In addition, doses one fourth that of normal human doses have caused prolonged labor in rats.[48] Finally, ketoconazole inhibits gonadal and adrenal steroid synthesis in humans. This inhibition could potentially alter sex organ differentiation in the human fetus.[48] Thus in view of the theoretical risk, it is not recommended to be used during pregnancy.

To summarise (Table 14.4), it is advisable ~eat dermatophytoses with only topicals

Table 14.4: Treatment of dermatophytoses in pregnancy	
Topicals	*First line:* Clotrimazole,[13,14] miconazole[7,8] *Second line:* Terbinafine[19] *For OM:* Ciclopirox[21], Amorolfine[22]
Systemic	Avoid all systemic antifungals Terbinafine is category B but very limited human safety data to recommend use[19]

throughout pregnancy. Amongst these, clotrimazole and miconazole have most well established safety profiles and should be preferred (Table 14.4). Dermatophytic nail infections can be treated with topical ciclopirox or amorolfine as these have favorable safety profiles during pregnancy. All oral antifungals should ideally be avoided throughout pregnancy. Terbinafine is the only systemic antifungal with no deleterious effects in animal studies, but human data are too scant to recommend its use.

PEDIATRIC AGE GROUP

Pediatric antifungal use has been most widely described with respect to tinea capitis, and has been covered in the respective section in this manual. There are reports and a few good reviews[49–52] available on pediatric onychomycosis (OM), while dermatophytoses of the glabrous skin in children is scantly covered in literature.

Pediatric OM is being increasingly recognized and several studies from around the world have estimated a prevalence ranging from 0.2 to 2.6% (significantly less than adults).[53–55] Children are less likely to develop onychomycosis than adults due to their faster nail growth, smaller nail surface area, reduced time spent in environments containing pathogens, reduced likelihood of trauma and subsequent colonization, reduced prevalence of tinea pedis and rarity of co-morbid predisposing conditions like pre-existing nail disorders and impaired circulation.[53] It is commoner in children with Down syndrome and HIV/AIDS or other immune deficiencies. Similar to adults, the most common presentation in children is distal subungual onychomycosis and toenails are affected more commonly than fingernails.

The most likely causative organism is the dermatophyte *Trichophyton rubrum*, followed by other dermatophytes including *Trichophyton mentagrophytes, Microsporum canis, Trichophyton tonsurans*, and rarer dermatophytes such as *Trichophyton equinum*.[56–58] *Candida* is a less common cause and generally associated with perionyxis.[49]

It is important to perform laboratory confirmation of OM in children, and to examine affected children for concomitant tinea pedis. As familial disease often occurs, it is important to check parents and siblings as well as for onychomycosis and tinea pedis.

Treatment options are the same as adults with topical (ciclopirox and amorolfine) and systemic (terbinafine, itraconazole and fluconazole) drugs. There is no data on the use of newer topical drugs tavaborole and efinaconazole in children. Children are more likely to respond to topicals as their nails are thin and grow faster than adults.[59] Oral therapy is often required when multiple nails are involved, more than 50% of the distal nail plate is affected, or when topical penetration may be suboptimal. Complete cure rates obtained for the systemic antifungals (terbinafine/itraconazole) in children are largely similar or slightly higher than rates observed in the adult population.[52] Addition of topical treatment to systemic drugs, increases the cure rate of pediatric OM from 70.8 to 80%, according to a recent meta-analysis, and may be added in older children who are more likely to adhere to this.[52] However, OM in children recurs more often than in adults.[59] None of the treatments is currently US FDA-approved for onychomycosis in children.

Terbinafine is FDA-approved for the treatment of pediatric tinea capitis. Fluconazole is used off-label to treat onychomycosis in adults and children, but is FDA-approved for candidiasis in children and considered very safe to use. Although rarely significant, some experts recommend a complete blood count and liver function tests prior to starting systemic antifungals in children. Surgical modalities in terms of debridement and avulsion can be used in combination.[50] There is no data on the use of laser and other devices in pediatric OM.

Terbinafine: Dosing is weight based with a dose of 62.5 mg for children weighing less than 20 kg, 125 mg for children between 20 and 40 kg, and 250 mg for children weighing more than 40 kg.[60] The clearance of terbinafine is about 40% higher in children compared to adults.[61] It has been used in the same durations as in adults, in continuous dosing for 6 weeks for fingernails and 12 weeks for toenails.

A systematic review of pediatric OM reported a pooled complete clearance rate of 78.8% with oral terbinafine, higher than that reported in adults.[52] The pooled efficacy of terbinafine combined with a topical antifungal (ciclopirox or amorolfine) was 90%.[52] The drug has a good safety profile in children with only occasional adverse events like acute urticaria, anorexia, epigastric pain, tiredness, vesiculopustular eruption, and agranulocytosis.[52] In adults, there have been rare reports of serious hepatic toxicity, which usually occurred in patients with pre-existing liver disease. Therefore, by extension systemic terbinafine is not recommended in a child with underlying liver disease.

Itraconazole: This has been used in the doses of 3–5 mg/kg/day, as a continuous therapy for 2–4 months, or in a pulsed regimen (in doses ranging from 3 to 7 mg/kg/day) similar to adults (1 week/month, 2–3 pulses).[52] In children weighing more than 50 kg, an adult dose of 200 mg/day is given.[62] It has a broader spectrum of activity than terbinafine and is useful in candidal and non-dermatophytic mould infections as well.

A systematic review of pediatric studies on OM found the complete cure rate for itraconazole to be 68.4% in the pulsed regimen and 85.7% for the continuous regimen.[52]

Itraconazole is well tolerated in the pediatric patients, with most reported adverse effects being transient and mild. The reported adverse effects include fatigue, gastritis, headache, dizziness, sleepiness and liver function test abnormalities. Itraconazole's potential for drug interactions, though less significant in children, must be kept in mind. It is advisable to order a liver function test in case of continuous dosage for more than one month, with concomitant use of other hepatotoxic drugs. Finally, by extrapolation from the adult literature, use in the setting of congestive cardiac failure is to be avoided.

Other systemic drugs used less often are **griseofulvin** (daily dosing) and **fluconazole** (daily/weekly/alternate day). Griseofulvin has been used in doses of 10 mg/kg/day or conventional dosing of 250 mg/day, for 2–12 months, with pooled efficacy of 6.3%.[52] Fluconazole has been used in very few reports, in doses of 50–100 mg/day or 300 mg once weekly or 100 mg on alternate days, and durations ranging from 40 days (with continuous dosing) to 4 months (with weekly dosing) with a pooled complete clearance rate of 66.7%. Fluconazole is relatively safe in pediatric patients, gastrointestinal toxicity being the most common adverse event. Hepatotoxicity, renal dysfunction, and rash have been reported rarely. It is important to be aware of drug interactions with fluconazole in pediatric patients being co-prescribed other systemic drugs.[49]

Tinea of the glabrous skin, hitherto considered uncommon is being increasingly seen over the past few years (Fig. 14.1). We

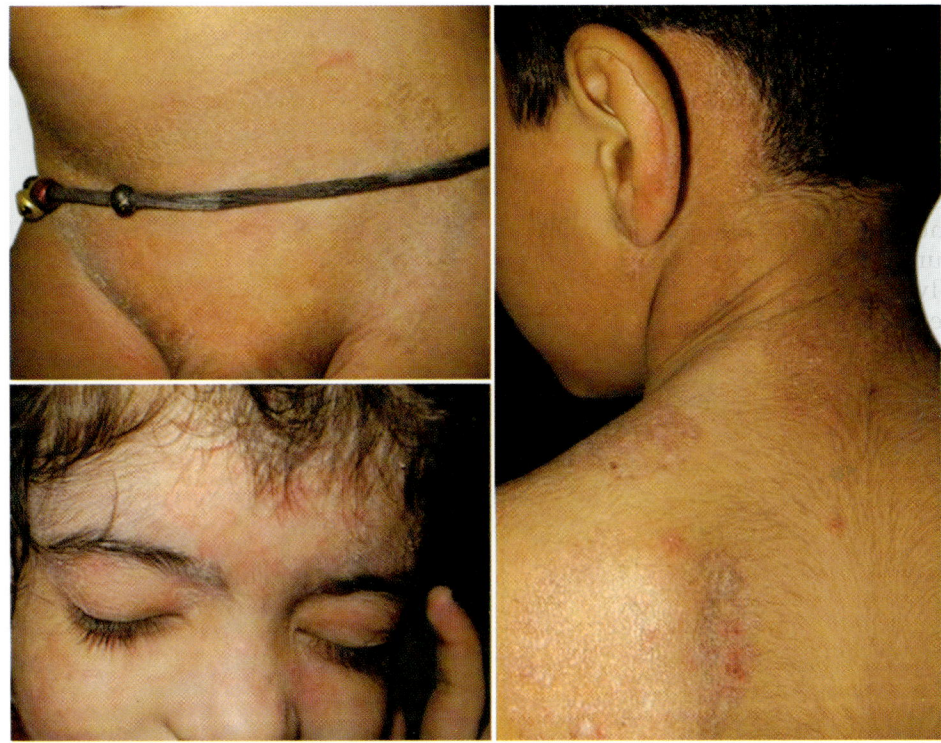

Fig. 14.1: The spectrum of dermatophytoses being commonly seen in the pediatric age group in the recent times

have been seeing tinea corporis/cruris in children as young as 6 months. Affected children mostly have affected parents and hence family history should be asked for specifically. Although the presentation is generally classical, difficulties may arise in the setting of atopic eczema. Further, tinea corporis in atopics may have staphylococcal superinfection.[63]

Tinea cruris can occur in both sexes but is more frequent in teenage boys.[64] It often occurs in conjunction with tinea pedis, because the fungus is autologously spread upwards while putting on pants and undergarments. Other risk factors include obesity, excessive sweating or participation in athletics. Tinea pedis, or athlete's foot, commonly presents in adolescents but is rare in prepubertal children. Occlusive footwear may be a predisposing factor.

There are not many reports dealing with tinea corporis/cruris/pedis in the pediatric age group, but the treatment remains essentially the same. There is often a history of self-medication using the topicals prescribed to adults in the household. In general, children are likely to respond better with topical alone due to their rapid skin turnover. Azoles and terbinafine may be used in the same way as adults.[64] Systemic antifungals may be added if there is extensive involvement (Table 14.5). Related safety concerns have been previously addressed in OM section. The drugs need to be continued for as long as it takes for clearance to be achieved.

Table 14.5: Use of antifungal drugs in children (for onychomycosis and tinea corporis/cruris/pedis)

Drug	Dosage
Terbinafine	<20 kg: 62.5 mg 20–40 kg: 125 mg >40 kg: 250 mg or 3–6 mg/kg/day
Itraconazole	3–5 mg/kg/day
Fluconazole	6 mg/kg/day [65]
Griseofulvin	10–20 mg/kg/day

LIVER DISEASE

Hepatic dysfunction alters the metabolism of certain drugs and further drugs with propensity to cause hepatic damage are to be avoided/used with caution in this setting. Hepatotoxicity has been consistently reported for all dermatologically important antifungal agents and may range from mild abnormalities in liver function tests to fatal fulminant hepatic failure. But, the risk of liver injury requiring or not requiring treatment discontinuation is generally low (<2%) for all treatment regimens.[66]

Terbinafine: The clearance of terbinafine is decreased by approximately 50% in cirrhotics, compared to normal volunteers. However, the C_{max}, T_{max} and absorption half-life of terbinafine in patients with liver dysfunction were identical to healthy volunteers. For dermatologic view point, terbinafine use should be avoided in the setting of a pre-existing liver disease due to its potential to cause a severe drug-induced liver injury (DILI). Minor elevations in serum transaminases may develop in <1% of patients, which may be asymptomatic and can resolve without stopping the drug.[67] DILI due to terbinafine is a rare and idiosyncratic reaction which usually occurs within the first 6 weeks of therapy. It has an incidence of 1 in 50,000 to 120,000 prescriptions.[68] The reaction can be hepatocellular or cholestatic. But it typically evolves into a usually prolonged cholestatic pattern and may progress to the vanishing bile duct syndrome.[69] The reaction is potentially organ and life-threatening and hence it is a good practice to inform the patients about it at the time of starting treatment.[70]

The US FDA and the British National Formulary (BNF) both recommend a baseline LFT prior to starting treatment with terbinafine and the BNF further recommends repeat measurements every 4–6 weeks of treatment. However, a recent critical appraisal of existing literature reported that DILI due to terbinafine is generally symptomatic, with presenting complaints of jaundice/icterus, flu-like symptoms or pruritus, and hence recommended a change in the BNF guidelines of performing repeat LFTs at 4–6 weeks.[68] We would like to mention here that we have observed marked elevations of liver enzymes without any clinical symptoms and hence routinely perform LFTs when the use of drug exceeds 4 weeks.[70]

Itraconazole: Liver dysfunction has rarely been reported with dermatologic use in other-wise healthy people. Tucker et al administered itraconazole in doses up to 400 mg/day for durations up to 1 year, for deep and superficial mycoses and reported mild (<2-fold) transient increase in liver enzymes in 4 patients, but the treatment was not discontinued in any.[72] In patients receiving pulse itraconazole, an asymptomatic increase in liver enzymes has been reported in 1.7–2% of patients.[73] The elevated enzymes usually return to normal either spontaneously or following disconti-nuation of treatment. There are rare isolated reports of symptomatic hepatotoxicity with continuous dosing for dermatological indications and in most of these symptoms resolved within several weeks to months after discontinuation.[74] There is only one such report with pulsed regimen.[75]

As itraconazole is predominantly meta-bolized in the liver, it is recommended that liver function monitoring be done in patients with pre-existing hepatic function abnor-malities or those who have experienced liver toxicity with other medications.[76] Further in such cases, treatment with itraconazole is discouraged unless there is a serious or life-threatening situation where the expected benefit exceeds the risk of exacerbating hepatic dysfunction.

Fluconazole: A cautious use is advised in patients with liver dysfunction.[77] It has a low incidence of hepatotoxicity, as with other azoles. Instances of fatal hepatic reactions were noted to occur primarily in patients with serious underlying medical conditions (predominantly AIDS or malignancy) and often while taking multiple concomitant medications. Its hepatotoxicity has usually, but not always, been reversible on disconti-nuation of therapy.

Ketoconazole: Use of ketoconazole is contraindicated in a patient with acute or chronic liver disease. Liver toxicity of this antifungal azole is well documented with an overall rate of 3.6–4.3%, but there is no clear correlation with dosing and lower rates (1.4%) are reported in children.[78]

Due to its hepatotoxic side effects (along with endocrine dysregulation, and drug interactions), oral ketoconazole was withdrawn from the European and Australian markets in 2013. Similarly, strict restrictions and cautionary advisements for hepatic function monitoring, have been added to oral ketoconazole labelling in the US and Canada.

Comparison of hepatotoxicity of the various antifungals: There have been few comparative analyses on relative hepatotoxicity of antifungals. A meta-analysis of the safety of oral antifungals in the treatment of superficial dermatophytosis and onychomycosis estimated the pooled probability of discontinuing terbinafine (250 mg per day) because of DILI at **0.34%** (95% CI: 0.09–0.6); the corresponding rates were **0.70** (95% CI: 0.33–1.06) for conti-nuous itraconazole (200 mg/day) and **1.22** (95% CI: 0.00–5.30) for continuous fluconazole at 50 mg/day.[79]

In another meta-analysis, among dermatolo-gically important antifungals, most cases of DILI were attributed to *terbinafine* (n = 422; 27 with LF), followed by *fluconazole* (n = 412; 31 with LF), *itraconazole* (n = 182; 4 with LF) and *ketoconazole* (n = 94; 6 with LF).[80] The corres-ponding reporting odds ratios for liver failure were highest among ketoconazole users (4.22; 95% CI: 1.88–9.45), followed by fluconazole (3.46; 2.42–4.93), and terbinafine users (3.39; 2.32–4.96).[81]

Thus, it is not advisable to use a systemic antifungal for treatment of dermatophytoses in patients with pre-existing liver disease. Further, dermatologist must keep the inherent hepatotoxicity of antifungals in mind, especially during prolonged use, and monitor the patients appropriately.

KIDNEY DISEASE

Terbinafine: In patients with renal impairment (creatinine clearance <50 ml/min), the clearance of terbinafine is decreased by approximately 50% compared to normal volunteers. Appropriate dose adjustments are advised.[82]

Itraconazole: It is primarily metabolized in liver. Not much data is available on its use in renal insufficiency. Drug exposure may be reduced in uremic patients, but is unaffected in those on dialysis.[76]

Fluconazole: The pharmacokinetics of fluconazole are markedly affected by reduction in renal function. There is an inverse relationship between the elimination half-life and creatinine clearance.[77] However, there is no need to adjust single dose therapy for vaginal candidiasis because of impaired renal function. In patients with impaired renal function who will receive multiple doses, an initial loading dose of 50 to 400 mg should be given. After the loading dose, the daily dose (according to indication) should be based on the creatinine clearance (ml/min); with normal regular dosing with clearance of >50 ml/min and in patients on dialysis and 50% of the dose if clearance <50 ml/min and patient is not on dialysis.[77]

CARDIAC DISEASES

There are cardiac concerns with the use of the following antifungals:

Itraconazole: It should not be administered in patients with evidence of ventricular dysfunction such as congestive heart failure (CHF) or a history of CHF.[76] Reversible edema of the extremities is reported in 0.4–3.5% of patients, and mild hypertension has been reported with high doses (60 mg/day) in several patients.[83,84] There are isolated reports of Conn's syndrome (hypokalemia, edema and hypertension) and ventricular fibrillations due to hypokalemia.[85]

Ketoconazole: It can prolong the QT interval leading to dysrhythmias. Co-administration of the following drugs with ketoconazole is contraindicated: Dofetilide, quinidine, pimozide, cisapride, methadone, disopyramide, dronedarone, ranolazine. Ketoconazole can cause elevated plasma concentrations of these drugs which may prolong the QT interval, sometimes resulting in life-threatening ventricular dysrhythmias such as torsades de pointes.[86]

Fluconazole: It can increase the plasma levels of terfenadine, astemizole, quinidine, pimozide and cisapride, leading to QT interval prolongation and hence co-administration is to be avoided.[77]

GERIATRIC AGE GROUP (Table 14.6)

Use of antifungals in the elderly must take into account their co-morbidities and other drugs the patient is on. Pharmacokinetics of

Table 14.6: Treatment of dermatophytoses in the elderly	
Prefer • Topicals over systemic • Terbinafine over azoles • Pulsed regimens over continuous	**Consider** • Reduced renal function (altered fluconazole PK) • Peripheral vascular compromise (may complicate treatment for OM) • Co-morbidities
Watch out for • Drug interactions • Toxicities	

fluconazole have been shown to be altered in elderly with higher values of C_{max}, AUC and mean terminal half-life compared with normal young male volunteers, possibly due to the decreased kidney function expected in the elderly.[77] Azoles have prominent drug interactions based on inhibition of CYP3A4 enzymes and hence terbinafine may be a better drug to use. Pulsed regimens should be preferable over continuous wherever appropriate. And needless to say topicals must be preferred wherever possible.

Prominent and clinically significant drug interactions with the three most commonly used antifungals are as follows:

Fluconazole: It has been shown to increase the levels of the following drugs which geriatric patients may commonly be on: Oral hypoglycemic tolbutamide, glipizide and glyburide; rifabutin; tacrolimus; cisapride; terfenadine (at $\geq$400 mg); voriconazole; midazolam; zidovudine; cyclosporine and warfarin. Interestingly, fluconazole co-administration can increase the C_{max} of terbinafine by 52% and its AUC levels by 69%.[77] The diuretic hydrochlorthiazide drugs can increase fluconazole's serum levels.[77]

Itraconazole: Concomitant administration of itraconazole with with cisapride, oral midazolam, nisoldipine, pimozide, quinidine, dofetilide, triazolam and levacetylmethadol (levomethadyl) is contraindicated.[75] HMG CoA-reductase inhibitors metabolized by CYP3A4, such as lovastatin and simvastatin as well as ergot alkaloids metabolized by CYP3A4 such as dihydroergotamine, ergometrine (ergonovine), ergotamine and methylergometrine are also contraindicated with itraconazole.[76]

Terbinafine: Drug interactions are much less with terbinafine. However, terbinafine is an inhibitor of the CYP450 2D6 isozyme and drugs predominantly metabolized by the CYP450 2D6 isozyme should not be used. These drugs include: Tricyclic antidepressants, selective serotonin reuptake inhibitors,

β-blockers, antiarrhythmics class 1 C (e.g. flecainide and propafenone) and monoamine oxidase inhibitors Type B.[82]

References

1. Chow AW, Jewesson PJ. Pharmacokinetics and safety of antimicrobial agents during pregnancy. Rev Infect Dis 1985; 7: 287–313.

2. Forfar JO, Nelson MM. Epidemiology of drugs taken by pregnant women: drugs that may affect the fetus adversely. Clin Pharmacol Ther 1973; 14: 632–42.

3. Hebert MF, Ma X, Naraharisetti SB, et al. Are we optimizing gestational diabetes treatment with glyburide? The pharmacologic basis for better clinical practice. Clin Pharmacol Ther 2009; 85: 607–14.

4. Tracy TS, Venkataramanan R, Glover DD, et al. Temporal changes in drug metabolism (CYP1A2, CYP2D6 and CYP3A activity) during pregnancy. Am J Obstet Gynecol 2005; 192: 633–9.

5. Millsop JW, Heller MM, Murase JE. Safety classification systems used in dermatological medication risk counseling of pregnant and lactating patients: a case for an evidence-based approach. Dermatol Ther 2013;26:347–53.

6. Wilmer E, Chai S, Kroumpouzos G. Drug safety: Pregnancy rating classifications and controversies. Clin Dermatol 2016;34:401–9.

7. Czeizel AE, Kazy Z, Puho E. Population-based case-control teratologic study of topical miconazole. Congenit Anom (Kyoto) 2004;44:41–5.

8. Rosa F, Baum C, Shaw M. Pregnancy outcomes after first trimester vaginitis drug therapy. Obstet Gynecol 1987;69:751–5.

9. Schering Corporation. *Lotrisone cream package insert.* 2009. Available at:http://www. accessdata. fda.gov/drugsatfda_docs/label/2009/020010s021lbl. pdf. (last accessed 2016 October 25).

10. Tan C, Good C, Milne L, Loudon J. A comparative trial of six day therapy with clotrimazole and nystatin in pregnant patients with vaginal candidiasis. Postgrad Med J 1974;50:102–5.

11. Haram K, Digranes A. Vulvovaginal candidiasis in pregnancy treated with clotrimazole. Acta obstetricia et gynecologica Scandinavica 1978;57: 453–5.

12. Frerich W, Gad A. The frequency of Candida infections in pregnancy and their treatment with clotrimazole. Curr Med Res Opin 1977;4:640–4.

13. Hale EK, Pomeranz MK. Dermatologic agents during pregnancy and lactation: an update and clinical review. Int J Dermatol 2002;41:197–203.

14. King CT, Rogers PD, Cleary JD, Chapman SW. Antifungal therapy during pregnancy. Clin Infect Dis 1998;27:1151–60.

15. PharmaDerm. *Oxistat package insert*. 2014. Available at: https://dailymed.nlm.nih.gov/dailymed/drugInfo.cfm?setid=b87a89d2-6e45-4eb8-be2c-7f55f34d61e5.

16. (https://www.accessdata.fda.gov/drugsatfda_docs/label/2013/204153s000lbl.pdf, accessed on 24/10/2017).

17. https://www.accessdata.fda.gov/drugsatfda_docs/label/2013/018533s040lbl.pdf. (accessed 2017 October 5).

18. Lind J. Limb malformations in a case of hydrops fetalis with ketoconazole use during pregnancy. Arch Gynecol 1985;237:398.

19. Sarkar M, Rowland K, Koren G. Pregnancy outcome following gestational exposure to terbinafine: A prospective comparative study. Clin Mol Teratol 2003;67:390.

20. Merz Pharmaceuticals. Naftin package insert. 2013. Available at: Http://www.naftin.com/wpcontent/uploads/NAFTIN-Cream-2-PI.pdf.

21. Leachman SA, Reed BR. The use of dermatologic drugs in pregnancy and lactation. Dermatol Clin 2006;24:167–97.

22. Pilmis B, Jullien V, Sobel J, Lecuit M, Lortholary O, Charlier C. Antifungal drugs during pregnancy: an updated review. J Antimicrob Chemother 2015; 70:14–22.

23. Briggs G. Drugs in Pregnancy and Lactation: A Reference Guide to Fetal and Neonatal Risk. 10th ed. Philadelphia, PA: Lippincott Williams & Wilkins, 2014.

24. Rosa F, Baum C, Shaw M. Pregnancy outcomes after first trimester vaginitis drug therapy. Obstet Gynecol 1987;69:751–5.

25. Culbertson C Monistat. A new fungicide for treatment of vulvovaginal candidiasis. Am J Obstet Gynecol 1974;120:973–6.

26. Davis J, Frudenfeld J, Goddard J. Comparative evaluation of Monistat and Mycostatin in the treatment of vulvovaginal candidiasis. Obstet Gynecol 1974;44:403–6.

27. Wallenburg HC, Wladimiroff JW. Recurrence of vulvovaginal candidosis during pregnancy: comparison of miconazole vs nystatin treatment. Obstet Gynecol 1976;48:491–4.

28. Patel VM, Schwartz RA, Lambert WC. Topical antiviral and antifungal medications in pregnancy: a review of safety profiles. J Eur Acad Dermatol Venereol 2017;31:1440–6.

29. Morra P, Bartle WR, Walker SE, Lee SN, Bowles SK, Reeves RA. Serum concentrations of salicylic acid following topically applied salicylate derivatives. Ann Pharmacother 1996;30:935–40.

30. Schwarb F, Gabard B, Rufli T, Surber C. Percutaneous absorption of salicylic acid in man after topical administration of three different formulations. Dermatology 1999;198:44–51.

31. Slone D, Siskind V, Heinonen OP, Monson RR, Kaufman DW, Shapiro S. Aspirin and congenital malformations. Lancet 1976;1:1373–5.

32. Klebanoff MA, Berendes HW. Aspirin exposure during the first 20 weeks of gestation and IQ at four years of age. Teratology 1988;37:249–55.

33. Lam J, Polifka JE, Dohil MA. Safety of dermatologic drugs used in pregnant patients with psoriasis and other inflammatory skin diseases. J Am Acad Dermatol 2008;59:295–315.

34. Briggs GG, Freeman RK, Yaffe SJ. Drugs in Pregnancy and Lactation: A Reference Guide to Fetal and Neonatal Risk. Philadelphia: Lippincott Williams & Wilkins, 2011.

35. Bar-Oz B, Moretti ME, Bishai R, et al. Pregnancy outcome after *in utero* exposure to itraconazole: a prospective cohort study. Am J Obstet Gynecol 2000; 183: 617–20.

36. De Santis M, Di Gianantonio E, Cesari E, et al. First trimester itraconazole exposure and pregnancy outcome: a prospective cohort study of women contacting teratology information services in Italy. Drug Saf Int J Med Toxicol Drug Exp 2009;32: 239–44.

37. Vlachadis N, Iliodromiti Z, Vrachnis N. Oral fluconazole during pregnancy and risk of birth defects. N Engl J Med 2013;369:2061.

38. Aleck KA, Bartley DL. Multiple malformation syndrome following fluconazole use in pregnancy: report of an additional patient. Am J Med Genet 1997;72:253–6.

39. Lee BE, Feinberg M, Abraham JJ, Murthy AR. Congenital malformations in an infant born to a woman treated with fluconazole. Pediatr Infect Dis J 1992;11:1062–4.

40. Lopez-Rangel E, Van Allen MI. Prenatal exposure to fluconazole: an identifiable dysmorphic phenotype. Birth Defects Res A Clin Mol Teratol 2005;73:919–23.

41. Pursley TJ, Blomquist IK, Abraham J, Andersen HF, Bartley JA. Fluconazole-induced congenital anomalies in three infants. Clin Infect Dis 1996; 22:336–40.

42. Tiboni GM, Marotta F, Del Corso A, Giampietro F. Defining critical periods for itraconazole-induced cleft palate, limb defects and axial skeletal malformations in the mouse. Toxicol Lett 2006; 167:8–18.

43. Mineshima H, Fukuta T, Kato E, et al. Malformation spectrum induced by ketoconazole after single administration to pregnant rats during the critical period—comparison with vitamin A-induced malformation spectrum. J Appl Toxicol 2012;32: 98–107.

44. Tiboni GM, Giampietro F. Murine teratology of fluconazole: evaluation of developmental phase specificity and dose dependence. Pediatr Res 2005;58:94–9.

45. Food and Drug Administration. Use of long-term, high-dose Diflucan (fluconazole) during pregnancy may be associated with birth defects in infants. 2011 (http://www.fda.gov/Drugs/Drug Safety/ucm266030.htm).

46. Rosa FW, Hernandez C, Carlo WA. Griseofulvin teratology, including two thoracophagus conjoined twins. Lancet 1987; 1: 171.

47. Czeizel AE, Me´tneki J, Kazy Z, et al. A population-based case-control study of oral griseofulvin treatment during pregnancy. Acta Obstet Gynecol Scand 2004; 83: 827–31.

48. Cottreau JM, Barr VO. A review of antiviral and antifungal use and safety during pregnancy. Pharmacotherapy 2016;36:668–78.

49. Solís-Arias MP, García-Romero MT. Onychomycosis in children. A review. Int J Dermatol. 2017;56:123–30.

50. S, Totri C, Friedlander SF. Antifungal therapy for onychomycosis in children. Clin Dermatol 2015; 33:333–9.

51. Totri CR, Feldstein S, Admani S, Friedlander SF, Eichenfield LF. Epidemiologic analysis of onychomycosis in the San Diego pediatric population. Pediatr Dermatol 2017;34:46–49.

52. Gupta AK, Paquet M. Systemic antifungals to treat onychomycosis in children: a systematic review. Pediatr Dermatol 2013;30:294–302.

53. Gupta AK, Sibbald RG, Lynde CW, et al. Onychomycosis in children: prevalence and treatment strategies. J Am Acad Dermatol 1997; 36:395–402.

54. Kim DM, Suh MK, Ha GY. Onychomycosis in children: an experience of 59 cases. Ann Dermatol 2013;25:327–34.

55. Gunduz T, Metin DY, Sacar T, et al. Onychomycosis in primary school children: association with socioeconomic conditions. Mycoses 2006;49:431–3.

56. Aly R, Hafeez ZH, Rodwell C, et al. Rapid response to Trichophyton tonsurans induced onychomycosis after treament with terbinafine. Int J Dermatol 2002; 41: 357–9.

57. Ploysangam T, Lucky AW. Childhood white superficial onychomycosis caused by Trichophyton rubrum: report of seven cases and review of the literature. J Am Acad Dermatol 1997; 36: 29–32.

58. Nicholls DS, Midgley G. Onychomycosis caused by Trichophyton equinum. Clin Exp Dermatol 1989; 14: 464–5.

59. Eichenfield LF, Friedlander SF. Pediatric onychomycosis: The emerging role of topical Therapy. J Drugs Dermatol 2016;16:105–109.

60. Gupta AK, Skinner AR. Onychomycosis in children: a brief overview with treatment strategies. Pediatr Dermatol 2004;21:74–79.

61. Nejjam F, Zagula M, Cabiac MD, Guessous N, Humbert H, Lakhdar H. Pilot study of terbinafine in children suffering from tinea capitis: evaluation of efficacy, safety and pharmacokinetics. Br J Dermatol 1995; 132: 98–105.

62. Gupta AK, Cooper EA, Ginter G. Efficacy and safety of itraconazole use in children. Dermatol Clin 2003;21:521–35.

63. Veraldi S, Schianchi R, Pontini P, Gorani A. The association of isoconazole-diflucortolone in the treatment of pediatric tinea corporis. J Dermatolog Treat 2017;19:1–2.

64. Hawkins DM, Smidt AC Superficial fungal infections in children. Pediatr Clin North Am 2014;61:443–55.

65. Paloni G, Valerio E, Berti I, Cutrone M. Tinea Incognito. J Pediatr 2015;167:1450–2.

66. Chang CH, Young-Xu Y, Kurth T, Orav JE, Chan AK. The safety of oral antifungal treatments for superficial dermatophytosis and onychomycosis: a meta-analysis. Am J Med 2007;120:791–8.

67. Liver toxicity: clinical and research information on drug-induced liver injury: drug record:

terbinafine. http://livertox.nlm.nih.gov/Terbinafine. htm accessed on 2/11/2017.

68. Kramer ON, Albrecht J. Clinical presentation of terbinafine-induced severe liver injury and the value of laboratory monitoring: a Critically Appraised Topic. Br J Dermatol 2017 Aug 1. doi: 10.1111/bjd.15854. [Epub ahead of print].

69. Ajit C, Suvannasankha A, Zaeri N, Munoz SJ. Terbinafine-associated hepatotoxicity. Am J Med Sci 2003;325:292–5.

70. Khurana A, Sardana K, Bhardwaj V. Response to 'Clinical presentation of terbinafine-induced severe liver injury and the value of laboratory monitoring: a critically appraised topic'. Br J Dermatol 2017 Nov 18. doi: 10.1111/bjd. 16134.

71. Guidance for industry, drug-induced liver injury: Premarketing clinical evaluation. (2009).

72. Tucker RM, Williams PL, Arathoon EG, Stevens DA. Treatment of mycoses with itraconazole. Ann NY Acad Sci 1988;544:451–70.

73. De Doncker P. Itraconazole and terbinafine in perspective: from Petri dish to patient. J Eur Acad Dermatol Venereol 1999 Sep;12 Suppl 1:S10–6; discussion S17.

74. Pettit NN, Pisano J, Weber S, Ridgway J. Hepatic failure in a patient receiving itraconazole for pulmonary histoplasmosis—case report and literature review. Am J Ther 2016;23:e1215–21.

75. Srebrnik A, Levtov S, Ben-Ami R, Brenner S. Liver failure and transplantation after itraconazole treatment for toenail onychomycosis. J Eur Acad Dermatol Venereol 2005;19:205–7.

76. https://www.accessdata.fda.gov/drugsatfda_docs/label/2009/020083s040s041s044lbl.pdf accessed 3/11/2017.

77. https://www.accessdata.fda.gov/drugsatfda_docs/label/2011/019949s051lbl.pdf (accessed 4/11/2017).

78. Yan JY, Nie XL, Tao QM, Zhan SY, Zhang YD. Ketoconazole associated hepatotoxicity: a systematic review and meta-analysis. Biomed Environ Sci 2013;26:605–10.

79. Phillips P, Shafran S, Garber G, et al. Multicenter randomized trial of fluconazole versus amphotericin B for treatment of candidemia in non-neutropenic patients. Canadian Candidemia Study Group. Eur J Clin Microbiol. Infect Dis 1997;16:337–45.

80. Chang CH, Young-Xu Y, Kurth T, Orav JE, Chan AK. The safety of oral antifungal treatments for superficial dermatophytosis and onychomycosis: a meta-analysis. Am J Med 2007;120:791–8.

81. Raschi E, Poluzzi E, Koci A, Caraceni P, Ponti FD. Assessing liver injury associated with antimycotics: Concise literature review and clues from data mining of the FAERS database. World J Hepatol 2014;6:601–12.

82. https://www.accessdata.fda.gov/drugsatfda_docs/label/2012/020539s021lbl.pdf (accessed 5/11/2017).

83. Grant SM, Clissold SP. Itraconazole. A review of its pharmacodynamic and pharmacokinetic properties and therapeutic potential in superficial and systemic mycoses. Drugs 1989;37:310–44.

84. Rosen T. Debilitating edema associated with itraconazole therapy. Arch Dermatol 1994;130: 260–71.

85. Nelson MR, Smith D, Erskine D, et al. Ventriculae fibrillation secondary to itraconazole-induced hypokalemia. J Infect 1993;26:348.

86. https://www.accessdata.fda.gov/drugsatfda_docs/label/2014/018533s041lbl.pdf (accessed on 5/11/2017).

Special Procedures: Laser, PDT Treatment for Dermatophytoses

Ananta Khurana

LASERS AND PDT IN ONYCHOMYCOSIS

Treatment of onychomycosis (OM) is often unsatisfactory with the currently available measures. Newer drugs with improved nail penetration have been introduced, but cure rates are not comparable to standard oral treatment. Different laser devices have been tried but so far lack thorough scientific evidence. The advantages over conventional treatments are few side effects and lesser contraindications, apart from compliance with infrequent treatment sessions. Currently 5 lasers, all utilizing neodymium-doped yttrium aluminum garnet (Nd:YAG) as their source, have received US FDA clearance for "temporarily increasing clearance" in the infected nails. However, the reader must be aware that this approval is based on equivalence to other legally marketed devices rather than clinical trial data.[1] Temporary improvement in clear nail does not require any mycological testing beyond baseline, emphasizing the temporary nature of the esthetic outcome and potential incomplete eradication of fungus with device use.

The parameters of lasers that have been US FDA/other international authorities cleared or tested and supported by publications for onychomycosis are summarized in Table 15.1.

Mechanism of Action

The exact mechanisms by which different laser systems may work in OM are not elucidated so far. Different mechanisms have been postulated and evaluated in *in vitro* trials for different laser systems.[2]

Nd:YAG Lasers

These lasers may act by a direct heating effect on the fungi. Since chitin surrounding the fungal mycelium is slow to dissipate heat, accumulation of heat and rising temperature can occur within the fungi creating a fungicidal effect.[3] However, Paasch et al found, while irradiating fungal pathogens cultured in liquid media, that complete clearance was achieved only when the temperature exceeded 50°C.[4] When the temperatures were not high enough, they observed stimulation in the growth of fungi, especially in case of *Microsporum gypseum* and *T. rubrum*. But temperatures over 45°C result in pain and tissue necrosis in humans.[5–7]

Thus, lasers should be delivered in pulses with durations shorter than the thermal relaxation time of the fungus.[8,9] This can allow for the accumulation of heat inside the fungal cell and prevent severe pain/necrosis in surrounding tissues. Further, to be able to produce these effects, the wavelength of a

Table 15.1: Laser systems approved for treatment of onychomycosis							
Laser system	Type of laser	Wavelength (nm)	Energy fluence (J/cm²)	Spot size (mm)	Pulse length	Pulse frequency (Hz)	International approvals for onychomycosis
Dualis SP™, Fotona	Long pulse Nd:YAG	1064	35–40	4	35 ms	1	EU
Q-Clear™ Light Age, Inc.	Qs Nd:YAG	1064	14	2.5–6	3–10 nanosecond	—	US, EU
FootLaser™, Nuvolase	Short pulse Nd:YAG	1064	25.5	2.5	100–3000 µs	1	US, Canada, EU, Australia
GenesisPlus™, Cutera	Short pulse Nd:YAG	1064	16	5	300 µs	2	US, Canada, EU
VARIA™, CoolTouch	Short pulse Nd:YAG	1064	—	—	600 µs	—	US, EU
LightPod® Neo™, Aerolase	Short pulse Nd:YAG	1064	223	2	650 µs	—	—
JOULE ClearSense™, Sciton	Short pulse Nd:YAG	1064	13	—	0.3–200 ms	6	US
CoolTouch CT3 Plus™, CoolTouch	Short pulse Nd:YAG	1320	—	2–10	450 µs	—	EU
Mira® 900, Coherent Laser Group	Mode locked Ti:Sapphire	800	10^{31} to 10^{33} m^2 s^{-1}	0.12–0.45	200 fs	76 MHz	—
Noveon®, Nomir Medical Technologies	Diode	870, 930	212/424	15	—	—	EU
V-Raser®, ConBio/ Cynosure	Diode	980	—	—	—	—	—

laser needs to selectively target the fungi and be able to penetrate the nail plate.[8,9]

Wavelengths of lasers that penetrate the nail range from 750 to 1300 nm.[10] The thermal relaxation time can be approximated to the square of the diameter of the target. The thermal relaxation time of hyphae (2–10 mm) is 0.004–0.1 milliseconds, of macroconidia (4–50 mm) is 16 microseconds to 2.5 milliseconds, and of microconidia (2–4 mm) is in the 0.004–0.016 milliseconds range. Thus, selective targeting of dermatophytes likely requires pulse durations in the nanosecond to very low millisecond range. [1]

The possible chromophores include xanthomegnin, chitin and melanin. The Qs Nd:YAG at 532 nm is absorbed by the large amount of xanthomegnin in *T. rubrum* and this explains the inhibitory effects of the laser on *T. rubrum*. Qs Nd:YAG at 1064 nm is however beyond the absorption spectrum of xanthomegnin but still shown to suppress the organism.[12] This wavelength may be absorbed by the great amount of melanin in cell wall of

Trichophyton species and act thereof. Targeting these fungal protective pigments could also render the organism more susceptible to host immune response and reactive oxygen species.[13]

Another postulated mechanism is that there only occurs a nonspecific tissue heating with a subsequent increase in circulation due to vasodilatation and stimulation of the host immunological processes.[14] This is supported by some *in vitro* studies which found no effect of laser irradiation on fungal colonies.[14,15] Carney et al found no growth inhibition of *T. rubrum* even on visibly pigmeted colonies.[15] Kozarev et al consider that 1064 nm long-pulsed Nd:YAG laser is mainly dependent on the thermal effect of the laser.[16]

Ghavam et al demonstrated that low-power laser systems modified colonies, but did not have any inhibitory effects on the fungal colonies, while in the high power laser category, the Q-switched Nd:YAG 532 nm in 8 J/cm², Q-switched Nd:YAG 1064 nm laser at 4 to 8 J/cm², and pulsed dye laser (PDL) in 8 J/cm 2595 nm to 14 J/cm² significantly inhibited the growth of *T. rubrum* and could significantly change the microstructure of *T. rubrum*.[17–19]

Carbon Dioxide (CO₂) Laser

The mechanism of action of CO_2 laser is partially based on a photothermal effect: The fungal tissue is heated; the water within the fungal tissue is converted into steam, which causes swelling and increased pressure within the fungal body, leading to micro-explosions and, eventually, catabolism. Higher local temperatures can directly kill the fungus. On the other hand, micro-holes made by fractional CO_2 laser may improve the penetration of the topical antifungal agent into the nail bed.[20]

Diode Lasers

Near-infrared diode laser is a two-wavelength laser, which can emit 870 and 930 nm near-infrared light. It likely acts through thermal effects.[21] Diode laser also cause a decreased mitochondrial membrane potential and increased production of reactive oxygen species, which play a role in the killing effect on *Candida albicans* and *Trichophyton rubrum*, confirmed by *in vitro* experiments.[22, 23]

A special case for use of lasers is for the disruption of fungal biofilms (dermatophytomas) which render oral and topical antifungal therapies ineffective, as these target freely suspended (planktonic) fungi and are unable to penetrate through the protective extracellular matrix covering of the biofilms.[24,25]

Laser Systems Tried

Most studies have used short pulse and long pulse 1064 nm Nd:YAG lasers, with lesser papers to the credit of near-infrared diode lasers, dual diode lasers, fractional CO_2 lasers and Q-switched Nd:YAG laser.

Cure Rates Reported

There are gross inconsistencies in studies evaluating different laser systems for OM. The response has been reported in terms of magnitude of clear nail, mycological cure, clinical cure and complete cure in different studies. The units of analysis also vary, with some reporting on patients and others on individual nails. Comparisons with topical and oral drugs are also lacking.

Francuzike et al in their 2016 review reported that 45.45% (10/22) of included laser studies demonstrated an improvement as evident in clinical outcome and/or mycological tests.[26] They found a complete cure rate in 36% (8/22) of their included laser studies with rates exceeding 50% when patients were used as the unit of analysis.[26] Most studies utilized Nd:YAG lasers and were small and uncontrolled. A total of 47.37% of the reviewed studies using a 1,064 nm device reported that all treated patients had a positive response, and 60% of studies reported complete clinical and mycologic cure in at least half of the treated patients.

But, given the heterogeneity of data, it was not possible to make comparisons between studies. In a more recent literature review, Gupta et al[27] concluded that laser studies, to date, provide preliminary evidence of clinical improvement and clear nail growth in toenail onychomycosis, consistent with the FDA clearance for aesthetic endpoints. But they do not provide efficacy rates for medical endpoints that equate or exceed those found with traditional therapies (oral and topical treatments). The authors included RCTs, non-randomized, uncontrolled and retrospective studies that included at least one of the following measures: Complete cure, mycological cure, clinical improvement, and clinical cure. Of the included studies, mycological cure (negative culture and negative microscopy) was evaluated in two studies using patients as the unit of analysis with an average rate of 11%, increasing to 63% when nails were used as the unit of analysis (3 studies). Clinical cure (100% clear nail) was evaluated in 6 studies with a rate of 13% using nails as the unit of analysis and 13% when patients were used as the unit of analysis (2 studies). Clinical improvement (at any time point) was found in 36% of patients (5 studies) and 67% of nails (9 studies). Nail clarity as measured by clear nail growth and/or nail plate/bed clearance at 12 weeks was found to be 2.6 mm across onychomycotic nails.

Laser Specific Data

Prominent data from individual laser studies is presented below.

Short-pulsed (SP) Nd:YAG[28–34]

Most of the approved devices, and of available literature, belongs to this class of lasers. Negative mycologic cure rates with SP Nd:YAG lasers have ranged from 51 to 95%.[1] But, these rates have been reported in small studies (Table 15.2) with varying parameters, number of treatment sessions and time between treatments. It is noteworthy that the

2 RCTs[28,29] demonstrated no benefit of the laser versus placebo. Results of a company-sponsored Phase III efficacy study, registered in 2010, under the title 'PinPointe™ and Foot-Laser™ for the treatment of onychomycosis' are yet to be published.[30]

Traditional 1064 nm lasers utilize a pulse duration between 5 and 30 milliseconds (ms), in excess of the approximately 0.7 ms thermal relaxation time of skin tissue. Thus, continuous cooling is required to avoid treatment-related pain and injury to the surrounding skin. Hochman et al used a 0.65 ms pulsed 1064 nm laser with a handpiece that does not come into contact the treatment site and does not require tissue cooling, to circumvent this issue.[31] They proposed this to be a practical approach for onychomycosis given the uneven surface geometry and thickness of the affected nail.

Long-pulsed (LP) Nd:YAG[35–38]

LP Nd:YAG laser has been used by a few, with widely varying results (Table 15.3). Ortiz et al used the 1,320 nm Nd:YAG laser on the grounds of deeper penetration compared with 1064 nm laser.[35] Hypothetically, this may result in more effective heating of the nail plate. However, greater improvement of onychomycosis from deeper light penetration is yet to be elucidated.[35] Further, the outcome in this RCT was not clearly positive. The culture negativity was achieved in a higher number of patients in the control group rather than the laser treated group. Few other studies showed positive outcomes and Kozarev et al[37] demonstrated a positive outcome in the *in vitro* arm of their study (with LP 1064 nm Nd:YAG) as well, with evident growth inhibition and colony decay after single irradiation session. Another RCT (El-Tatawy et al) demonstrated a positive outcome over topical terbinafine.[38]

Q-switched (Qs) Lasers[39–44]

Qs Nd:YAG lasers have been reported to be beneficial in dermatophytic OM in a few

Table 15.2: Summary of papers on short-pulsed Nd:YAG laser in onychomycosis			
Authors	*Patients*	*Parameters*	*Outcome*
Hollmig et al, 2014[28] **RCT**	27 (125 affected nails) vs placebo	1064 nm Nd:YAG (Joule ClearSense™); 5 J/cm², 6 Hz, 0.3 ms PD, 6 mm SS (to achieve measured target temperature of 40°C)	At 3 months and 12 months: No statistically significant difference between proximal nail plate clearance and negative culture between laser and placebo arm
Karsai et al, 2016[29] **RCT**	20 patients (82 nails)	Randomized to SP 1064 nm Nd:YAG laser (PinPointe™, Footlaser™) or control group (no laser treatment) Laser parameters: 20 J/cm²; 0.1 ms PD; 1.5 mm SS; 30 Hz PR; 4 sessions, 4–6 weeks apart Both groups applied topical antifungal to the soles	No mycological cure in any group OSI score worsened in both groups after 12 months
Hochman et al, 2014[31]	8 patients	0.65 ms (650 µs) pulsed 1064 nm Nd:YAG laser (Aerolase, LightPod Neo) 2 mm SS, 223 J/cm², 2–3 session at least 3 weeks apart	7/8 culture negative (done after 2nd or 3rd treatment) Clinical improvement in most treated nails
Kimura et al, 2012[32]	13 patients (37 nails)	Submillisecond 1064 nm Nd:YAG; 5 mm SS, 14 J/cm², 0.3 ms PD; 1–3 sessions/4–6 weeks apart	81% nails had "moderate" to "complete" clearance. 51% cleared completely with negative KOH. 19% had significant clearance and 11% had moderate clearance
Harris et al, 2009[33] (PinPointe™, FootLaser™ phase I/II clinical trial data)	17: Randomized into treated (11) and untreated (6) groups	1064 nm (PinPointe™, FootLaser™), 0.1–3 ms PD, 2.5 mm SS, 25.5 J/cm², 1 Hz; single treatment	79% treated toes improved in terms of clear linear growth. Improvement ranged from 2.1 to 6.1 mm over 90 days (average 3.9 mm, or 1.3 mm clearing per month) No mycological data reported

PD: Pulse duration; SS: Spot size; ms: millisecond; PR: Pulse rate; OSI: Onychomycosis severity index.

Table 15.3: Summary of papers on long-pulsed Nd:YAG lasers in onychomycosis			
Authors	Patients	Parameters	Outcome
Ortiz et al, 2014[35] **RCT**	10 patients with culture proven bilateral great toenail OM randomized to receive laser or sham treatment	1,320 nm LP Nd:YAG laser (CoolTouch CT3 Plus) 5 mm SS, 350 microsecond PD, 20 Hz, and 3W at a target temperature of 38°C; 4 treatments on days 1, 7, 14, and 60	At 6 months, the treated toenails improved from an average rating of severe involvement (>67% involvement) to moderate involvement (34–66% involvement) Treated arm: 50% culture negative at 3 months However, in the control group, 70% of cultures were negative at this time
Moon et al, 2014[36]	13 patients (43 nails)	1,064 nm LP Nd:YAG laser (ClearSense™): 6 mm SS, 5 J/cm², 0.3 ms PD and 5 Hz PR 5 sessions at 4-week intervals	Only 4 (9.3%) nails "cured" with complete clearance and negative KOH; 8 (18.6) nails had >80% clearance; and 31 (72%) nails had 50–80% clearance
Kozarev et al, 2010[37]	72 patients (194 nails)	LP Nd:YAG 1064 nm laser light (Dualis SP, Fotona, Slovenia); 35–40 J/cm², 35 ms PD, 4 mm SS, 1 Hz PR; to achieve nail plate temperature of 45° ± 5°C 4 sessions with one week gap between each	On 6 and 12 months follow up all patients (100%) were "clear of infection". Positive response in in vitro arm as well
El-Tatawy et al, 2015[38] **RCT**	40 patients	Laser arm: 1064 nm Nd:YAG laser (Dualis SP, Fontana); 35–40 J/cm², 4 mm SS, PD 35 ms, PR 1 Hz 4 sessions, weekly Topical terbinafine arm: Six months, twice daily application after abrasion of the nail by abrasive stick to improve transungual delivery	At 6 months: All patients in laser group showed marked improvement, while only 50% in terbinafine group showed mild to moderate improvement, 80% patients in laser group showed mycological clearance, 0% in terbinafine group

PD: Pulse duration; SS: Spot size; ms: millisecond; PR: Pulse rate

Table 15.4: Results with Qs Nd:YAG lasers in onychomycosis			
Authors	*Patients*	*Parameters*	*Outcome*
Garcia et al, 2014[40]	120 patients	Qs Nd:YAG 1064 nm; 600 mJ/cm², 3 mm SS, 3 Hz PR Single session	At 9 months: 100% clinical and mycological response (KOH negative)
Kalokasidis et al, 2013[39]	131 patients	*First pass:* Qs 1064 nm (Q clear), 14 J/cm², 5Hz PR, 2.5 mm SS, 9 billionths of a second PD *Second pass:* Same laser at 532 nm setting, 14 J/cm², 5 Hz PR, 2.5 mm SS, 9 billionths of a second PD 2 minutes gap between the two passes 2 sessions at day 0 and 30	At 3-month follow-up, 125 patients (95.42%) showed mycological cure (negative microscopy and culture)
FDA 510 (k) Summary K110370, 2011 (Q clear trial)[42]	100 patients	Single session with 2–14 J/cm² fluence, 2.5–6 mm SS, 3–10 ns PD	95% mycological cure rate

PD: Pulse duration; SS: Spot size; PR: Pulse rate; ns: Nanosecond

previous reports (Table 15.4). Q-switched lasers might target melanin or chitin in the fungal cell wall leading to photomechanical or photothermal effects. Kalokasidis et al reported a mycological cure of 95.42% after 3 months of treatment with 2 sessions of Qs Nd:YAG.[39] Garcia (2014) reported a clinical response rate of 93%, which increased to 100% after 6 months.[40] *In vivo* studies with Qs Nd:YAG have however been conflicting. While Vural et al[41] demonstrated significant inhibition of growth in irradiated colonies of *T. rubrum*, Hees et al 14 did not find any change after using various energy doses of Qs Nd:YAG, long-pulsed Nd:YAG and KTP laser.

We have used a protocol similar to Kalokasidis et al with successful outcomes in dermatophytic OM (Fig. 15.1) and one case of *Fusarium solani* complex OM (Fig. 15.2).[43]

Diode Laser

The approved diode equipment (Noveon laser, Nomir Medical Technologies, Inc., Woodmere, NY, USA) is a dual wavelength 870 and 930 nm laser. In a single clinical trial of individuals with toenail onychomycosis confirmed by culture and PAS microscopy,[45] 26 participants received four laser treatments on days 1, 14, 42, and 120. At 180 days follow-up, 85% of participants showed an improvement in clear nail linear extent; 65% showed at least 3 mm and 26% showed at least 4 mm of clear nail growth. Simultaneous negative culture and periodic acid–Schiff was noted in 30% at 180 days. In a follow-up paper, review of 270-day mycological data showed a further decrease in both measures with 38% of the treated population having negative culture and microscopy, qualifying as "mycological cures".[46] The status of the phase II and II/III trials for the Noveon laser in onychomycosis (NCT00771732 and NCT00776464) remains unknown till date.[47, 48]

Fractional Carbon Dioxide (CO₂) Lasers

Recent publications have demonstrated beneficial effects of fractional CO_2 along with topical therapies. Lim et al hypothesize that

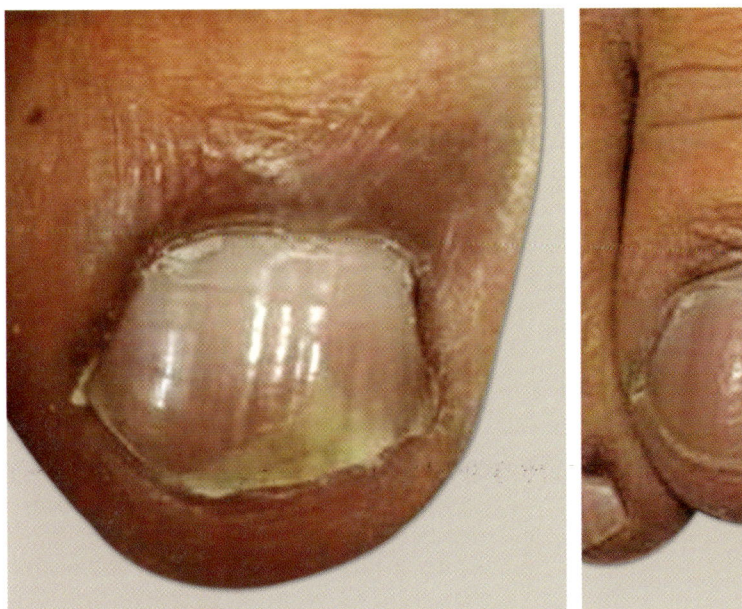
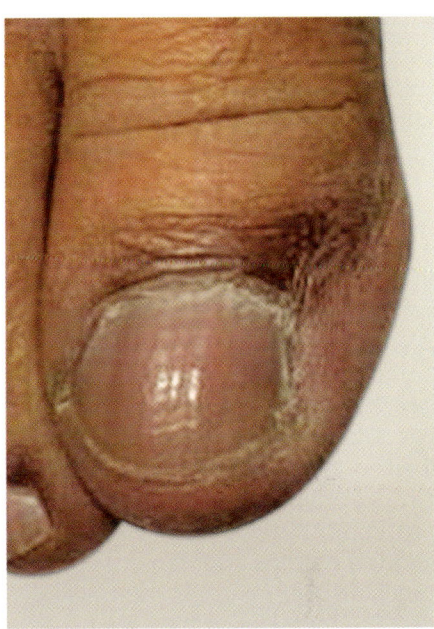

Fig. 15.1: KOH positive case of dermatophytic OM, failed 3 months of terbinafine 250 mg OD, completed one year before. The patient was treated with a single session of Qs 1064 nm (9.3 J/cm^2, 4 mm SS, 1 Hz), combined in the same session with Qs 532 nm (5 J/cm^2, 2 mm SS, 1 Hz). Complete clearing with negative microscopy after one year

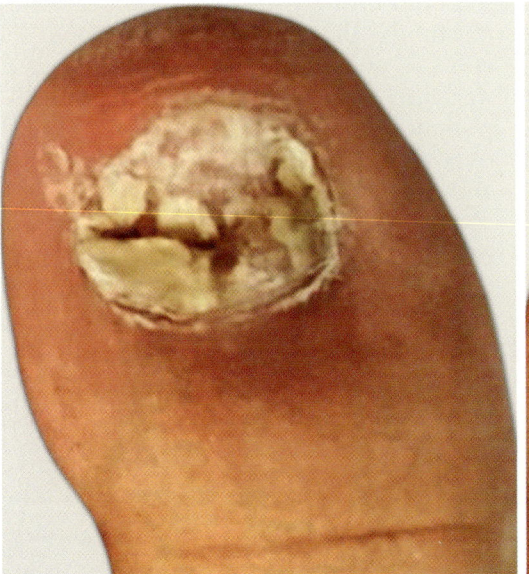
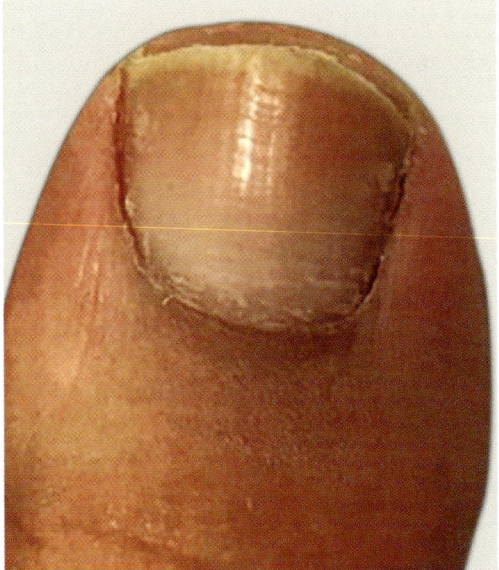

Fig. 15.2: A culture positive case of *Fusarium solani* OM, previously failed multiple adequate oral antifungal treatments. The patient was given 2 sessions with combined Qs Nd:YAG 532 nm and 1064 nm (as mentioned in Fig. 15.1). Complete clinical and mycological cure at one year. (Khurana A, Chowdhary A, Sardana K, et al. Dermatol Ther. 2017 Nov 28)

the tissue ablation process caused by fractional CO_2 laser induces direct fungicidal effects and that the multiple columns created by the laser enhance the penetration of topical antifungal agents into the nail bed or matrix.[49] After 3 CO_2 treatments at 4-week intervals along with daily topical amorolfine cream, 50% of their patients had a complete response with negative microscopy, while 92% showed a clinical response.[49] In another series of 75 patients 50 fractional CO_2 was similarly given along with daily application of terbinafine cream. The authors reported 84% KOH and 80% culture negativity at 6-month follow-up. Zhou et al used fractional CO_2 laser treatment (12 two weekly sessions over 6 months) alone and in combination with 1% luliconazole cream for 6 months and demonstrated higher efficacy in the combination treatment group.[51]

The laser is simple and cost-effective, with good patient compliance. Nevertheless, there is no standard protocol for energy density, depth and breadth of the wavelength. It remains to be further explored and summarized with its proper mechanism of action.

Others: Er:YAG lasers have been used with topical amorolfine with favorable outcomes, where one study (*n* = 9) reported mycological cure of 75% and complete cure of 60% of nails treated (35– 62 J/cm^2 fluence), compared with 20% of those treated with amorolfine alone.[52]

CONCLUSION

To summarize, as per the scientific evidence available so far, there is no evidence of unequivocal benefit with lasers as mono-therapy/combination therapy. However, a few trials are encouraging. While in the SP Nd:YAG group, both RCTs done so far are negative, there is one positive RCT to the credit of LP Nd:YAG. Qs Nd:YAG has all positive results to its credit, though the available literature is scant so far. A single trial on diode laser shows beneficial response. Fractional CO_2 has demonstrated benefit in combination with topicals compared to topicals alone.

Going by the proposed mechanisms and available data, Qs lasers seem to hold promise. The likely chromophores are abundantly present within the common causative dermato-phytic species and the laser is thus capable of producing a selective action damaging fungal cells. However, confirmation from *in vitro* studies is not absolute and the best parameters are yet to be defined.

PHOTODYNAMIC THERAPY

Photodynamic therapy involves the absorption of light energy by a photosensitive molecule, which transforms the ground state photo-sensitiser to a short-lived excited singlet state. From here, the excited PS can either lose energy via light or heat emission, and thus return to its ground state, or it will undergo a change in electron spin, converting it to an excited triplet state. The latter can return to its singlet state via phosphorescence, or react with molecular oxygen (O_2) to create excited oxygen radicals, via either a Type 1 or Type 2 photochemical pathway.[53]

Photosensitizers which have been used in antifungal PDT include porphyrinoid mole-cules [5 aminolevulinic acid (ALA) and its derivative methyl aminolevulinate (MAL)], phthalocyanine molecules, phenothiazinium dyes (methylene blue and toluidine blue O) and xanthene dyes (e.g. rose Bengal).[53]

Several reports have demonstrated improve-ment in onychomycosis treated with PDT.[54–57] In these studies, patients were pretreated with 20 to 40% urea ointment under occlusion for 10 hours to 10 days prior to treatment. In some cases, the entire nail plate was removed. Cure rates reported have been between 32 and 80%.[54–57]

References

1. Wiznia LE, Quatrano NA, Mu EW, Rieder EA. A clinical review of laser and light therapy for nail psoriasis and onychomycosis. Dermatol Surg 2017;43:161–72.

2. Bhatta AK, Keyal U, Wang X, Gellén E. A review of the mechanism of action of lasers and

photodynamic therapy for onychomycosis. Lasers Med Sci 2017;32:469–74.

3. Lahiri K, De A, Sarda A. Textbook of Lasers in Dermatology. 1st ed. Jaypee Brothers Medical Publishers; 2016: 249–253.

4. Paasch U, Mock A, Grunewald S, Bodendorf MO, Kendler M, Seitz AT, et al. Antifungal efficacy of lasers against dermatophytes and yeasts *in vitro*. Int J Hyperthermia 2013;29:544–50.

5. Anderson RR, Parrish JA. Selective photo-thermolysis: precise microsurgery by selective absorption of pulsed radiation. Science 1983; 220(4596):524–7.

6. Hashimoto T, Blumenthal HJ. Survival and resistance of *Trichophyton mentagrophytes* arthrospores. Appl Environ Microbiol 1978; 35: 274–7.

7. Carney C, Cantrell W, Warner J, Elewski B. Treatment of onychomycosis using a submillisecond 1064 nm neodymium: yttrium-aluminum-garnet laser. J Am Acad Dermatol 2013; 69:578–82.

8. Landthaler M, Brunner R, Braun-Falco O, Haina D, Waidelich W. Effects of argon, dye, and Nd: YAG lasers on epidermis, dermis, and venous vessels. Lasers Surg Med 1986;6:87–93.

9. Gupta AK, Simpson FC, Heller DF. The future of lasers in onychomycosis. J Dermatol Treat 2016;27:167–72.

10. Lee K, Onwudiwe O, Farinelli W, Garibyan L, Anderson RR. Absorption Spectra of Onycho-mycotic Nails. In: Laser 2015 ASLMS Conference. Kissimee, FL; 2015: p. LB13.

11. Sardana K. Miscellaneous Laser Responsive Disorders. In Sardana K (ed). Lasers in Clinical Practice. Jaypee Publishers, New Delhi, 2015.

12. Gupta AK, Ahmad I, Borst I, Summebrbell RC. Detection of xanthomegnin in epidermal materials infected with *Trichophyton rubrum*. J Invest Dermatol 2000;115:901–5.

13. Gomez BL, Nosanchuk JD. Melanin and fungi. Curr Opin Infect Dis 2003;16:91–6.

14. Hees H, Raulin C, Bäumler W. Laser treatment of onychomycosis: an *in vitro* pilot study. J Dtsch Dermatol Ges 2012;10: 913–8.

15. Carney C, Cantrell W, Warner J, Elewski B. Treatment of onychomycosis using a submillisecond 1064 nm neodymium:yttrium-aluminum-garnet laser. J Am Acad Dermatol. 2013; 69:578–82.

16. Kozarev J, Mitrovica S. Laser treatment of nail fungal infection. Berlin conference of the European Academy of Dermatology and Venereology, 2009.

17. Ghavam SA, Aref S, Mohajerani E. Laser irradiation on growth of *Trichophyton rubrum*: an *in vitro* study. J Lasers Med Sci 2015;6:10–16.

18. Gupta AK, Nakrieko KA. *Trichophyton rubrum* DNA strain switching increases in onychomycosis patients failing antifungal treatments. Br J Dermatol 2015;172:74–80.

19. Gupta AK, Nakrieko KA. *Trichophyton rubrum* DNA strain switching increases in onychomycosis patients failing antifungal treatments. Br J Dermatol 2015;172:74–80.

20. Bhatta AK, Keyal U, Huang X, Zhao JJ. Fractional carbon dioxide (CO_2) laser-assisted topical therapy for onycomycosis. J Am Acad Dermatol 201;74: 916–23.

21. Harris DM, Mc Dowell BA, Strisower. Laser treatment for toenail fungus. Proc of SPIE, 2009; 7161:71610M1-M7.

22. Landsman AS, Robbins AH, Angelini PF, et al. Treatment of mild, moderate, and severe onychomycosis using 870 and 930 nm light exposure. J Am Pediatr Med Assoc 2010; 100:166–77.

23. Bornstein E, Hermans W, Gridley S. Near-infrared photoinactivation of bacteria and fungi at physiologic temperatures. Photochem Photobiol 2009;85:1364–74.

24. Gupta A, Daigle D, Carviel J. The role of biofilms in onychomycosis. J Am Acad Dermatol 2016; 74:1241–6.

25. Pierce CG, Thomas DP, Lopez-Ribot JL. Effect of tunicamycin on *Candida albicans* biofilm formation and maintenance. Antimicrob Chemother 2009;63:473–9.

26. Francuzik W, Fritz K, Salavastru C. Laser therapies for onychomycosis—critical evaluation of methods and effectiveness. J Eur Acad Dermatol Venereol 2016;30:936–42.

27. Gupta AK, Versteeg SG. A critical review of improvement rates for laser therapy used to treat toenail onychomycosis. J Eur Acad Dermatol Venereol 2017;31:1111–8.

28. Hollmig ST, Rahman Z, Henderson MT, Rotatori RM, Gladstone H, Tang JY. Lack of efficacy with 1064 nm neodymium:yttrium-aluminum-garnet laser for the treatment of onychomycosis: a randomized, controlled trial. J Am Acad Dermatol 2014;70:911–7.

29. Karsai S, Jäger M, Oesterhelt A, Weiss C, Schneider SW, Jünger M, Raulin C. Treating onychomycosis with the short-pulsed 1064 nm Nd:YAG laser:

results of a prospective randomized controlled trial. J Eur Acad Dermatol Venereol 2017;31:175–80.

30. Evaluation Study for the Efficacy and Safety of PinPointe and FootLaser in Treatment for Onychomycosis. [WWW document]. URL http://clinical trials.gov/ct2/show/NCT00935649? term= onychomycosis+laser&rank=4 (last accessed: 26 December 2017).

31. Hochman LG. Laser treatment of onychomycosis using a novel 0.65 millisecond pulsed Nd:YAG 1064 nm laser. J Cosmet Laser Ther 2011;13:2–5.

32. Kimura U1, Takeuchi K, Kinoshita A, Takamori K, Hiruma M, Suga Y. Treating onychomycoses of the toenail: clinical efficacy of the sub-millisecond 1,064 nm Nd:YAG laser using a 5 mm spot diameter. J Drugs Dermatol 2012;11:496–504.

33. Harris D, McDowell B, Strisower J. Laser treatment for toenail fungus. Proc of SPIE. 2009 Feb 19; 7161: 7161M1–7.

34. Gupta A, Simpson F. Device-based therapies for onychomycosis treatment. Skin Therapy Lett. 2012; 17:4–9.

35. Ortiz AE, Truong S, Serowka K, Kelly KM. A 1,320 nm Nd:YAG laser for improving the appearance of onychomycosis. Dermatol Surg 2014;40:1356–60.

36. Moon SH, Hur H, Oh YJ, Choi KH, Kim JE, Ko JY, Ro YS. Treatment of onychomycosis with a 1,064 nm long-pulsed Nd:YAG laser. J Cosmet Laser Ther 2014;16:165–70.

37. Kozarev JVZ. Novel laser therapy in treatment of onychomycosis. J Laser Health Acad; 2010:1–8.

38. El-Tatawy RA, Abd El-Naby NM, El-Hawary EE, Talaat RA. A comparative clinica l and mycological study of Nd: YAG laser versus topical terbinafine in the treatment of onychomycosis. J Dermatolog Treat 2015;26:461–4.

39. Kalokasidis K, Onder M, Trakatelli MG, Richert B, Fritz K. The effect of Q-switched Nd:YAG 1064 nm/532 nm laser in the treatment of Onychomycosis *in vivo*. Dermatol Res Pract 2013;2013: 379–725.

40. Galvan Garcia HR. Onychomycosis: 1064 nm Nd:YAG Q-switch laser treatment. J Cosmet Dermatol 2014 ;13:232–5.

41. Vural E, Winfield HL, Shingleton AW, Horn TD, et al. The effects of laser irradiation on *Trichophyton rubrum* growth. Lasers Med Sci 2008; 23: 349–53.

42. FDA 510(k) Summary K110370. Q-Clear, Light Age, Inc., 2011.

43. Khurana A, Chowdhary A, Sardana K, Gautam RK, Sharma PK. Complete cure of *Fusarium solani* complex onychomycosis with Qs Nd:YAG treatment. Dermatol Ther 2017 Nov 28. doi: 10.1111/dth.12580.

44. Gupta AK, Simpson FC. Medical devices for the treatment of onychomycosis. Dermatol Ther 2012;25:574–81.

45. Landsman AS, Robbins AH, Angelini PF, Wu CC, et al. Treatment of mild, moderate, and severe onychomycosis using 870 and 930 nm light exposure. J Am Podiatr Med Assoc 2010;100:166–77.

46. Landsman AS, Robbins AH. Treatment of mild, moderate, and severe onychomycosis using 870 and 930 nm light exposure: some follow-up observations at 270 days. J Am Podiatr Med Assoc 2012;102:169–71.

47. Nomir Medical Technologies. Using light therapy to treat toenail fungus. In: Clinical Trials.gov editor: US NIH, 2008.

48. Nomir Medical Technologies. Treating onychomychosis. In: ClinicalTrials.gov editor: US NIH, 2008.

49. Lim EH, Kim HR, Park YO, et al. Toenail onychomycosis treated with a fractional carbon dioxide laser and topical antifungal cream. J Am Acad Dermatol 2014;70:918–23.

50. Bhatta AK, Keyal U, Huang X, Zhao JJ. Fractional carbon dioxide (CO_2) laser-assisted topical therapy for the treatment of onychomycosis. J Am Acad Dermatol 2016;74:916–23.

51. Zhou BR, Lu Y, Permatasari F, Huang H, Li J, Liu J, Zhang JA, Luo D, Xu Y. The efficacy of fractional carbon dioxide (CO_2) laser combined with luliconazole 1% cream for the treatment of onychomycosis: A randomized, controlled trial. Medicine (Baltimore). 2016;95:e5141.

52. Zhang J, Lu S, Huang H, Li X, Cai W, Ma J, Xi L. Lasers Med. Sci 2016, 31:1391–6.

53. Houang J, Perrone G, Mawad D, Boughton PC, Ruys AJ, Lauto A. Light treatments of nail fungal infections. J Biophotonics 2017 Dec 11.

54. Sotiriou E, Koussidou-Eremonti T, Chaidemenos G, Apalla Z, Ioannides D. Acta Derm. Venereol 2010;90: 216–7.

55. Gilaberte Y, Robres MP, Frias MP, Garcia-Doval I, Rezusta A, Aspiroz CJ Eur Acad Dermatology Venereol 2017;31:347–54.

56. Figueiredo Souza LW, Souza SVT, Botelho CC. Dermatol Ther 2014;27:43–7.

57. Tardivo JP, Wainwright M, Baptista MJ. Photochem Photobiol B Biol 2015;150:66–68.

16

Scenarios

A MANAGEMENT PROTOCOL IN CLINICAL PRACTICE

Shyam Verma

A 23-year-old college student consulted me for widespread tinea cruris et corporis and tinea faciei which he was battling with for the past one year. He had widespread erythematous, scaly annular lesions diffusely over both his lower limbs and buttocks (Figs 16.1 to 16.3). Many lesions on his buttocks and thighs showed central clearing with concomitant disease activity in the cleared areas.

He was initially prescribed 'Castor NF cream' containing clobetasol propionate, clotrimazole and neomycin by a GP which he later continued to buy and had applied about 75–80 tubes of 15 gm each on an average of 5–6 tubes per week. He had a strong history of allergic rhinitis, the father had bronchial asthma and he had 'dry skin'. The skin of the areas unaffected by dermatophytosis was dry. In fact the skin over the treated areas in places was more dry than unaffected areas. A clinical diagnosis of 'steroid modified tinea' in a patient with atopic diathesis was made after getting a KOH mount positivity adding Chicago sky blue stain, a procedure that we follow in our affiliated laboratory.

I prescribed 100 mg of itraconazole for two weeks with topical luliconazole once daily. Upon 2 weeks follow-up visit he showed new

lesions on neck and beard area (Figs 16.4 and 16.5). The dose of itraconazole was increased to 200 mg per day and luliconazole was advised to be applied twice daily. An 8 am

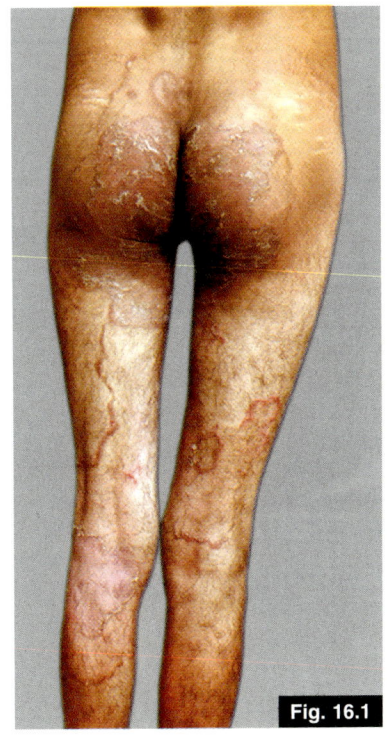

Fig. 16.1

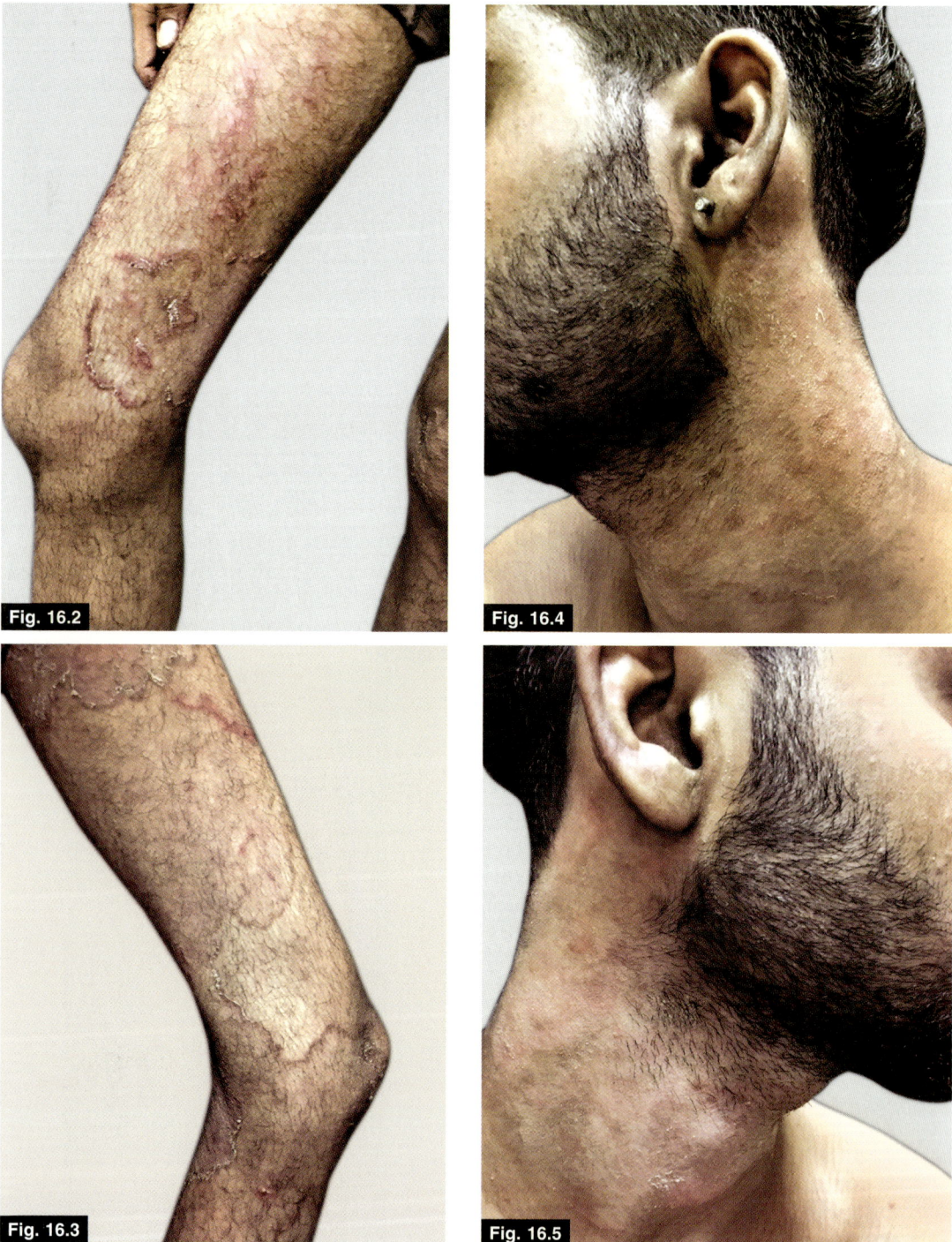

Fig. 16.2

Fig. 16.4

Fig. 16.3

Fig. 16.5

Figs 16.1 to 16.3: Extensive lesions over lower limbs and buttocks at initial presentation

Figs 16.4 and 16.5: New lesions over neck and beard at 2 weeks follow-up

and 4 pm serum cortisol was ordered at this point which were 1 µg and 1.75 µg/dl respectively. The patient was called for follow-up every 2 weeks. Oral itraconazole was stopped after 2 months and luliconazole was continued for a total of 3 months which led to total clinical as well as microbiological cure (Figs 16.6 to 16.10).

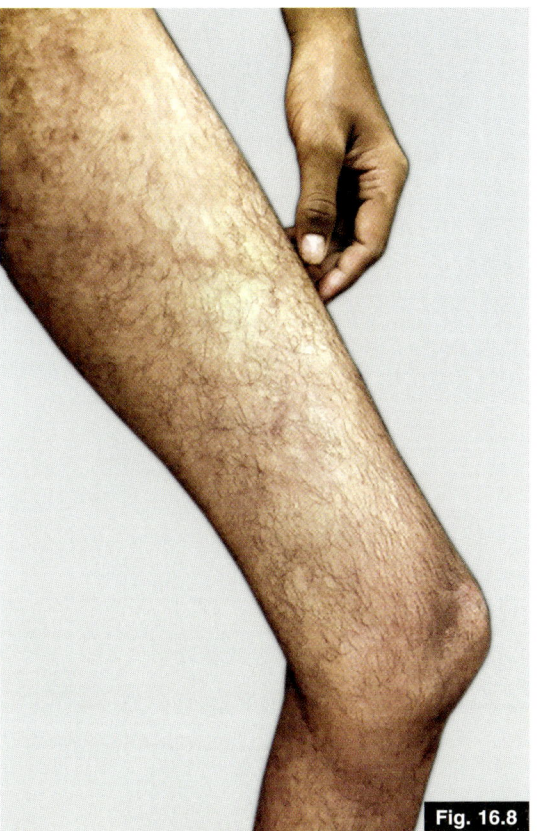

Fig. 16.8

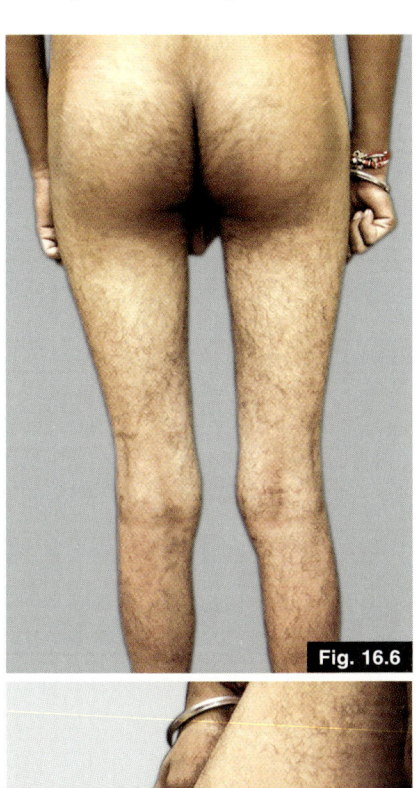

Fig. 16.6

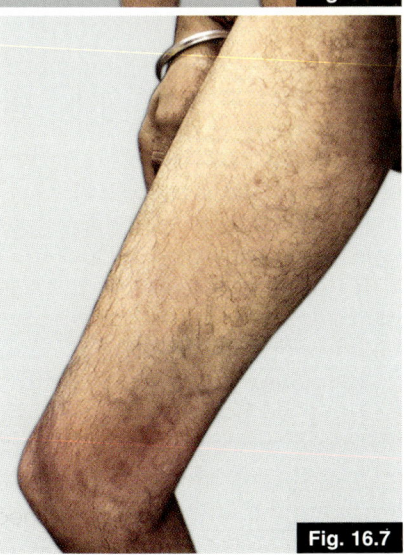

Fig. 16.7

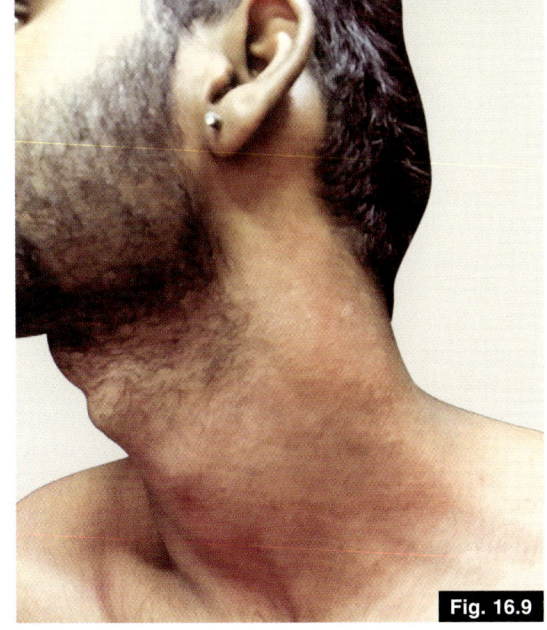

Fig. 16.9

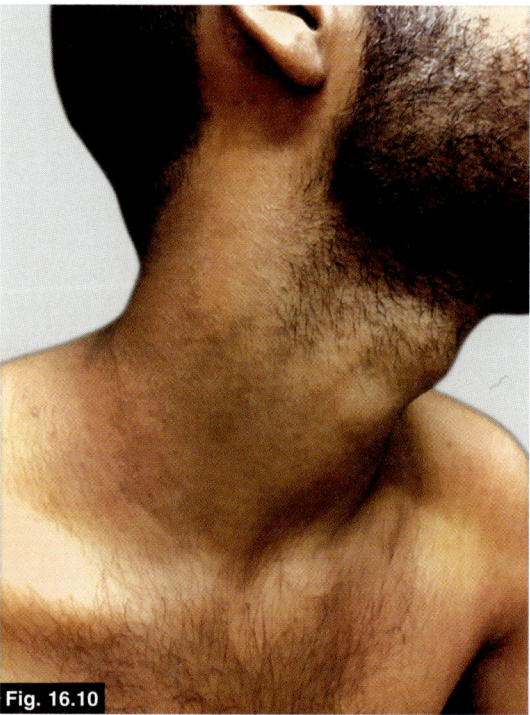

Fig. 16.10

Figs 16.6 to 16.10: Complete clearance following 2 months of oral itraconazole and 3 months of luliconazole

Discussion: Before sharing my prescription preferences with other colleagues a disclaimer is necessary. This is just 'an opinion', an opinion of a private practitioner who does not have the luxury of time to experiment with the patient or be driven primarily by textbooks and guidelines, both of which have so far cited Western literature. While I would insist on following broad recommendations and pay heed to evidence, I do not believe in being tied down by shackles of Western recommendations which are clearly not relevant to the current Indian dermatophyte scenario. We need Indian standardization of doses and treatment regimens backed by multicentric studies.

It is my personal belief that a detailed first consultation with examination is a worthwhile investment in the long run. I also do not take for granted my patient's ability to understand and remember what I tell him in those few minutes. Patients often do not fully register all that we explain and instruct. And therefore I often repeat my instructions.

I do not subscribe to treating with only oral antifungals or only topical antifungal agents with some exceptions. I have witnessed good outcome with only local therapy in patients with limited lesions, especially in very young children and when no other family member is affected. First three months of pregnancy are another exception.

Itraconazole is my favorite oral antifungal. I have drastically reduced giving terbinafine because I have seen patients taking a very long time to achieve significant clinical clearance and cure. When I compare the two groups of patients on itraconazole and terbinafine in the first two-week follow-up I have seen less clinical benefit in patients on terbinafine. Itraconazole, on the other hand, works faster in my personal opinion. I do not have the luxury of time to advise my terbinafine patients to wait for a longer time and then assess the benefit and compare it with those on itraconazole. This is one of the pressures of private practice where one deals with patients who expect quick recovery and the physician would therefore be hesitant to experiment for the fear of losing him/her to another colleague.

My oral drug of choice is itraconazole. An exception is when there is a significant drug interaction with other drugs that the patient is taking. That is, when I give terbinafine 250 mg per day or fluconazole 150 mg three times a week for 6–8 weeks. Having said that, my experience with oral terbinafine plus topical terbinafine or azoles in pregnant patients has been fairly satisfactory even if I have to give it for a few weeks more to achieve comparable clinical clearance. I usually warn and explain to my patients the possibility of a longer disease clearance time due to the pregnancy induced lowering of cell-mediated immunity.

I keep in mind that the best of itraconazole brands are poorly absorbed. Therefore, I give

200 mg per day and I continue for 4 to 6 weeks in a majority of cases. Many cases of chronic widespread dermatophytosis, especially those with lower serum cortisol levels, need treatment for 8–12 weeks. In cases of chronic widespread dermatophytosis, especially those who give a history of applying a large number of steroid containing combination creams I have started ordering 8 am and 4 pm serum cortisol studies. It is not uncommon to see lowering of endogenous cortisol in patients who have applied large quantities of potent topical steroid containing creams which corrects itself in due course of time after completely stopping their application. Though I do not do baseline liver function tests I order them after a month and then 2 months of therapy by which time the patient is released from oral treatment. I look for yellowing of sclera, ask for loss of appetite and malaise, yellow discoloration of urine and use that to order relevant hepatic investigations.

I like to prescribe antifungals manufactured by reputed companies. I tell patients that sometimes 'success comes at a cost'. I have learnt this from the poor performance of significantly cheaper brands that the patient has used unsuccessfully. A reliable brand from a reputed company inspires confidence and also ensures compliance by the rapid clearance it provides. I tell the patients to apply anti-fungals for at least 3–4 weeks after stopping the oral drugs and I personally feel the newer azoles work faster than the older ones like clotrimazole and miconazole. I tell patients to keep their bed linen separate for the first week of treatment and towels separate always. I instruct the patient to dry clothes and towels separately and sun them as far as possible. A dry ironing of underclothes is also a good idea.

I try to probe for history of tinea in household contacts and am surprised with how misleading it often is. The initial denial of the disease in household contacts very often changes and other members start appearing one by one. Therefore, I tell patients to come for follow-up once in 3 months after complete cure for a period of one year and also report a new case in the family. Though it is unusual for patients to follow-up for such a long time I do see them coming back once in a while, sometimes with another household contact in tow just because of the parting advice about the importance of follow-up.

CASE SCENARIO 2

MICROSPORUM CANIS: AN UNUSUAL CAUSE OF TINEA CORPORIS

Manjunath Shenoy M

A 23-year-old girl presented with intensely pruritic skin lesions on her shoulder, chest and thighs for the past 4 days. She has been a healthy girl without any history of previous skin diseases and any medications. Examination revealed multiple polymorphous erythematous scaly papule and plaques measuring about half centimeter up to an inch in sizes over the back, chest and thighs (Figs 16.11 and 16.12). On detailed history she revealed that she had contact with a Persian cat. It had areas of reddish patches with loss of hair in the ears, trunk and tail (Fig. 16.13).

KOH mount of scales revealed spores and branching hyphae on direct microscopic examination (Fig. 16.14). Culture in SDA revealed yellow colonies that microscopically

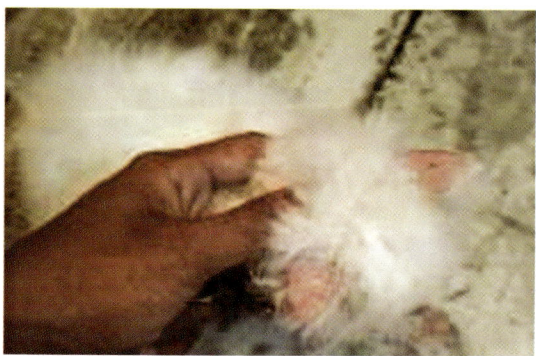

Fig. 16.13: The patient's cat with reddish patches with hair loss

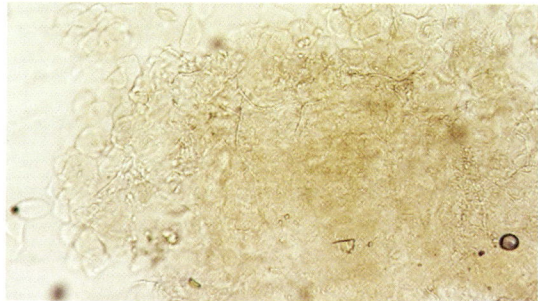

Fig. 16.14: Septate hyphae and spores on KOH mount

revealed thick-walled macroconidia with a few microconidia.

Diagnosis: Tinea corporis due to *Microsporum canis*.

Discussion: Tinea corporis is a common glabrous skin infection caused by dermatopyhytes. Zoophilic infections can rarely occur in humans. Common pets like cats and dogs are the source of the infection. Lesions can be atypical and highly inflammatory. Suspicion should arise when lesions appear all of a sudden following contact with pets. Treatment does not differ from other forms of dermatophytoses and the disease responds to the topical and systemic antifungals.

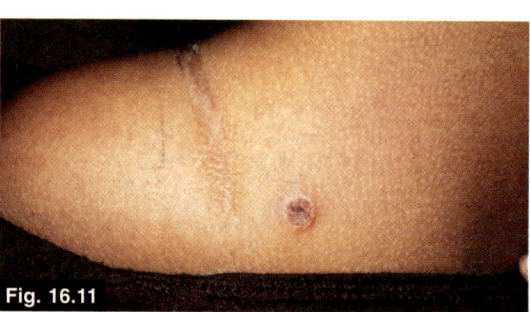

Fig. 16.11

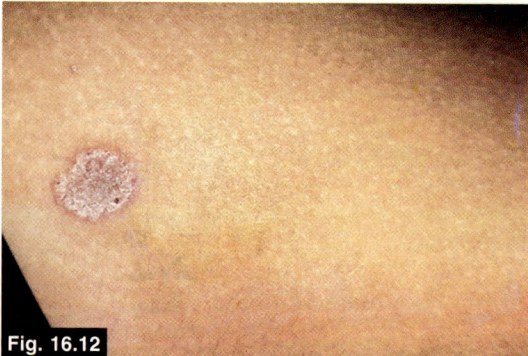

Fig. 16.12

Figs 16.11 and 16.12: Erythematous scaly lesions involving back and chest

CASE SCENARIO 3

A DIFFERENT ORAL AZOLE AND ITS RESULTS

Madhu Rengasamy

A 6.5 years old boy from a town 250 km from Chennai was brought by his mother with complaints of itchy skin lesions over the face, trunk and legs since 1 year (Figs 16.15 and 16.16). History of irregular application of topical antifungal steroid combination creams and systemic therapy was present. Last application was 1 month back. His parents and maternal grand mother had similar lesions since 2 years and 1 year respectively. There was no H/o pet animals. There was no other positive history.

General and systemic examination was normal. Dermatological examination revealed multiple annular scaly plaques over the face, front and nape of neck and well-defined scaly patches with papules in the periphery and center interspersed with areas of clearing over the thighs and lower legs. Diagnosis of extensive tinea corporis, tinea faciei and glabrous type of tinea capitis was made. Potassium hydroxide mount revealed fields full of hyaline, long branching septate hyphae with arthrospores.

He was started on short contact therapy with ketoconazole lotion for 15 minutes before bath, luliconazole cream once a day after bath and tab. fluconazole 75 mg biweekly for 8 weeks, at the end of which there was complete resolution of all the skin lesions (Figs 16.17 and 16.18). Topical luliconazole application and fluconazole tablet was continued for 2 more weeks. He is on follow-up and there is no recurrence.

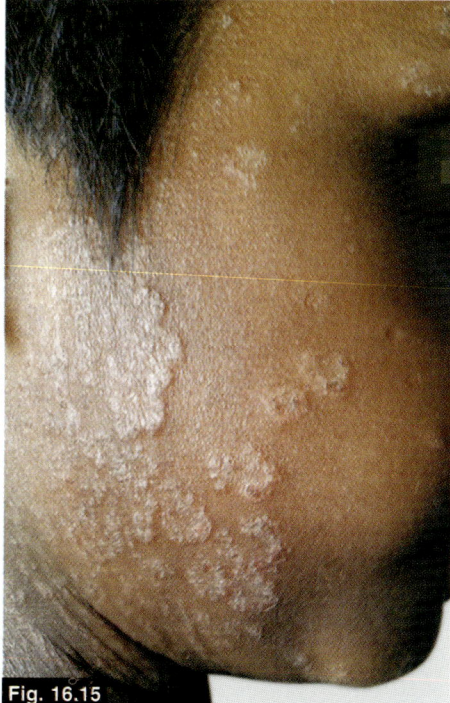 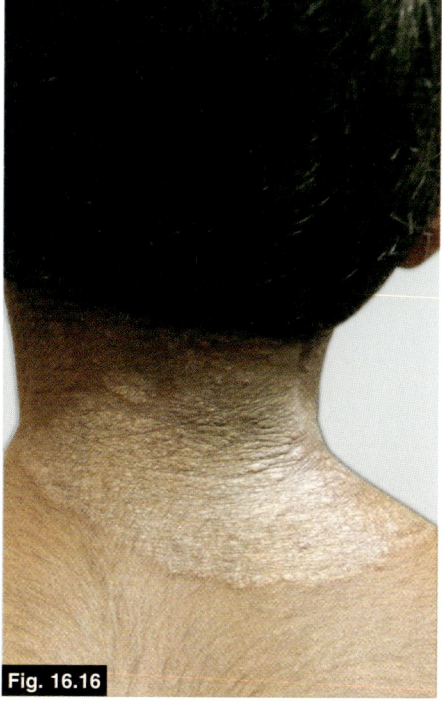

Fig. 16.15

Fig. 16.16

Figs 16.15 and 16.16: Annular scaly plaques over face and neck in a 6.5 years old boy with history of application of combination creams off and on

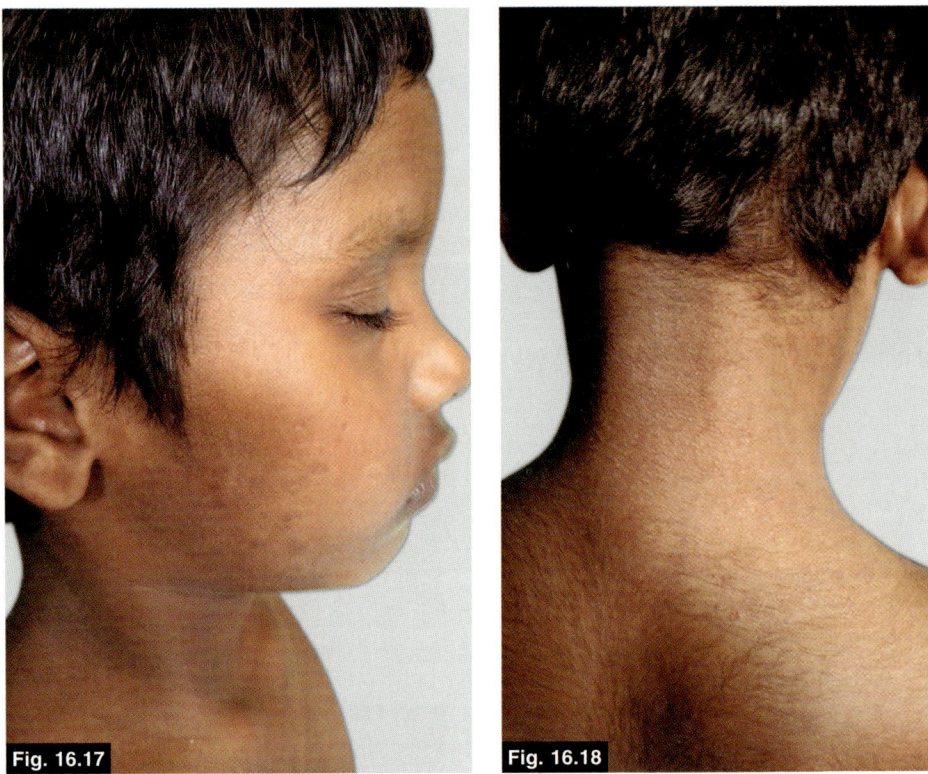

Figs 16.17 and 16.18: Post-treatment with topical ketoconazole (short contact), luliconazole and oral fluconazole 75 mg twice a week for 8 weeks

AN UNUSUAL CAUSE OF ONYCHOMYCOSIS

Chander Grover, Prachi Kawthekar

Total dystrophic onychomycosis (TDO) as a presenting manifestation of chronic mucocutaneous candidiasis (CMC) with polyendocrinopathy.

A 12-year-old girl presented with recurrent redness, swelling and pain over the proximal nail fold of right ring finger, accompanied with episodic pus discharge. Over the past year, the nail had become thickened and dystrophic (Fig. 16.19a). There were no similar complaints in family. She also had history of chronic diarrhea and failure to thrive. On examination, there was exquisite tenderness, swelling and erythema of the nail fold, with pus discharge, loss of cuticle and rounded appearance. Nail-plate was thickened and discolored, with uneven surface and subungual hyperkeratosis (Fig. 16.19b). It was only loosely adherent and pus was exuding from the bed.

Potassium hydroxide (KOH) mounts showed presence of fungal elements. Culture of pus grew *Staphylococcus aureus*, as well as *Candida albicans* on appropriate media. Histopathology revealed necrotic debris with serum exudates under the nail plate with deep pink stained (viable) as well as lightly stained, ill-defined (dead) fungal elements within

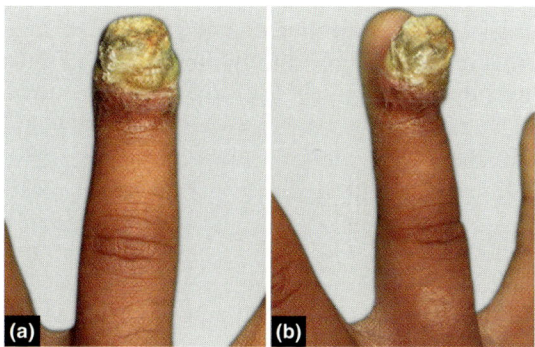

Figs 16.19a and b: (a) Total dystrophic onychomycosis with acute-on-chronic paronychia involving the right ring finger. (b) Pus can be seen exuding from under the nail plate surface and from nail folds

subungual debris and nail plate (PAS stain) (Figs 16.20a and b). A diagnosis of chronic paronychia with candidal total dystrophic onychomycosis (TDO) was entertained and oral fluconazole was initiated with visible improvement over 6 months.

However, TDO in a young child being atypical, we suspected CMC and investigated further. The child was underweight, short-statured and had triangular facies with clinodactyly. There were sparse scalp hair and

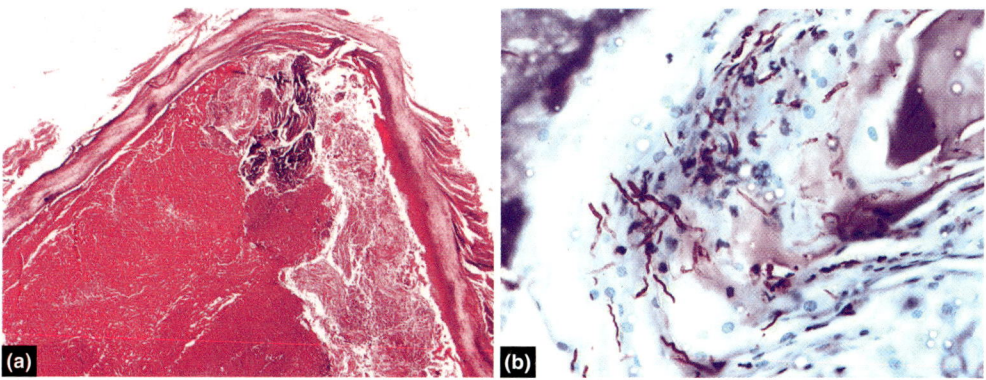

Figs 16.20a and b: Histopathological examination shows (a) necrotic debris, neutrophilic infiltrate and serum exudates (H&E 40X), with (b) fungal elements within the nail plate structure (PAS stain 400X)

left eye cataract. Routine hematological and biochemical investigations were normal except for extremely raised random blood sugar (436 mg/dl). Anti-tissue transglutaminase (tTG) IgA antibodies were significantly raised. HIV serology was non-reactive. She was diagnosed with juvenile onset diabetes mellitus and coeliac disease.

Thus, in view of her atypical candidal onychomycosis, autoimmune endocrinopathy (diabetes mellitus) and autoimmune non-endocrinological disease (coeliac disease), a diagnosis of CMC with polyendocrinopathy was considered. Further investigations for evaluating cell-mediated immunity; genetic testing for mutational analysis; or hormonal evaluation (parathormone, ACTH, etc.) could not be done due to resource constraints. Patient was advised gluten-free diet and insulin injections and has done well over the past one year.

Chronic mucocutaneous candidiasis (CMC) is a symptom complex characterized by varied manifestations including immunodeficiency and autoimmune endocrine abnormalities. This child presented with chronic paronychia and total dystrophic candidal onychomycosis (TDO), was investigated and diagnosed with endocrinal and non-endocrinal autoimmune disease on further evaluation. The bizarre cutaneous and nail manifestations prodded us to suspect and evaluate the underlying pathology.[1]

CMC is a clinically heterogeneous syndrome characterized by chronic, treatment-resistant, candidal infection of skin and appendages. Various types of endocrinopathy have been associated with CMC varying from familial polyendocrinopathy to isolated hypothyroidism.[3] According to Mazza et al, presence of resistant and relapsing candidiasis, especially before 3 years of age, should prompt physicians to check for underlying immunodeficiency including various variants of CMC like autoimmune polyendocrine syndromes.[4] Autoimmune polyendocrine syndrome (APS) is a heterogeneous group of rare disorders characterized by autoimmunity against endocrine glands. APS Type-1 or autoimmune

polyendocrinopathy-candidiasis-ectodermal dystrophy/dysplasia (APECED) syndrome is a rare autosomal recessive disorder presenting with diverse features of endocrine failure, CMC and involvement of nail and dental enamel. Associated non-endocrinological autoimmune disease include hepatobiliary disease, pernicious anemia, etc. Classically its diagnosis requires presence of 2 of the 3 major components of the 'Whitaker's triad' [autoimmune adrenocortical insufficiency, hypoparathyroidism and CMC]. Recently defined criteria for APECED by Husebye et al has even allowed definitive diagnosis in a broader spectrum of manifestations including isolated or atypical components, proving that the disorder is truly heterogeneous.[2]

Though, due to resource constraints, we could not attempt genetic testing (AIRE gene mutation); hormonal testing; or serology (adrenal cortex auto-antibodies, anti-interferon antibodies).[5] Our case serves to highlight that a high index of suspicion should be maintained with atypical manifestations of candidal infection and further evaluation to rule out endocrinal and non-endocrinal autoimmune disease is warranted.

References

1. Goldsmith L, Katz S, Gilchrest B, Paller A, Leffell D, Wolff K, editors. Fitzpatrick's Dermatology in General Medicine, 8th ed. McGraw-Hill, 2012. 2303–2307.

2. Husebye ES, Perheentupa J, Rautemaa R, Kämpe O. Clinical manifestations and management of patients with autoimmune polyendocrine syndrome type I. J Intern Med 2009; 265:514–529.

3. Griffiths C, Barker J, Bleiker T, Chalmrs R, Creamer D, editors. Rook's Textbook of Dermatology, 9th ed. Oxford: Wiley-Blackwell, 2016.

4. Mazza C, Buzi F, Ortolani F, Vitali A, Notarangelo LD, Weber G et al. Clinical heterogeneity and diagnostic delay of autoimmune polyendocrinopathy candidiasis ectodermal dystrophy syndrome. ClinImmunol2011;139(1):6–11.

5. Meager A, Visvalingam K, Peterson P, Möll K, Murumägi A, Krohn K, et al. Anti-interferon autoantibodies in autoimmune polyendocrinopathy syndrome type 1.PLoS Med. 2006; 3(7): e289. Available from: http://doi.org/10.1371/journal. pmed.0030289.

TINEA WITH STEROID INDUCED ULCERS

Shilpa Garg

A 27 years female presented with painful ulcers in both inguinal regions, along with complaints of itching and stretch marks. Ulcers were present since the past 1 month. Patient gave history of applying combination of beclomethasone dipropionate and clotrimazole cream on and off for past 6 months, which was given by her doctor and even chemist for the treatment of her "fungal infection of groins". She was also given multiple courses of oral antifungals for her infection.

She gave history of responding to treatment while she was taking the tablets and applying the creams, however, the fungal infection recurred once the treatment was stopped. No one else in her family had similar infection. She gave history of appearance of a painful ulcer which first appeared on the right groin and in the next few weeks she noticed appearance of similar painful ulcers adjoining the first ulcer and appearance of ulcer in the left groin also. Examination revealed presence of 4 oval-shaped ulcers close to each other present on the right inguinal region ranging in size from 1.5 cm × 0.5 cm to 0.5 cm × 0.5 cm (Fig. 16.21). All 4 ulcers had punched out appearance and bluish margins. The floor was covered with pus in three ulcer and with red granulation tissue in one ulcer. Patient also had a single oval ulcer measuring 1.5 cm × 1 cm with purulent floor and erythematous margins present on her left groin. The base of all the ulcers was slightly indurated and the ulcers were slightly tender on touch.

Single erythematous to hyperpigmented scaly plaque with active advancing margins and central clearing measuring around 7 cm × 5 cm was present on the left upper thighs and extended on the perineal region (Fig. 16.21). Bilateral erythematous striae were present on the inguinal region and extended to the level of lower one-third of both thighs.

Skin scraping with potassium hydroxide examination under microscope was positive for fungus.

Diagnosis of tinea incognito with steroid-induced ulcers and striae was made. She was told to stop application of steroid containing preparations and explained that her ulcers and

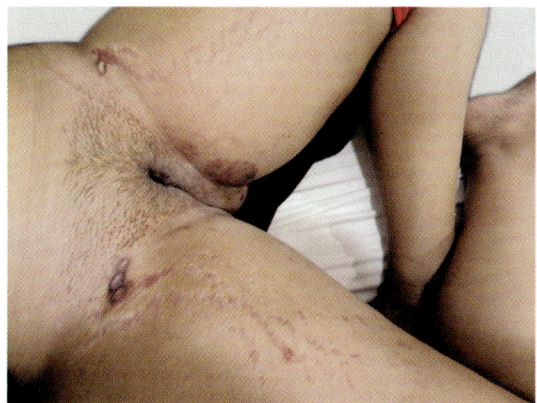

Fig. 16.21: Annular scaly plaque left thigh with punched out ulcers with bluish margins in right inguinal region

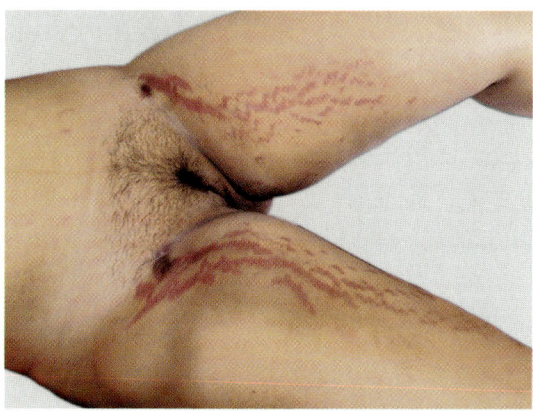

Fig. 16.22: Complete healing of ulcers and tinea following topical antibiotics and oral itraconazole

striae were caused by steroid application and her fungal infection was worsened by it.

Patient was started on oral itraconazole 100 mg twice a day after meal for 21 days along with topical application of eberconazole cream for 45 days. She was advised to cover her ulcers with fucidic acid antibiotic cream and tegaderm dressing changed every third day. She was advised to use tretinoin cream 0.25% at night on her striae. Her ulcers healed completely after 20 days with hyperpigmentation after which fucidic acid application was stopped and she was advised to continue her antifungals and tretinoin cream (Fig. 16.22). This is a classic case of steroid abuse which landed the patient with resistant and relapsing fungal infection, multiple ulcers and extensive striae.

CICLOPIROX: RECALLING A FORGOTTEN ALLY IN OUR FIGHT AGAINST CUTANEOUS MYCOSES IN THE ERA OF RAMPANT ANTIFUNGAL THERAPEUTIC FAILURE AND RISING AZOLE RESISTANCE

Sidharth Sonthalia

The rising crisis of rampant antifungal therapy failures challenging the Indian Dermatology fraternity has stemmed from multiple factors such as the injudicious use of topical as well as oral antifungals, indiscriminate use of topical steroids (alone or fixed drug combination (FDC) of an antifungal and a topical corticosteroid) by prescription of practitioners and/or self-use by patients.[1] Although, persistence of predisposing factors such as excessive sweat retention, comorbidities such as uncontrolled diabetes, recurrent infection, use of inappropriate choice and/or inadequate duration of antifungal agent, parasitization of the vellus hair with dermatophytes, and self-medication with steroid-containing preparations are major contributors to the majority of antifungal therapy failures, the rising incidence of true resistance to antifungal drugs is also becoming a nuisance in this regard.

Several biochemical mechanisms are involved in the acquisition or development of drug resistance in fungi, which include decrease in drug uptake, structural alterations in the antifungal drug target, enhanced drug efflux, and stress adaptation.

Although resistance (*in vitro* as well as *in vivo*) to allylamines like terbinafine remains low, resistance of dermatophytes to multiple clinical azoles is assuming epidemic proportions. In contrast to the cidal allylamines, azoles including flucanozole and itraconazole permit the occurrence of mutations in enzymes involved in ergosterol biosynthesis, and unlike squalene, the accumulation of which renders terbinafine fungicidal the ergosterol precursors accumulating as a consequence of azole action are not toxic.[2] More importantly, unlike allylamines, the azole antifungals, potentiate resistance development in dermatophytes.

In vitro study by Gupta and Kohli has shown that the initial minimal inhibitory concentration (MIC) value of 0.125 µg/ml of itraconazole and ketoconazole for *Trichophyton rubrum* demonstrated a 256-fold increase to 32 and 4 µg/ml, respectively after 15 months of antifungal therapy; suggesting the development of azole resistance in dermatophytes after repeated exposure.[3]

This case report shall not only highlight a clinical scenario of failure of long term oral itraconazole, but also emphasize on the urgent need to bring back a highly effective antifungal topical drug into our therapeutic arsenal. Ciclopirox olamine (CPO) 1% cream is an apparently forgotten ally that could be the answer to our struggle against antifungal therapeutic failure.

A 47-year old Indian man with controlled diabetes of 8-year duration presented with multiple large non-annular erythematous patches with mild scaling involving the buttocks, lower back (Fig. 16.23a), groins, lower abdomen, and lower regions of the thighs. He had been applying 'Fourderm®' a proprietary cream consisting of chlorhexidine, clobetaosol propionate, miconazole and neomycin off and on for at least 2–3 months when the eruption started around 9 months back. With temporary improvement in his symptoms followed by relapse within days of stopping the cream and having been told by his general physician that he should not be using that combination cream, he stopped applying it 6 months back.

Since then he had received topical clotrimazole (1%), sertaconazole nitrate (2%) and luliconazole (1%) creams for twice-a-day application sequentially (each cream given for 3–4 weeks followed by a gap of 1–2 weeks) with concomitant oral terbinafine (250 mg OD) for

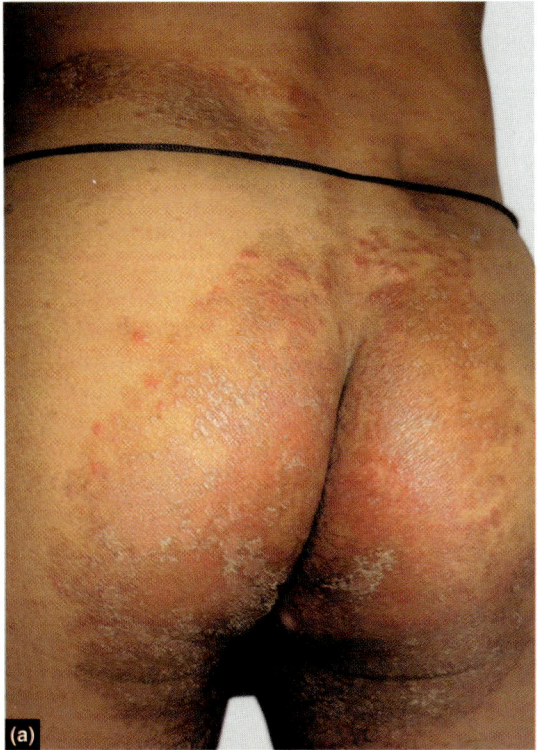

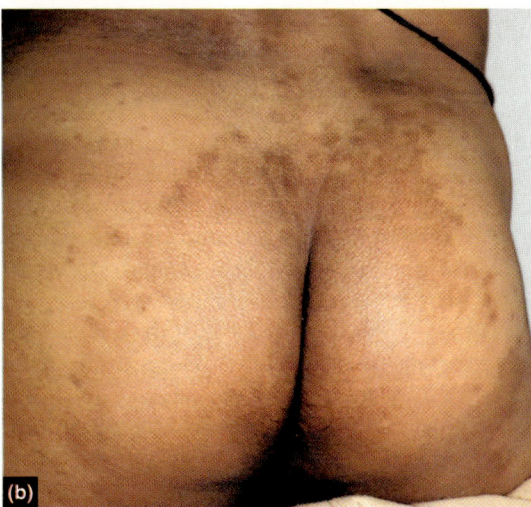

Figs 16.23a and b: Clinical image of the patient with: (a) Steroid-modified tinea at the time of presentation displaying multiple large non-annular erythematous patches with mild scaling involving the buttocks and lower back; and (b) Complete healing with post-inflammatory hyperpigmentation after 6 weeks of BD application of ciclopirox cream 1% cream

3 weeks, followed by oral itraconazole 200–400 mg/day (capsule Sporanox®) which was started 3 months ago and continued till date. He reported that the period of symptomatic remission lasting for 7–10 days became shorter and shorter while on itraconazole, followed by full blown relapse each time. He admitted to additionally applying CANDID-B® cream, a dual combination of clotrimazole (1%) and beclomethasone around 10 days prior to seeking my consultation.

A diagnosis of steroid modified tinea (extensive) was made clinically, and confirmed by dermoscopy that revealed diffuse erythema, mild scaling, morse-code hairs, broken hair shafts and multiple linear branching vessels and telangiectasis (Figs 16.24a and b). Although a 10% KOH smear was negative, PAS stain revealed fungal elements. Fungal culture from the skin scrapings confirmed *T. rubrum* with MIC value of 16 µg/ml and 8 µg/ml for itraconazole and clotrimazole respectively. MIC values to other antifungals could not be ascertained.

I stopped all the topicals and oral itraconazole, and started the patient on oral loratadine 10 mg/day and Synpirox®, which is CPO 1% cream for BD application for 6 weeks, in addition to general advice on maintaining hygiene and avoiding risk factors for a relapse. The lesional improvement was visible within 10 days and complete healing with post-inflammatory hyperpigmentation was observed at the 6th week (Fig. 16.23b) confirmed by dermoscopy (Fig. 16.24c) and a negative PAS stain and fungal culture, without any adverse effects. The patient has remained in complete remission for the last 6 months at least.

The patient presented to me with complicated and extensive steroid-modified and clinically azole resistant tinea corporis and cruris caused by *T. rubrum*. Although the fungal culture and MIC values of azoles were not done prior to the initiation of topical azoles or oral itraconazole, the history of progressively

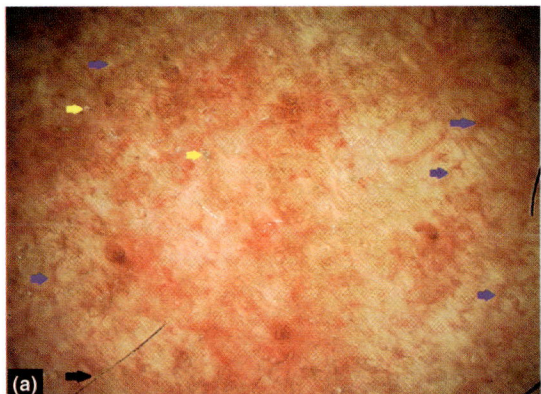

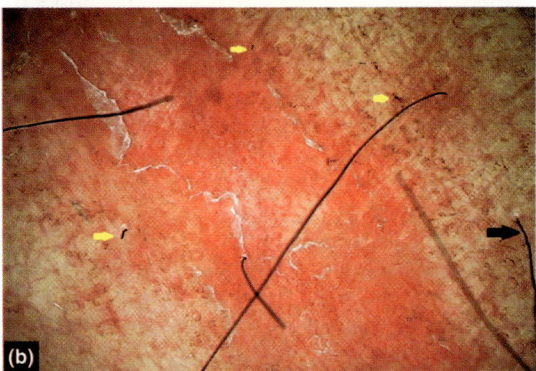

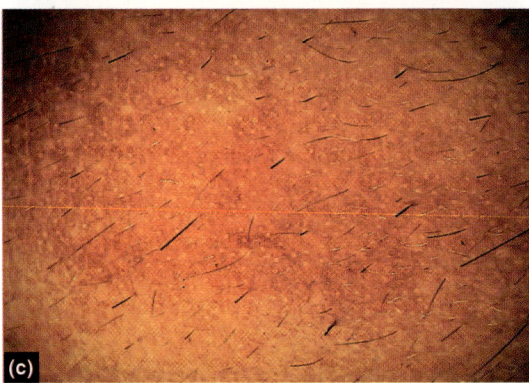

Figs 16.24a to c: Dermoscopic image from the buttocks of the patient: (a and b) At presentation revealing diffuse background of erythema with mild scaling, morse-code hairs (black arrows), broken hair shafts (yellow arrows) and multiple linear branching vessels and telangiectasias (blue arrows) consistent with steroid-modified tinea corporis; and (c) On complete healing after 6 weeks revealing disappearance of erythema, scaling, abnormal hairs and prominent dark brown post-inflammatory pigmentation [Escope, videodermatoscope, X30, polarized]

shortening periods of remission while on oral itraconazole and some topical azole and the high MIC values to clotrimazole and itraconazole convincingly suggest that *T. rubrum* may have developed resistance to multiple azoles due to the prolonged and repeated exposure to that group of antifungal agents. Abuse of topical steroids, of course played their part in persistence of the infection for so long. It must be noted that many times failure to oral itraconazole therapy is attributed to low dose, short duration, improper intake and using a low-grade drug that is not bioequivalent to the innovator brand. However, my patient was taking the innovator brand of itraconazole,[4] in proper dose, for no less than 3 months, and as per the general instructions of taking the capsules with an acidic beverage and after a meal. Thus, the case represents the prototype of development and potentiation of resistance to azoles in the dermatophyte due to repeated and continuous exposure to that group of drugs.

More importantly, this case highlights the potential of CPO as a highly efficacious and safe topical agent for not only dermatophytes in general, but even azole-resistant species (Table 16.1).

This stems from the mechanism of action of CPO against the superficial mycoses, which is unique and totally different from the major groups of antifungals, i.e. azoles and allylamines, both of which target ergosterol biosynthetic pathway. Ciclopirox is thought to act through the chelation of polyvalent metal cations, such as ferric (Fe^{3+}) and aluminium (Al^{3+}), thereby causing inhibition of metal dependent enzymes (cytochromes, catalase, peroxidase) leading to disruption of cellular activities such as mitochondrial electron transport processes, energy production, and nutrient intake across cell membrane.[5] Many other mechanisms have also been postulated that have been summarized in Table 16.2.[6–8] Another unique property of ciclopirox is that it exerts fungicidal activity

Table 16.1: The unique properties of cicloprox that make it a near-ideal topical antifungal

- One of the broadest antifungal spectrum coverage-dermatophytes, yeasts, moulds
- Unique mechanism of antifungal action
- Cidal effect even against non-growing fungal cells
- Lowest MIC values for dermatophytes compared to practically all azoles*
- Lowest MIC values for yeasts compared to practically all azoles as well as terbinafine*
- Highly effective against multiple-azole resistant species of dermatophytes and Candida*
- High inhibitory activity against multiple non-fungal organisms including many significant Gram-positive and Gram-negative bacteria
- High anti-inflammatory activity, equivalent to 2.5% hydrocortisone
- No resistance reported till date and theoretical possibility of fungi developing resistance to ciclopirox extremely remote
- Excellent safety profile with practically no adverse effects
- Safe for use during pregnancy (category B)

*Data from the West

Table 16.2: Postulated antifungal mechanisms of action of ciclopirox

- Chelation of polyvalent metal cations, especially iron (Fe^{3+}) leading to inhibition of metal dependent enzymes (cytochromes, catalase, peroxidase) followed by disruption of cellular activities such as mitochondrial electron transport processes, energy production, and nutrient intake across cell membrane
- Alteration of membrane permeability causing blockage of intracellular transport of precursors
- Disruption of DNA repair, cell division signals and disorganization of internal structures (mitotic spindles) of the fungi.
- Compromising the integrity of the cell membrane of susceptible organisms followed by leakage of potassium ions and other intracellular material.

against dormant hyphae as well. For practically all types of superficial mycoses, the MIC value of ciclopirox is consistently lower than the concentrations attained *in vivo* after topical application. According to the results of Gupta and Kohli,[9] for dermatophytes, ciclopirox was considerably more effective against all species tested (110 strains of dermatophytes) than itraconazole and ketonazole, being only minimally inferior to terbinafine. For yeasts (14 strains of Candida) and nondermatophyte moulds (9 strains), ciclopirox was the most potent with lowest MIC values for these fungi, compared to ketoconazole, itraconazole and terbinafine.

Ciclopirox additionally possesses activity against many Gram-positive (GP) and Gram-negative (GN) bacteria.[7,10] The combined broad-spectrum antifungal and antibacterial activity of ciclopirox is of particular advantage in the treatment of macerated tinea pedis and "dermatophytosis complex", both conditions being symptomatic intertriginous fungal affections secondarily infected by bacteria. What makes ciclopirox a highly attractive candidate in our fight against antifungal therapeutic failure is its impressive anti-inflammatory activity exerted through inhibition of prostaglandin (especially PGE_2) and leukotriene synthesis, decrease in reactive oxygen species (ROS) production by chelating transition metals such as iron and copper, and a direct and potent scavenging effect over the hydroxyl radical. Reported to be as potent an anti-inflammatory agent as indomethacin, desoximetasone, and 2.5% hydrocortisone, many *in vivo* studies have reported its anti-inflammatory activity to be superior to most of the other topical antifungals (naftifine, terbinafine, econazole, ketoconazole, miconazole, fluconazole, oxiconazole).[7,8,10] This property adds to the anti-pruritic effect of ciclopirox and renders needless the desire for adding a topical steroid even for inflamed tinea.

Last but not the least, ciclopirox olamine could be the answer to the emerging antifungal resistance. Till date, there is no report of resistance to ciclopirox (*in vitro* or *in vivo*). The postulated reasons of almost impossibility of dermatophytes and yeasts developing resistance to CPO include its steep dose-response curve, irreversible binding to intracellular structures and lack of effect of drug resistance pumps.[7,8,10] The excellent safety profile, including during pregnancy (category B) further make CPO a near-ideal topical antifungal.

Its high time that we bring back CPO, a molecule that has been approved by the Drug Controller General of India's (DCGI) for treatment of superficial cutaneous fungal infections of the skin and vagina since October 1985, to the frontier of our fight against cutaneous mycoses.

References

1. Shivanna R, Inamadar AC. Clinical failure of antifungal therapy of dermatophytoses: Recurrence, resistance, and remedy. Indian J Drugs Dermatol. 2017;3:1–3.

2. Ghannoum M. Azole Resistance in Dermatophytes: Prevalence and Mechanism of Action. J Am Podiatr Med Assoc 2016;106:79–86.

3. Gupta AK, Kohli Y: Evaluation of *in vitro* resistance in patients with onychomycosis who fail antifungal therapy. Dermatology 2003;207:375–80.

4. https://www.accessdata.fda.gov/drugsatfda_docs/label/2009/020083s040s041s044lbl.pdf [Last accessed on 6 February 2018].

5. Markus A. Hydroxy-pyridones. Outstanding biological properties. In: Shuster S, ed. Hydroxy-pyridones as Antifungal Agents with Special Emphasis on Onychomycosis. Berlin: Springer-Verlag, 1999: 1–10.

6. Jue SG, Dawson GW, Brogden RN. Ciclopirox olamine 1% cream. A preliminary review of its antimicrobial activity and therapeutic use. Drugs. 1985;29:330–41.

7. Subissi A, Monti D, Togni G, et al. Ciclopirox: recent nonclinical and clinical data relevant to its use as a topical antimycotic agent. Drugs. 2010;70:2133–52.

8. Gupta AK. Ciclopirox: an overview. Int J Dermatol. 2001;40:305–10.

9. Gupta AK, Kohli Y. *In vitro* susceptibility testing of ciclopirox, terbinafine, ketoconazole and itraconazole against dermatophytes and nondermatophytes, and *in vitro* evaluation of combination antifungal activity. Br J Dermatol 2003;149:296–305.

10. Abrams BB, Hanel H, Hoehler T. Ciclopirox olamine: a hydroxypyridone antifungal agent. Clin Dermatol 1992; 9:471–7.

CASE SCENARIO 7

TINEA MANAGEMENT IN A CHILD

Shital Poojary

An 11-month-old girl presented with extensive tinea corporis and tinea cruris (Fig. 16.25). On examination, large plaques with no erythema, fine scaling were present, extending from bilateral mid-thighs to chest.

Patient was treated with topical amorolfine 0.25% cream applied once daily for 4 weeks with complete clearance of lesions (Fig. 16.26).

Rationale for treatment:

1. Topical treatment was opted for the child in view of very young age.
2. It is relatively difficult to administer oral antifungals in pediatric age group especially in very young children as in the above case.
3. It is difficult to titrate the dose according to weight of the child as formulations of varied doses of antifungals are not available.
4. Pediatric formulations of antifungals are not available in India.
5. Choice of topical antifungal, amorolfine, has a relatively unique mechanism of action as compared to azoles, allylamines: It inhibits $\delta14$-reductase and $\delta7$–$\delta8$-isomerase enzymes. Hence amorolfine was chosen in this case of extensive tinea corporis.

Alternative options which could have been used: Fluconazole dispersible tablet 50 mg/day can be administered for 2–4 weeks.

Lessons learnt: Topical antifungals are effective even in extensive dermatophyte infections and are a useful option in pediatric age group.

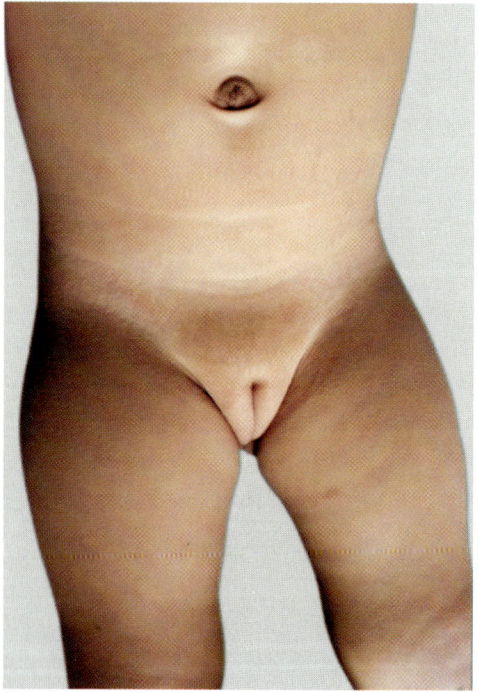

Fig. 16.25: Extensive tinea corporis and cruris in an 11-month-old infant

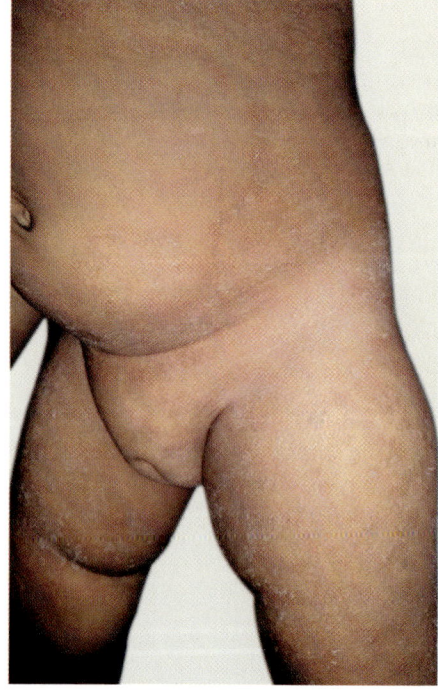

Fig. 16.26: Complete clearance with topical amorolfine 0.25% cream applied OD for 4 weeks

ITRACONAZOLE USE IN TINEA CORPORIS

Shital Poojary

A 20-year-old male presented with extensive tinea cruris and tinea corporis of 6 months duration (Figs 16.27 and 16.28). Patient had been applying steroid combination creams intermittently.

Patient was treated with cap itraconazole 200 mg per day for two weeks with complete clearance of lesions and post-inflammatory hyper-pigmentation (Figs 16.29 and 16.30). Itraconazole was continued for 2 weeks after clearance.

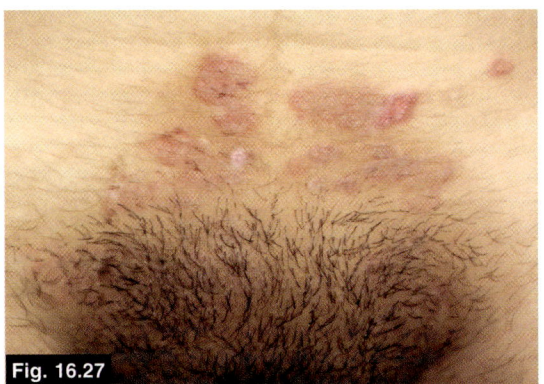

Fig. 16.27

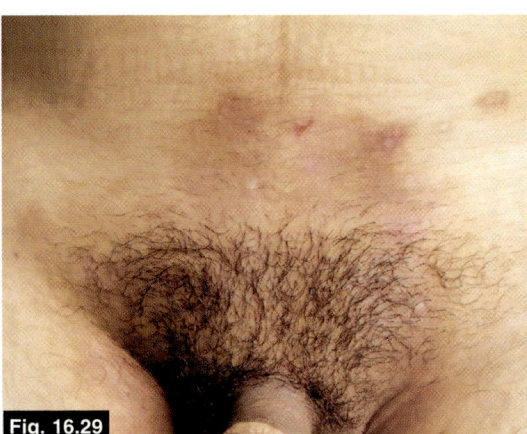

Fig. 16.29

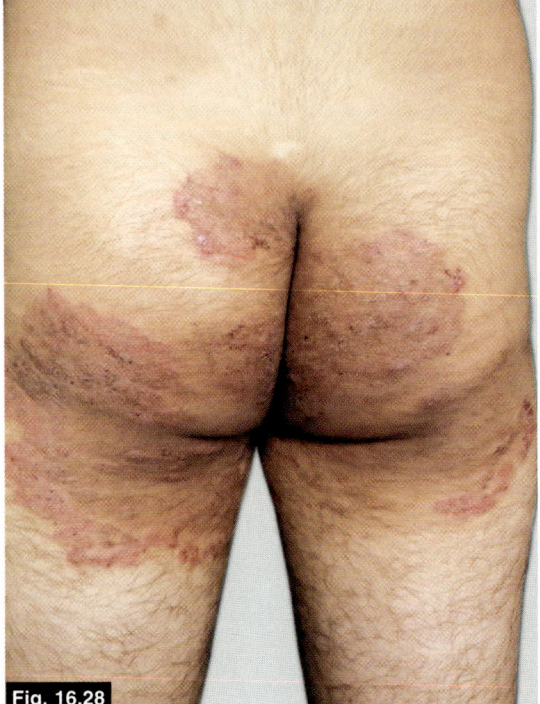

Fig. 16.28

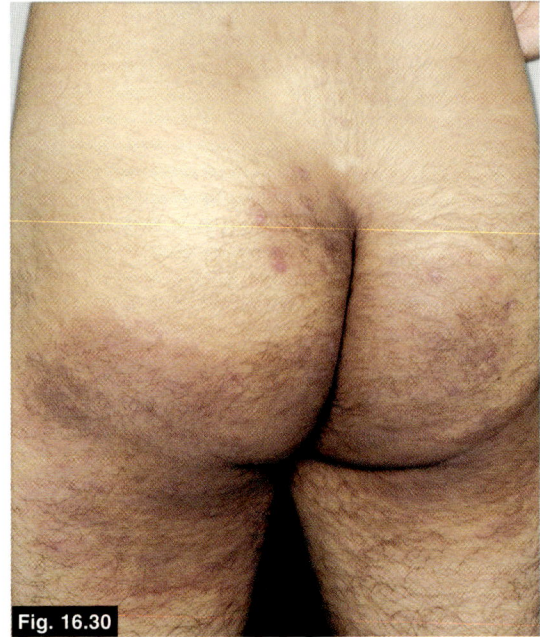

Fig. 16.30

Figs 16.27 and 16.28: Extensive tinea in a 20-year-old male

Figs 16.29 and 30: Complete clearance following treatment with itraconazole (200 mg/day)

Rationale for treatment:

1. In view of application of topical steroid-antifungal combination and long duration of the disease, itraconazole was the antifungal of choice as it is the most effective antifungal in the present scenario with MICs within the effective range.

2. Dose of itraconazole: 200 mg/day was given as 100 mg/day is not sufficient in the present scenario of recalcitrant dermatophytosis.

3. Duration of treatment was extended to 2 weeks after clinical cure to take care of any possible persistent spores and vellus hair involvement, thereby reducing possibility of recurrence.

Lessons learnt: Oral antifungals should be continued for at least 2 weeks after resolution of lesions so that epidermal turnover will result in shedding of residual fungi if any and vellus hair involvement requires longer duration of treatment.

CASE SCENARIO 9

MAJOCCHI'S GRANULOMA

Ananta Khurana

A 45-year-old female presented with extensive tinea cruris, corporis and faciei. She was put on oral terbinafine in the dose of 250 mg twice a day, along with emollients for local application. There was partial improvement in lesions but the patient noticed some persistent papulo-nodules over the right side of her face (Fig. 16.31). The erythema and scaling initially present at this site had decreased to reveal the papulo-nodules conspicuously. Dermoscopy revealed a patchy dusky coating over the hair shafts, akin to the described morphology of morse-code hair, apart from background erythema and scaling (Fig. 16.32). A clinical diagnosis of Majocchi's granuloma (MG) was made and a biopsy sent for histopathological examination. The biopsy revealed follicular plugging with spores and occasional hyphal fragments. The hair follicles visualised were filled with inflammatory cells with rupture of a follicle and surrounding

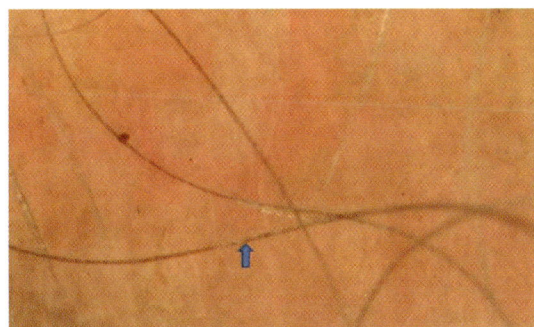

Fig. 16.32: Dermoscopy demonstrates involvement of facial hair with morse-code appearance (blue arrow)

dense lymphohistiocytic inflammatory infiltrate, consistent with the clinical diagnosis of Majocchi's granuloma (Fig. 16.33). As the patient had already received about 8 weeks of terbinafine with a suboptimal response, we decided to switch to itraconazole. It was started in the dose of 100 mg twice a day and complete clearance of all lesions was achieved in another 5 weeks (Fig. 16.34). The patient remains under follow-up and has not developed any recurrence till 5 months post-treatment completion.

Majocchi's granuloma was first described by Professor Domenico Majocchi as granuloma tricofitico in 1883. It is essentially a deep folliculitis caused by dermatophytic infection. Most cases have been attributed to *Trichophyton rubrum*, although *T. mentagrophytes*, *T. violaceum*, *T. verrucosum*, *T. tonsurans*, *M. gypseum*, *M. audouinii* and *E. floccosum* have also been implicated in fewer reports.

MG usually appears in one of the 2 settings. The *first* is a limited immunological defect, generally with topical steroid preparations, an important concern in our country. In this setting, the condition mostly presents with peri-follicular papules. More severe disease can present as extensive papulo-plaques or nodules, erythematous plaques studded with

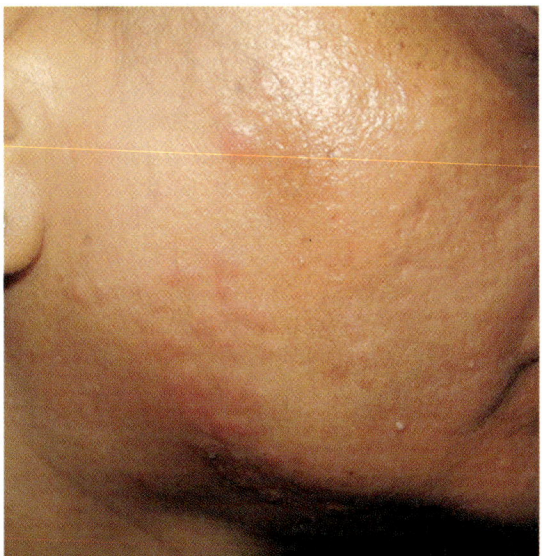

Fig. 16.31: Papulonodular lesions on face of a 45- year-old female. The patient presented with these at 8 weeks of treatment with terbinafine 250 mg BD

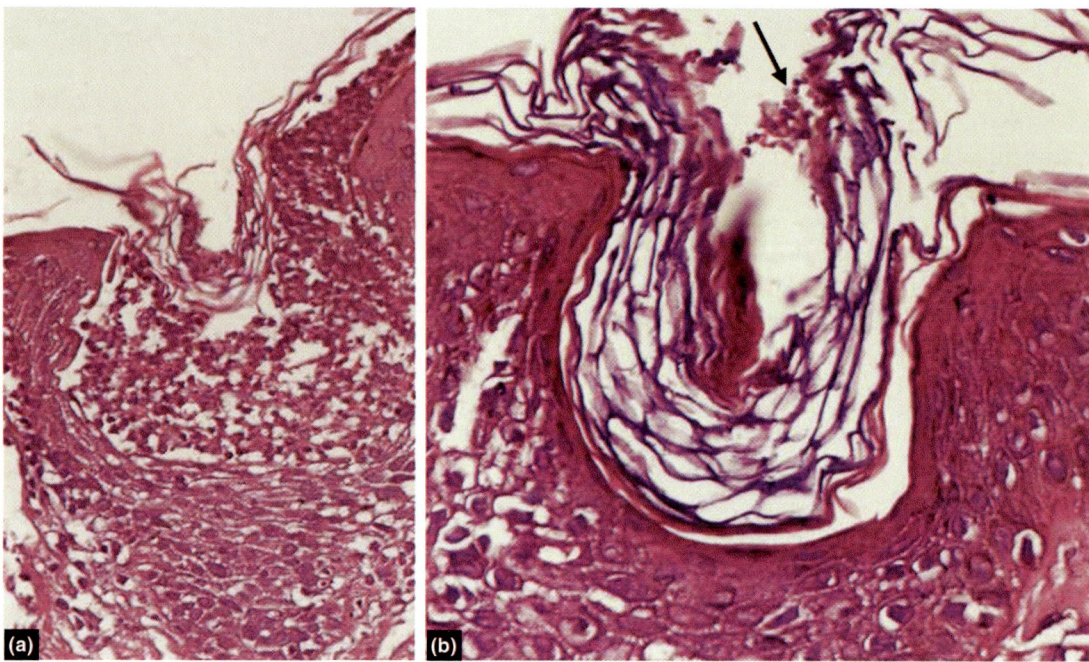

Fig. 16.33: Histopathology shows (a) suppurative folliculitis with follicular rupture (H&E, 200X) and (b) fungal spores (black arrow) (H&E, 400X) (*Courtesy:* Dr Arvind Ahuja)

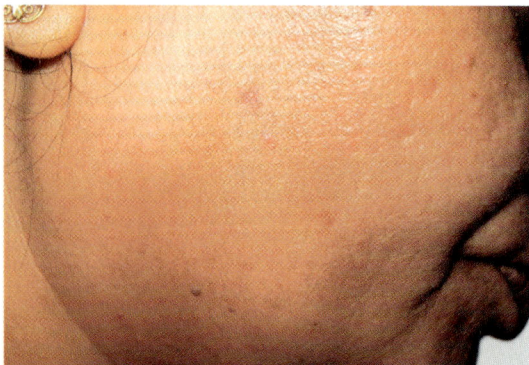

Fig. 16.34: Resolution of lesions following 5 weeks of oral itraconazole 100 mg BD

papules, pustule and nodules, and boggy swelling of the affected region. There may be associated lymphadenopathy in some cases. Many previous reports of MG have been associated with shaving or waxing of legs in females, with trauma to follicles being the proposing factor leading to lodging of the organism deeper into the dermis. Interestingly,

our patient did not have any of these predisposing factors—she had no history of using any hair removing techniques over face and denied using a steroid preparation. Absence of signs of steroid abuse on dermoscopy added weight to her denial. We believe that vigorous scratching on an accessible site may have been the predisposing factor in her, as has also been proposed by some other authors.[1]

The *second* scenario for development of MG is with underlying broader immunological defects like in organ transplant recipients, graft versus host disease, those on long-term systemic immunosuppressives or chemotherapeutic agents and those with HIV infection.[2] Such patients may present with more severe forms and subcutaneous nodules or abscesses. Majocchi's granuloma occurs mostly on the buttocks and lower legs of patients with AIDS and may mimic Kaposi's sarcoma.[2]

It is not clearly known how the dermatophytes, which require keratin as a substrate for survival, remain viable within the dermis. Also, the pH here is more alkaline than the epidermis, a further inhibitory factor for these fungi. One explanation suggested is that the keratinous material introduced into the dermis after follicular disruption can potentially provide a substrate for the organisms. And the resulting cellular destruction and increased amounts of stromal acid mucopolysaccharides, secondary to the associated inflammation, may lower the pH in the dermis and make the dermal environment more suitable for the survival of the dermatophytes.[3]

Diagnosis of MG requires a high index of clinical suspicion. Patients are often misdiagnosed and advised topical steroids. KOH is often falsely negative, because the fungi are located deeper. Histopathology, with the characteristic findings of follicular rupture and dense peri-follicular infiltrate, which is often granulomatous, however confirms the diagnosis.

Treatment is prolonged and topicals are generally ineffective as the organism is deeper, though these may be given in combination with systemic drugs.

Treatment options detailed in literature include:

1. *Terbinafine*: 250 mg OD[4]
2. *Itraconazole* as: 100 mg OD[3] or
   200 mg OD[5]/BD[6] or
   1–2 Pulses of 200 mg BD
   for 1 week, with a gap of
   2 weeks between pulses[7]
3. *Griseofulvin*[3,8]: 500 mg BD or 15 mg/kg/day
4. *Voriconazole:* There is a single report of successful use of voriconazole (IV for 2 weeks followed by oral 200 mg BD) for MG in an immunocompetent patient not responding to terbinafine and itraconazole.[1]

Length of treatment would be dependent on the clinical response, and complete clearance may take months. Time to clearance depends on the severity of presentation and the immune status of the patient.

As our patient had already received prolonged high dose terbinafine, we switched her to itraconazole which led to complete clearance in 5 weeks. Both the drugs exhibit similar pharmacokinetics with respect to hair and the drug response likely depends on local sensitivity patterns. There is a reported case of the opposite situation, with unresponsiveness to itraconazole followed by successful treatment with terbinafine, favoring this point.[9]

Conclusion: The learning point here is to look for subtle lesions suggesting follicular/deeper involvement. The lesions may often be hidden within the erythema and scaling of an untreated plaque, but clearance in the surrounding would make these prominent, as in the presented case. The scenario becomes especially important in our patients, where topical steroid abuse, a major risk factor for development of MG, is rampant. Such cases need to be treated with longer than otherwise courses of anti-fungals to achieve complete clearance. Missing such subtle lesions would invariably lead to treatment failure/recurrence.

Acknowledgment: Dr Arvind Ahuja MD. Associate Professor and Head of Histopathology Unit, Department of Pathology, PGIMER, Dr RML Hospital, New Delhi.

References

1. Liu HB, Liu F, Kong QT, Shen YN. Successful Treatment of Refractory Majocchi's Granuloma with Voriconazole and Review of Published Literature. Mycopathologia 2015;180:237–43.
2. Feng WW, Chen HC, Chen HC. Majocchi's granuloma in a 3-year-old boy. Pediatr Infect Dis J. 2006;25:658–9.
3. Elgart ML. Tinea incognito: an update on Majocchi's granuloma. Dermatol Clin 1996;14: 51–5.
4. Gupta AK, Prussick FR, Sibbald RG, et al. Terbinafine in the treatment of Majocchi's granuloma. Int J Dermatol 1995;34:489–90.

5. Liu C, Landeck L, Cai SQ, Zheng M Majocchi's granuloma over the face. Indian J Dermatol Venereol Leprol 2012;78:113–4.

6. Sequeira M, Burdick AE, Elgart GW, et al. New-onset Majocchi's granuloma in two kidney transplant recipients under tacrolimus treatment. J Am Acad Dermatol 1998;38:486–8.

7. Gupta AK, Groen K, Woestenborghs R, et al. Itraconazole pulse therapy is effective in the treatment of Majocchi's granuloma: a clinical and pharmacokinetic evaluation and implications for possible effectiveness in tinea capitis. Clin Exp Dermatol 1998;23:103–8.

8. Carter RL. Majocchi's granuloma. J Am Acad Dermatol 1980;2:75.

9. Rallis E, Katoulis A, Rigopoulos D. Pubic Majocchi's Granuloma Unresponsive to Itraconazole Successfully Treated with Oral Terbinafine. Skin Appendage Disord 2016;1: 111–3.

CASE SCENARIO 10

GRISEOFULVIN IN TINEA CAPITIS

Taru Garg

An 8-year-old boy presented with complaints of multiple patches of hair loss associated with minimal itching and scaling for two months. On examination he had five well-defined, irregularly-shaped patches of partial hair loss over the scalp (Fig. 16.35). Fine white, semi-adherent scaling was present within the patches not extending on to the normal scalp. Hair within the patches were rough, grey, dull looking and broken. A few black dots were also observed. Easily pluckable hair were present at the margin of the patches.

Clinically he was diagnosed with grey patch type of tinea capitis (Fig. 16.35). KOH examination from scalp scrapings and hair showed multiple spores and septate hyphae. Fungal culture was sent.

After clinical and microscopic confirmation of diagnosis he was treated with tab. griseofulvin (micronized formulation) 250 mg daily (weight = 18.10 kg) along with ketoconazole 2% shampoo twice a week for hair wash.

General measures were explained in detail. Follow-up was advised at 4 weeks. Patient reported for follow-up at 6 weeks with report of fungal culture which did not show any fungal growth. Minimal clinical improvement

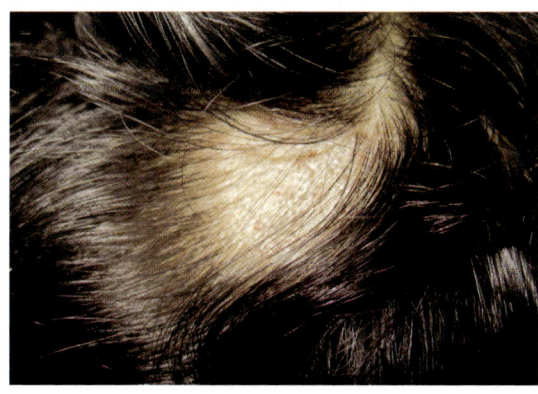

Fig. 16.35: Patch of partial hair loss and scaling in an 8-year-old boy

was present. KOH examination from hair and scalp scrapings was repeated and showed the previous findings. The dose of griseofulvin was hiked up to 250 mg 2 times a day and patient was followed up 4 weeks later. Significant improvement was present (around 70%). Treatment was continued for another 2 weeks with complete resolution of the patches. Hence antifungal given at higher dosage and for extended period in some of the non-responders (recalcitrant cases) of tinea capitis infection may lead to improvement.

CASE SCENARIO 11

TINEA INCOGNITO—A MANAGEMENT PROTOCOL

Pooja Arora Mrig

A 25-year-old male presented to the OPD with reddish itchy lesions in groins for the 3 months. He gave history of application of Fourderm cream (clobetasol, miconazole, neomycin) and clotrimazole dusting powder. He had also taken betamethasone tablets 1 mg

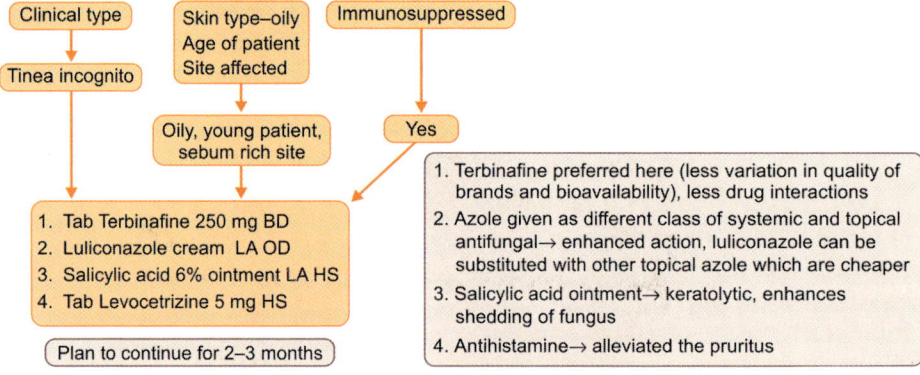

Fig. 16.36: Management of Indian case

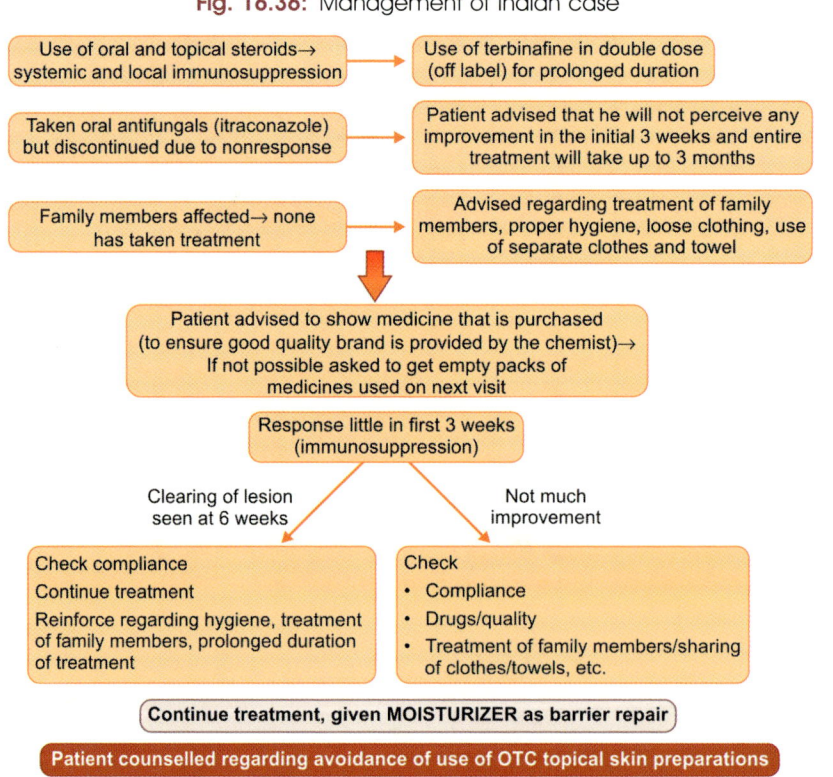

Fig. 16.37: Rationale for treatment and follow-up

daily and tab cefadroxyl 500 mg twice daily for 6 weeks followed by decrease in pruritus. The lesions reappeared on stopping the above treatment. He took capsule itraconazole 200 mg once daily for 2 weeks and stopped treatment as there was no relief in symptoms. There was history of similar lesions in all family members that included mother and five brothers. None had taken proper treatment from a dermatologist but all had taken the above medication without prescription. Examination revealed erythematous plaque on left side of lower abdomen with partial clearing of lesion and variable scaling. Similar lesions but non-scaly were seen in bilateral inguinal region. Scraping from the abdominal lesion showed hyphae on KOH examination. The proposed treatment plan for such a case is listed in Figs 16.36 and 16.37.

CASE SCENARIO 12

USING AN APPARENTLY INEFFECTIVE DRUG WITH EFFECTIVE RESULTS: TERBINAFINE, KETOCONAZOLE AND SYNERGISM

Kabir Sardana

A patient came to us with erythrodermic tinea corporis (Fig. 16.38). There was a history of use of multiple courses of generic ITR. Some of the doses were way beyond the approved doses including 400 mg BD.

The topical medications had a mixture of TCS and antifungals. Of note amorolofine, azoles and terbinafine had been used. There was no other comorbidity.

A KOH was positive while the culture, without molecular identification, revealed *T. rubrum*.

Treatment

The first concept that has to be understood is that we should not discard conventional drugs specially as the quality of ITR in India is variable and some are abysmal (pages 93, 98). Thus though we believe and practice the dictat that a normal dose of 100 mg to 100 mg BD would work, here was a patient who told us that he is sick of taking ITR as it is useless drug (patients know the brand by now)!

Here we may point that the MIC data is elegantly spoke of in conferences but it follows the classic hindsight view. It come so late that it is of a little practical value. Also the skin levels of antifungal drugs are enough to tackle most infections (*see* Chapter 9). Here we may point out that our own work has shown that the MIC of TER has risen to cross breakpoint levels. Thus we choose to double the dose to 250 mg BD which is more logical than 500 mg OD. This dose incidentally in the original articles is also 250 mg BD but a certain company did not obviously read the fine print!

I prescribe salicylic acid 6% in the initial stage and prefer topical ketoconazole as it is cheap with a high keratin adherence. Topical keratolytic agents with an appropriate base help to remove the stratum corneum, are non-selective antifungals and potentiate the penetration of the topical AF agents. Note that the KETs MIC is low.

Now a note on KET. Topical use achieves a level of >100 µg/gm and though we are currently on a different azole, I would like to highlight study of 119 patients with the following values (TER 0.001–0.64 µg/ml, ketoconazole MIC range 0.01–3.84 µg/ml, itraconazole MIC range 0.082–20.45 µg/ml, griseofulvin and fluconazole showed a high MIC range 0.32–5.12 µg/ml) There are colleagues who prescribe ketoconazole orally. Though a cautious LFT monitoring is mandated, the drug has a strong keratin adherence; delivery to skin occurs within 2 hours through eccrine sweat. Delivery occurs much

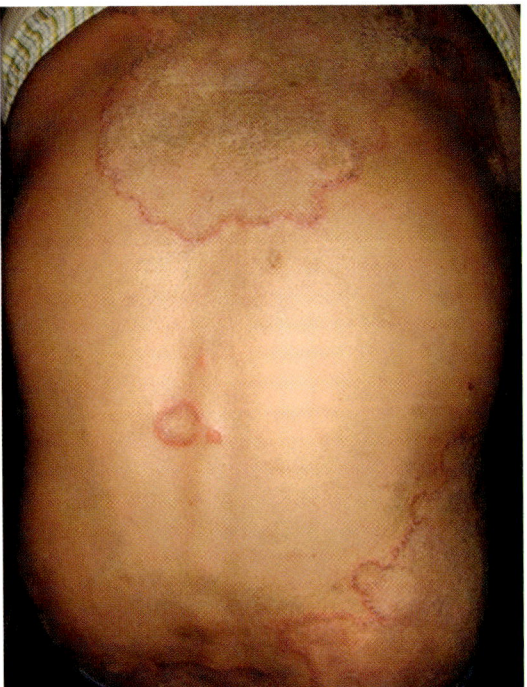

Fig. 16.38: Circinate conglomerate of tinea corporis involving the whole body

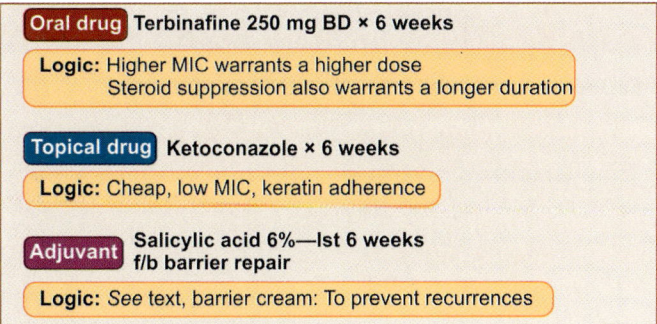

Oral drug Terbinafine 250 mg BD × 6 weeks

Logic: Higher MIC warrants a higher dose
Steroid suppression also warrants a longer duration

Topical drug Ketoconazole × 6 weeks

Logic: Cheap, low MIC, keratin adherence

Adjuvant Salicylic acid 6%—Ist 6 weeks
f/b barrier repair

Logic: *See* text, barrier cream: To prevent recurrences

Fig. 16.39: Therapy and the rationale (for barrier cream *see* Chapter 11, salicylic acid 6% to be used only for non-inflammatory tinea)

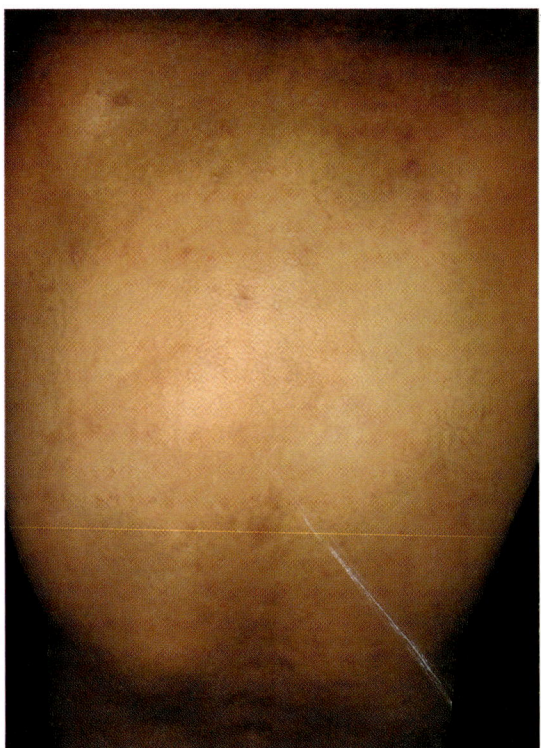

Fig. 16.40: Post-treatment at 6 weeks

more slowly (3–4 weeks) through the epidermal basal layer. Inhibitory concentrations of ketoconazole remain for at least 10 days following termination of the drug. Thus it is a good replacement oral drug only in recalcitrant cases and in others topical would suffice.

And lastly checkerboard studies have shown that an allylamines and azoles are synergistic and the results speak for themselves (Figs 16.39 and 16.40). The longer duration is consequent to topical, yes topical steroid, suppression documented in literature and explains the tepid response initially. Those who believe steroid suppression is a myth with topicals, can access US FDA trials on the same, to save the readers time we have it in the book! (Page 88–90).

Lesson learnt: TER is not a useless drug, it still works in fact nor is KET.

Bibliography

1. Indira Gadangi. Antifungal Susceptibility Testing of Dermatophytes. Springer India 2016A. Basak et al. (eds.), Recent Trends in Antifungal Agents and Antifungal Therapy.

2. Sardana K. Recalcitrant Dermatomycosis: Focus On tinea corporis/cruris/pedis in Fungal Infections Diagnosis and Treatment. Sardana K, Mahajan K, Mrig PA. CBS Publishers, 2017, Delhi. 104–26.

3. Khurana A, Sardana K. Reinterpreting minimum inhibitory concentration (MIC) data of itraconazole versus terbinafine for dermatophytosis—time to look beyond the MIC data? Indian J Dermatol Venereol Leprol. 2017; Dec 14.

4. Sardana K, Arora P, Mahajan K. Intracutaneous pharmacokinetics of oral antifungals and the irrelevance in recalcitrant cutaneous dermatophytosis: Time to revisit basics. Indian J Dermatol Venereol Leprol. 2017;83:730–32.

CASE SCENARIO 13

THE PATIENT WHO DID NOT RESPOND TO THE MOST EXPENSIVE BRAND OF ITRACONAZOLE

Kabir Sardana

This patient came with what looked like tinea faciei. He had annular mild scaling and had been using topical antifungals, tacrolimus and steroids (Fig. 16.41a).

It looked tinea atypica and ITR was prescribed. We decided to work on quality and gave him the best brand. We often call patients at 2 weeks as the compliance is an issue. There was no response. The patient went for a second opinion and granuloma annulare was opined. A Bx revealed PAS positive hyphae in the stratum corneum. We confronted the patient and he gave a telling two-point history

which is crucial for the companies that get costly medications and those who prescribe them for 6 weeks.

He said one, why would he come to a Government Hospital if he had to buy expensive medications. And secondly 6 weeks of a capsule costing so much is beyond his reach. Considering the options, we gave samples of ITR and a conventional dose. He responded in 3 weeks (Fig. 16.41b).

Lesson learnt: *Compliance is crucial*, call the patients back in *2 weeks*, with, if possible, empty strips of the medications (*see* page 95).

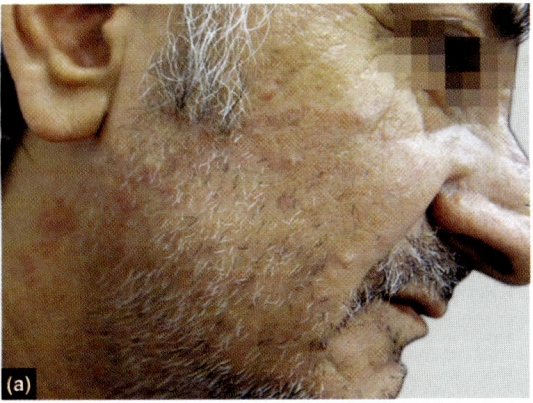 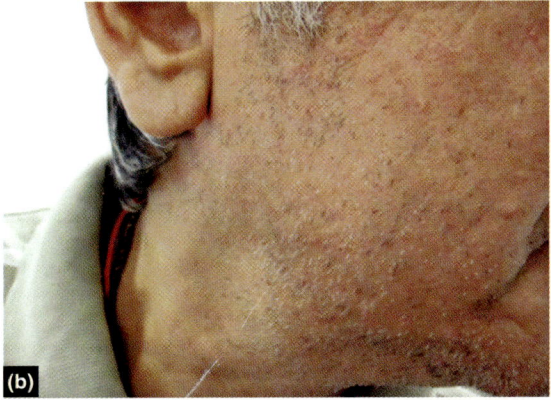

Figs 16.41a and b: (a) Expensive brand of ITR 100 mg × 3 weeks—no response, (b) Patient was not taking the medicine due to the cost, samples of the same salt cleared the eruption

CASE SCENARIO 14

THE NATIONAL PLAGUE-STEROID ABUSE. HOW TO TACKLE IT IN THE CONTEXT OF TINEA

Kabir Sardana

This patient was obviously cushingoid; he had striae, erythema and acne. He had taken amongst other things combo creams and 4 injections of Tricort 40 mg/ml from a famous GP in Bijnor! (Fig. 16.42). The diagnosis was tinea atypica, steroid modified.

The first step was to assess the cortisol levels (Page 90). They were predictably low (Fig. 16.43). In fact amazingly low. Our endocrinologist almost got a repeat done as it was really low (Fig. 16.43). Cortisol levels have some unique advantages.

1. It tells you how *bad is the immuno-suppression* and we forget that it is a very important cause for the mess that we face (86–88). The cortisol level is a surrogate marker of immunity. It is suppressed the first 3 weeks after stopping the steroid, thus there will be a "balancing" game and most anti-fungals do a little, initially, hence one needs to wait for a response.

2. It answers the vexing and irritating question of patients "why am I not getting alright?". We told this patient to go back and show the cortisol report to the legendary Bijnor GP! He refused to believe it, saying this test has no value! The reason why CMEs are important for our GP friends (not in the metros).

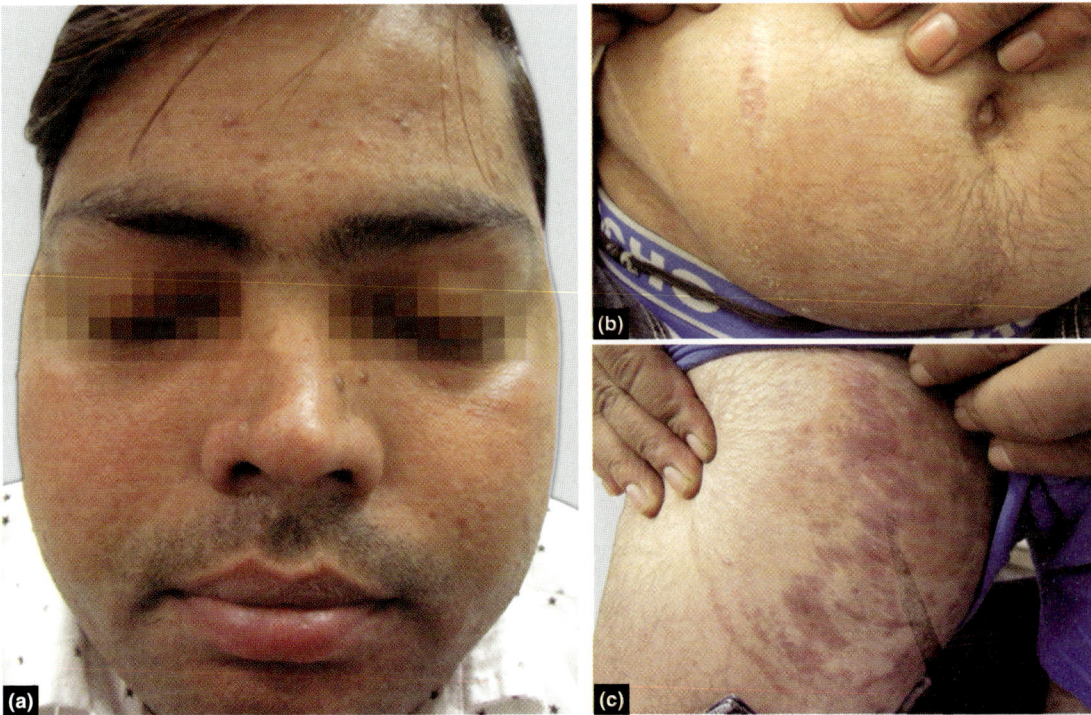

Figs 16.42a to c: Cushingoid habitus with acne and erythema, striae and tinea atypica on the trunk and extremities

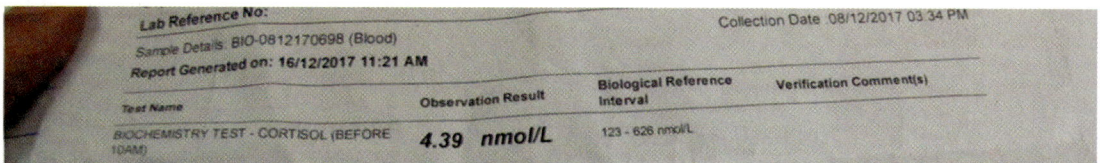

Fig. 16.43: Note the value 4.39 and the units. The books quote a figure of <10 μg/dl. This is 0.159 μg/dl. And he walked into the OPD with that level

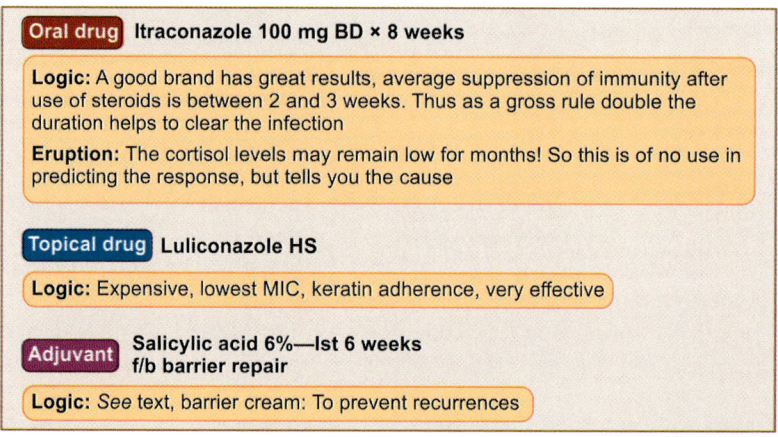

Fig. 16.44: Therapy and the rationale (barrier cream, *see* Chapter 11, salicylic acid 6% to be used only for non-inflammatory tinea)

3. Lastly for some peculiar reason ITR works in such cases and the topical drug I use is luliconazole here as it has the lowest MIC. So at least when the immunity is knocked off for some time give the patients the most powerful (MIC based) drugs (Table 11.2, Page 94).

Using a keratolytic is always a sensible option as it tends to potentiate the effect. A barrier cream is useful post therapy (Page 99). Also get a CXR, some of these cases actually have TB also. Here it is an issue as the ATT interacts with ITR, so may be one can use TER. Do not do a Mantoux; it is usually negative. Such cases take time to respond but they do. Interestingly the cortisol takes 3–4 months to normalize, but the patient gets better before!

Lesson learnt: Apart from telling the patient point blank why it happened, send him back to his provider. If 8000 dermatologists do it, very soon the patients will question these GPs, and this is more effective than legislation, believe me!

CASE SCENARIO 15

THEY DO NOT PROMOTE IT BUT IT HAS ITS ADVANTAGES: FLUCONAZOLE

Kabir Sardana

In India, therapies are largely driven by the industry and some mistruths. One is that fluconazole is a dated drug and has high MIC. True it has high MIC but that is its intrinsic property. Meaning even in a susceptible host FLU has a higher MIC. That is why we should use MIC data in clinical perspective and not the other way around.

Here is a boy with tinea (Fig. 16.45). If one goes back to page 69, Table 9.1, one will realise that FLU secretion does not depend on lipophilic secretion. TER and ITR do and in children there is hardly any sebum secretion. Also remember FLU (*see* Fig. 9.3) has high skin levels. Now this makes it a great drug in xerotic skin and children.

Now one may ask why do standard books mention a weekly dose, well simple, this is for adult patients, where there is also a element of sebum secretion (though not as much as direct diffusion), thus weekly would be enough. Yes there is a minor sebum secretion also. There is a reference in a book, if you wish to be more academic and less trusting, which I quote verbatim.

"**Dosages and suggested regimens:**
- Genital candidiasis: 150 mg as single oral dose.
- Oropharyngeal/esophageal candidiasis: 50 mg daily (100 mg maximum daily in recalcitrant infection) given for 7–14 days.
- Chronic atrophic candidiasis associated with dentures: 50 mg daily for 14 days.
- Esophageal and mucocutaneous candidiasis: 50 mg for 14–30 days. In unusually difficult cases of mucosal candidal infections the dose may be increased to 100 mg daily.
- Tinea pedis, tinea corporis, tinea cruris, pityriasis versicolor and dermal candidiasis: *50 mg daily for 2–4 weeks* (*up to 6 weeks in tinea pedis*).

Other reported regimens (*unlicensed*) include pulse dosing of 150 mg fluconazole

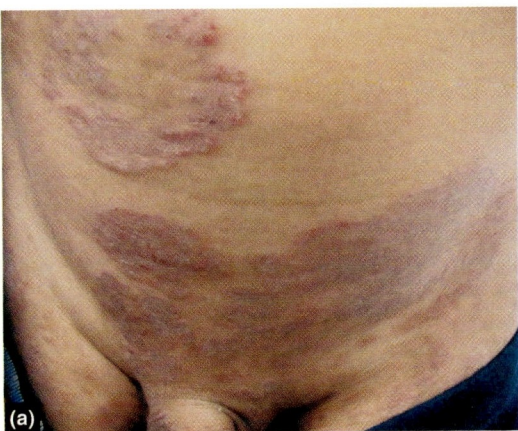
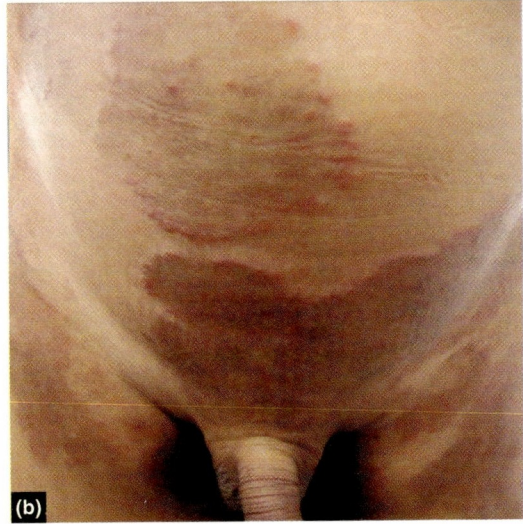

Figs 16.45a and b: A child with tinea, 3 weeks after fluconazole 100 mg given for a total of 4 weeks

once weekly for tinea corporis and tinea cruris, and 300 mg once weekly for 6–9 months for onychomycosis. However, fluconazole is not licensed for the treatment of nail disease and has lower efficacy than other licensed drugs, so should only be considered when these are contraindicated or not tolerated."

Fluconazole has other advantages. Although hydrophilic, long-term administration of fluconazole results in high levels of the drug in the skin and nails. Since higher levels are reached in eccrine sweat and in the dermis–epidermis than in serum, the drug reaches the stratum corneum both by sweat and by direct diffusion from the dermis–epidermis. Prolonged keratin levels result several months after discontinuation of fluconazole.

And it works in children (Figs 16.46 and 16.47). An important caveat, the levels dip down after stopping therapy, more than ITR and TER, hence it is not the preferred drug. It hits hard and withdraws, unlike ITR/TER which hit hard and keep hitting for 3–4 more weeks after stopping therapy (page 80).

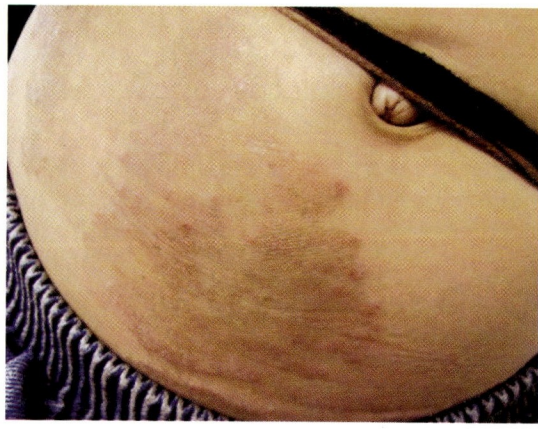

Fig. 16.46: Near complete resolution. Patient continued on salicylic acid 6% and topical ketoconazole

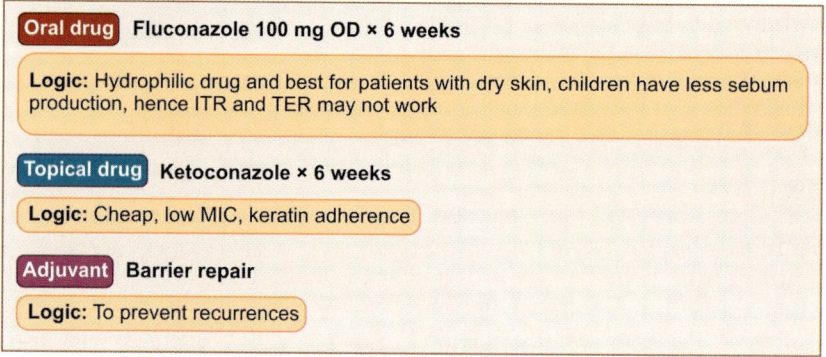

Oral drug	**Fluconazole 100 mg OD × 6 weeks**

Logic: Hydrophilic drug and best for patients with dry skin, children have less sebum production, hence ITR and TER may not work

Topical drug	**Ketoconazole × 6 weeks**

Logic: Cheap, low MIC, keratin adherence

Adjuvant	**Barrier repair**

Logic: To prevent recurrences

Fig. 16.47: Rationale of therapy

Now for those who doubt the drug, let us look at a pivotal meta-analysis of 15 trials ($n = 1438$) in T. pedis. As the sole has a little sebum secretion here is where FLU should be assessed. This study identified no significant difference between fluconazole and itraconazole, as well as terbinafine and itraconazole. However, terbinafine had a significantly higher rate of cure compared to griseofulvin.

Lesson learnt: Dry skin, lack of sebum, children—fluconazole works.

Bibliography

1. Handbook of systemic drug treatment indermatology, second edition. Sarah H. Wakelin © 2015 by Taylor & Francis Group, LLC.

2. Faergemann J, Godleski J, Laufen H, Liss R. Intracutaneous transport of orally administered fluconazole to the stratum corneum. Acta Derm Venereol (Stockh)1995; 75: 361–63.

3. Faergemann J, Laufen H. Levels of fluconazole in serum, stratum corneum, epidermis (without stratum corneum) and eccrine sweat. ClinExp Dermatol 1993; 18:102–6.

4. Faergemann J, Laufen H. Levels of fluconazole in normal and diseased nails during and after treatment of onychomycoses in toe-nails with fluconazole 150 mg once weekly. Acta Dermatol Venerol (Stockh) 1996; 76: 219–221.

5. Bell-Syer SE, Khan SM, Torgerson DJ. Oral treatments for fungal infections of the skin of the foot. Cochrane Database Syst Rev. 2012;10: CD003584.

CASE SCENARIO 16

GRISEOFULVIN AS AN ALTERNATIVE IN RESOURCE RESTRICTED SETUP

Yogesh S Marfatia

A 15-year-old boy presented to us with chief complaints of a dry reddish lesion on his face and groins for 2 months. The lesion progressively increased to the present size and was accompanied with itching. He gave history of application of over-the-counter medications with no relief. On further questioning, it was found that his mother had similar lesions on the face and trunk in the past but the same were not present on examination now.

On examination, there were well circumscribed, scaly, erythematous annular plaques on his ear and surrounding skin of face (Fig. 16.48) and over genitalia, with an inflammatory advancing margin. No central clearing was present. No other parts of the body showed similar lesions.

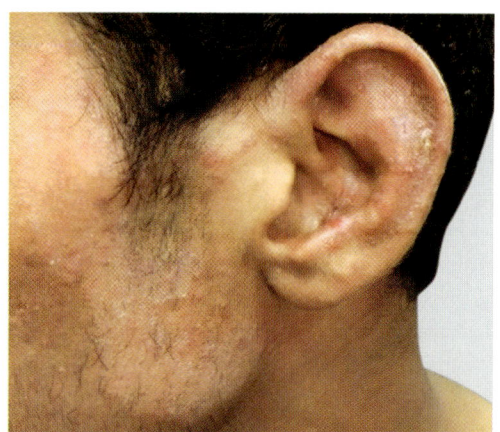

Fig. 16.48: Pre-treatment photograph depicting the plaque overlying left ear and adjoining part of the face

Skin scrapings were taken from the active margin of the lesions for examination. A direct potassium hydroxide (KOH) mount revealed thin hyaline septate hyphae.

Therapy was started with oral fluconazole 150 mg OD along with topical 1% clotrimazole cream for local application twice a day, as these are the only antifungal medications dispensed at our hospital. He was reviewed 6 weeks later but there was no response.

As he had not received griseofulvin in the past and there were resource constraints, he was prescribed tablet griseofulvin 250 mg twice a day along with twice daily topical application of sertaconazole cream. At the end of 6 weeks, there was marked clinical improvement with clearing of lesions. Erythema and scaling subsided completely (Fig. 16.2). KOH smear was negative. Patient was advised to continue treatment for another 2 weeks.

Currently there is trend to use itraconazole or terbinafine orally, but there are many cases not having resources to procure it. Though griseofulvin is not reported to work as efficaciously as itraconazole or terbinafine, it

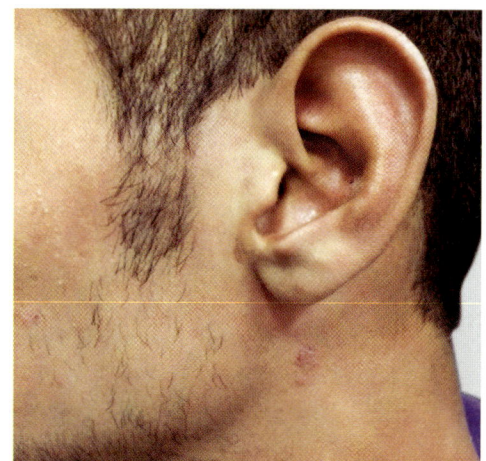

Fig. 16.49: Complete clearance following 6 weeks of griseofulvin and topical sertaconazole

is worth trying it in griseofulvin naïve cases in a resource restricted setup.

Limitations: Culture was not done.

Acknowledgments: Reema Baxi, PG student, Department of Skin and VD, Medical College, Vadodara.

Ashutosh Pal, PG student, Department of Skin and VD, Medical College, Vadodara.

CASE SCENARIO 17

LOOK FOR TINEA BEFORE AND AFTER YOU PRESCRIBE POTENT TOPICAL CORTICOSTEROIDS

Yogesh S Marfatia

A 22-year-old male, who was a known case of pemphigus vulgaris, was admitted to the Inpatient Department of Dermatology of Government Medical College Hospital, with chief complaints of itchy fluid filled blisters and crusted plaques in his right axilla, chest and back since 15 days.

Injectable dexamethasone (8 mg), antibiotics (inj metronidazole, inj amikacin, injectable cefoparazone + sulbactum), topical steroids (clobetasol propionate 0.01% + gentamycin cream) and other supportive treatment was given. Though there was an overall improvement with prescribed therapy, some lesions did not show any improvement even after 3 weeks of admission.

He had recalcitrant and non-healing lesions on right axilla (Fig. 16.50), chest (Fig. 16.51) and back. Some lesions had double edges suggestive of tinea. Tinea corporis was thus suspected and skin scrapings were taken from the active margin of the lesions. A direct potassium hydroxide (KOH) mount revealed thin hyaline septate hyphae confirming the diagnosis.

His topical steroid was stopped. Therapy was started with oral fluconazole 150 mg OD, continuing the treatment for pemphigus. Two weeks later, he showed significant clinical improvement with decrease in erythema and scaling (Figs 16.52 and 16.53). Oral fluconazole therapy was continued for 4 weeks.

In any chronic dermatoses or autoimmune bullous disease, potent topical steroids are often used. In recalcitrant resistant cases which are not responding to the usual line of management, it is essential to rule out an underlying dermatophytic infection. There is a need to monitor cases on steroid therapy, particularly topical for development of dermatophytic infections. Pre-treatment and

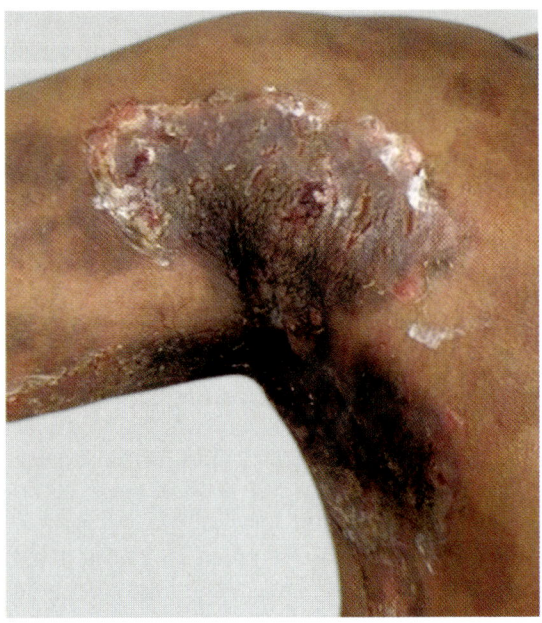

Fig. 16.50: Right axilla pre-treatment

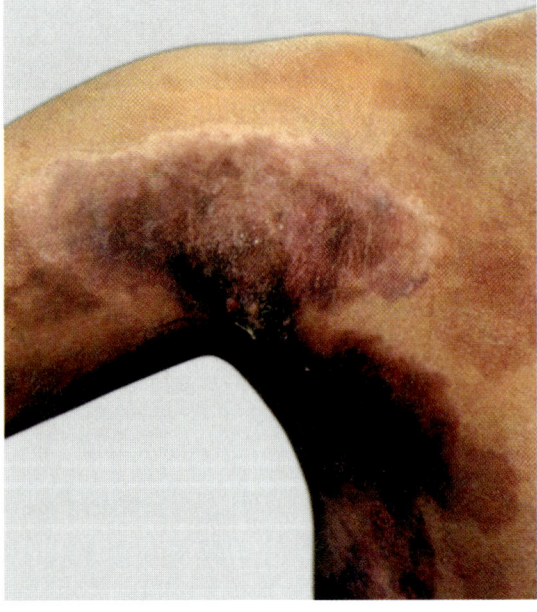

Fig. 16.51: Post-treatment with oral fluconazole

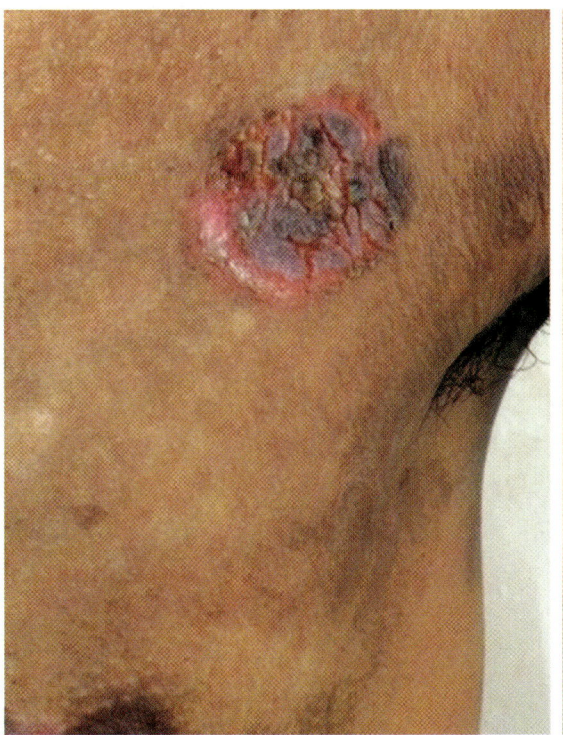

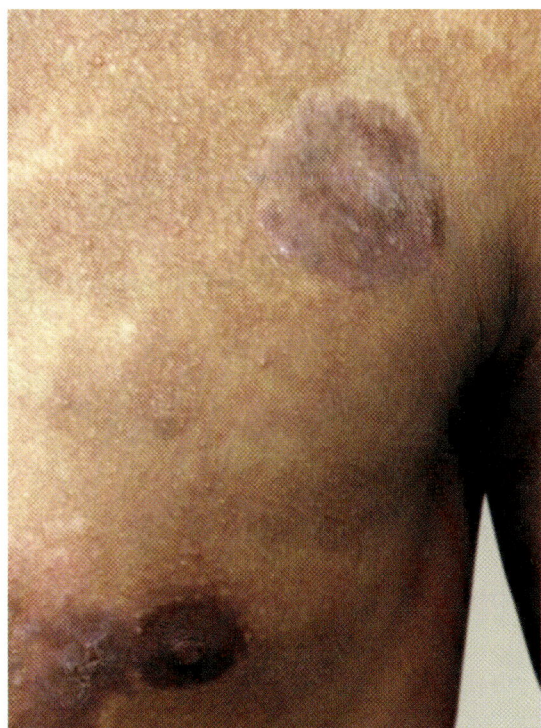

Fig. 16.52: Pre-photograph of left chest lesion   **Fig. 16.53:** Post-treatment with oral fluconazole

periodic skin examinations, including web spaces as well as nail, for evidence of dermatophytosis is essential. Such cases are susceptible to clinically atypical superinfections with dermatophytes, such as tinea incognito.

A high index of suspicion, immediate cessation of potent topical steroid application and institution of oral antifungal was of paramount help in this case. Clinical response confirmed the diagnosis of tinea incognito.

Limitations: Culture was not done.

Acknowledgments: Reema Baxi, PG student, Department of Skin and VD, Medical College, Vadodara.

Ashutosh Pal, PG student, Department of Skin and VD, Medical College, Vadodara.

CASE SCENARIO 18

A QUASI MULTIDRUG THERAPY WITH THE ANCHOR ORAL DRUG UPDOSED AND PROLONGED WITH A DIFFERENT CLASS OF TOPICAL AGENT ATTACKING THE DERMATOPHYTES UTILIZING A DIFFERENT MECHANISMS OF ACTION

Premanshu Bhushan

A 39-year-old male presented with unilateral red itchy plaque on right cheek of more than 6 months duration. The lesion was previously treated with terbinafine 250 mg daily for 6 weeks, itraconazole 200 mg twice daily for 6 weeks, topical steroid containing antifungal creams for many months. Only temporary and partial relief was reported. On examination a large, erythematous, plaque covering the entire right cheek was seen. There was some central clearing while the edges were indurated. Scaling was minimal (Fig. 16.54). However, a KOH mount showed abundant hyphae. A diagnosis of dermatophytosis of Majocchi's granuloma type was made.

Treatment given and rationale: Patient was started on oral terbinafine 500 mg once daily in the morning along with levocetrizine 5 mg at bedtime. Patient was asked to stop all previous topical agents. He was asked to apply luliconazole cream once every night. Patient was treated with this regimen for 6 weeks with complete resolution of the lesion (Fig. 16.55).

With growing clinical resistance of dermatophytes with or without microbiological evidence of the same, dermatologists are trying various methods to cope up with the challenge. I have found that the resistance is relative in most patients and updosing of standard drugs for longer periods of time (minimum 6 weeks) leads to significantly more cases getting cured than the usual. Further, terbinafine is an allylamine and is fungicidal compared to itraconazole which is fungistatic at usual concentrations. We can approach the cases like we do with resistant organisms like mycobacteria. Hence, addition of a topical agent with a different mechanism of action will further increase the efficacy of the treatment. In present case topical luliconazole was chosen because it has a significantly lower MIC amongst the azoles and inhibits the C-14 demethylase, whereas terbinafine inhibits the

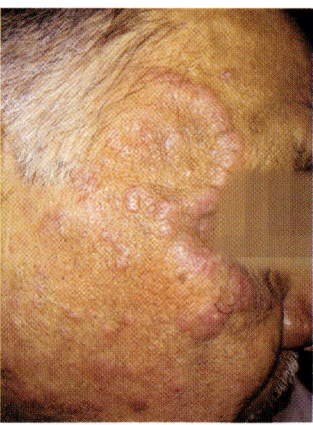

Fig. 16.54: Pre-treatment B

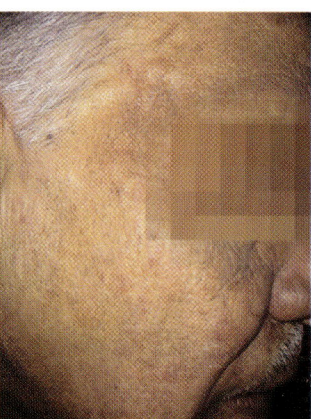

Fig. 16.55: Post-treatment B

squalene epoxidase. This combined attack works better than monotherapy as the resistant mutants to one drug are likely to be targeted with the other. While trying to give two different classes of antifungals orally may be unacceptable due to toxicity, adding a topical agent to an anchor oral antifungal is safe.

Lesson learnt: A quasi-multidrug therapy with updosed terbinafine at 500 mg daily with topical luliconazole is effective in treating apparently resistant dermatophytosis.

Index